C12

BEHAVIORAL SCIENCE
IN THE
PRACTICE OF MEDICINE

BEHAVIORAL SCIENCE
IN THE
PRACTICE OF MEDICINE

Editors

John E. Carr, Ph.D.

Professor and Acting Chairman,
Department of Psychiatry and Behavioral Sciences
University of Washington, Seattle, Washington

Harold A. Dengerink, Ph.D.

Professor and Director of Clinical Training, Department of Psychology
Washington State University, Pullman, Washington

ELSEVIER BIOMEDICAL
New York · Amsterdam · Oxford

Elsevier Science Publishing Co., Inc.
52 Vanderbilt Avenue, New York, New York 10017

Sole distributors outside the United States and Canada:
Elsevier Science Publishers B.V.
P.O. Box 211, 1000 AE Amsterdam, The Netherlands

Library of Congress Cataloging in Publication Data

Main entry under title:

Behavioral science in the practice of medicine.
    Includes index.
    1. Medicine and psychology. I. Carr, John E.
    II. Dengerink, H. A., 1943-   [DNLM: 1. Behavioral
    medicine. WB 100 B419]
R726.5.B428   1983   610'.1'9   83-5551
ISBN 0-444-00784-9

Manufactured in the United States of America

Contents

Foreword: **The Old and a New Testament
for Medical Education in Our Time**   ix
Charles E. Odegaard, Ph.D.

Preface   xix

Contributors   xxiii

    PART I **BEHAVIORAL SCIENCE MODELS AND RESEARCH**   **1**
              IN HEALTH CARE

Chapter 1 **The Behavioral Sciences in Medicine:
Introduction and Overview**   3
John E. Carr, Ph. D., and Harold A. Dengerink, Ph.D.

Chapter 2 **Behavioral Research in Health Care**   21
Harold A. Dengerink, Ph.D.,
and Cornelis B. Bakker, M.D.

Chapter 3 **The Interpretation and Treatment of Pathological
Behavior in Historical Perspective**   43
Charles Bodemer, Ph.D.

Chapter 4 **Brain–Behavior Relations and the Delivery
of Health Care**   67
George A. Ojemann, M.D.

Chapter 5 **Social Science in the Clinic: Applied Contributions
from Anthropology to Medical Teaching and
Patient Care**   85
Gary Rosen, M.D., and Arthur Kleinman, M.D.

Chapter 6   Somatization in Primary Health Care   105
             Wayne Katon, M.D., and Harold A. Dengerink, Ph.D.

Chapter 7   Communication Research and the Doctor–Patient
             Relationship   133
             John E. Carr, Ph.D., and Peter E. Maxim, M.D., Ph.D.

Chapter 8   The Unity of Biomedical and Psychosocial Issues
             in Individual and Family Health Care   163
             Gabriel Smilkstein, M.D.

Chapter 9   Behavioral Medicine: Basic Concepts
             and Clinical Applications   185
             John E. Carr, Ph.D., Dean Funabiki, Ph.D.,
             and Harold A. Dengerink, Ph.D.

Chapter 10   Self-Management of Health-Related Behaviors   201
             Thomas A. Brigham, Ph.D.,
             and Harold A. Dengerink, Ph.D.

             PART II BEHAVIORAL SCIENCE RESEARCH AND SOME
             MAJOR MEDICAL PROBLEMS   225

Chapter 11   The Relation of Stress to Health and Illness   227
             William M. Womack, M.D., Peter P. Vitaliano, Ph.D.,
             and Roland D. Maiuro, Ph.D

Chapter 12   Psychological Aspects of Hypertension   249
             George N. Aagaard, M.D.

Chapter 13   Biobehavioral Interactions and Hypertension   263
             Orville A. Smith, Ph.D.

Chapter 14   Biofeedback and Psychophysiological
             Disorders   283
             Jeffrey C. Steger, Ph.D.

Chapter 15   Behavioral Problems in Pediatric Practice   311
             Eric Trupin, Ph.D., Robin Beck, M.D.,
             and Peter Fehrenbach, Ph.D.

Chapter 16   Chronic Pain   331
             John D. Loeser, M.D., and Wilbert E. Fordyce, Ph.D.

Chapter 17   Depressive Illness and Medical Practice   347
             John A. Chiles, M.D., Nicholas G. Ward, M.D.,
             and Joseph Becker, Ph.D.

Chapter 18 Psychosocial Perspectives on Depressive Disorders   361
Joseph Becker, Ph.D., John A. Chiles, M.D.,
and Nicholas G. Ward, M.D.

Chapter 19 Anxiety and Insomnia in Medical Practice   385
Nicholas G. Ward, M.D., Joseph Becker, Ph.D.,
and John A. Chiles, M.D.

Chapter 20 Behavioral Aspects of Drug Misuse and Abuse   403
Albert S. Carlin, Ph.D., and Nicholas G. Ward, M.D.

Chapter 21 Alcohol Abuse in Medical Practice   419
James W. Smith, M.D., and Ruth E. Little, Sc.D.

Chapter 22 Problems of Aging in Medical Practice   442
Burton V. Reifler, M.D., M.P.H.,
and Suzanne Wu, Ph.D.

Index   463

Foreword
The Old and a New Testament
for Medical Education in Our Time*

Charles E. Odegaard, Ph.D.

I recently had the opportunity to read a document distributed in February 1982 by the American Association of Medical Colleges entitled, "An Overview of the General Professional Education of the Physician and College Preparation for Medicine," which raises questions about various aspects of premedical education and education for the M.D. degree and seeks responses from diverse types of individuals. There are many good and important questions raised by this document that deserve attention and which will be faced in the course of a three-year study under the general direction of a panel whose chairman is President Steven Muller of The Johns Hopkins University and whose vice-chairman is our own President Gerberding. However, I confess to disappointment at the constricted view of medical education, at the narrowness of its underlying ideology. The article reflects the established orthodoxy about medicine as articulated by Flexner (1910). It refers throughout to physicians as "biomedical scientists" and is content to refer to the preclinical phase of professional education as "didactic education in the biomedical sciences." It affirms that "six disciplines comprise the sciences basic to medicine: anatomy, biochemistry, physiology, pharmacology, microbiology, and pathology" (p. 27). It does recognize that "medical school faculties, already burdened by the quantity of information that they are attempting to teach their students, with increasing frequency are being asked to introduce new subjects such as nutrition, geriatrics, cancer, sexuality, alcoholism and drug abuse, etc." (p. 33). Behavioral science does get a mention at the end of a list of the traditional basic medical sciences as disciplines covered by

*University of Washington Conference on Medical Education, June 17, 1982.

questions on Part I of the examination of the National Board of Medical Examiners. The only new subjects singled out for mention in a question as to new subjects that should be incorporated into the general professional education of the physician are information science and computer literacy (p. 37).

It is only in the last paragraph of this document, after reaffirmation of the old testament of Flexner, namely; "scientific ability has been and will continue to be considered essential for the study of medicine," that we come upon something else that is needed in the profession; the words in the document and in the questionnaire with reference to the science of medicine are *knowledge, teaching, learning, instruction,* and *study skills*. Now listen carefully to the remainder of the final paragraph with its shifts in terminology:

> But the practice of medicine must combine scientific knowledge with an appreciation and respect for human needs. It seems unlikely that any combination of courses can ensure the acquisition of humane qualities or an appreciation and respect for human needs. Knowledge acquired from many fields can broaden the perspective of students as they progress through college and enlarge their understanding of the role they will play in society. College preparation should promote such breadth and provide an environment for personal development for all students regardless of what their future careers may be. It is important that the personal growth of students aspiring to a medical career be directed toward helping and concern for others. Unnecessary invidious competition for admission to medical school is a deterrent to the development of these qualities. Medical school and college faculties must cooperate in establishing an environment that promotes students' acquisition of caring attitudes.

Similarly, the final set of questions in the questionnaire is headed "Caring attitudes and respect for human needs are vital qualities for physicians," and the questions ask if the present educational environment in colleges and in medical schools nurture these qualities and emphasize their importance.

We have shifted from the acquisition of knowledge as in science to the acquisition of humane qualities such as appreciation and respect for human needs. We emphasize the construction of an environment for personal development and growth toward helping and concern for others, an environment that promotes the student's acquisition of caring attitudes. Who could be against the formation of such characters for the practice of medicine? I presume no one. But how are we to arrive at such a result? We are told that "it seems unlikely that any combination of courses can ensure the acquisition of humane qualities or an appreciation and respect for human needs." I suppose that it is true that one cannot ensure such a result. I doubt that by teaching courses in science one can ensure in students scientific thinking and habits of scientific analysis of relevant problems, but maybe we can encourage the development of such capacity for scientific thinking in a fair number of future physicians. At least the effort is made to do so by the provision of courses in bioscience subjects in medical school and by the requirement of courses in biology, physics, and chemistry in the undergraduate college.

We are also told in that final paragraph that "knowledge acquired from many fields can broaden the perspective of students and enlarge their understanding of the role they will play in society." If this is so, why should an effort not be made to provide physicians with systematic knowledge about human needs and desires so that they will know how to care for patients and demonstrate a caring and respectful attitude toward them? Why should the medical curriculum not deal responsibly with this aspect of the physician's responsibility if it is indeed a vital quality for him or her?

Please do not push the question aside, as I have often heard it dismissed, as though with a shrug of the shoulders toward "soft science." In the friendliest of spirits I urge you to be conscious of the possibility of a quick response attributable to the imprint of the physician's guild. Let me explain what I mean.

It is a commonplace now to note the recent development in our culture of a massive amount of material technology which shapes and patterns the operation of things that surround us in such great bounty. As my years have passed in institutions of higher education, I have become more and more aware of the increasing degree by which these things are accompanied by something less commonly noted, a burgeoning social technology which shapes human beings and patterns the way in which diverse groups of people operate in their daily transactions. The institutions of formal education are powerful influences on human beings in shaping characteristics and inculcating patterns of thought, language, skills, competencies, expectations, views, and values—and limitations, areas of ignorance, and distinctive prejudices. As I have moved from a professorship of history to the directorship of a humanities research council, to a deanship in arts and sciences, and to the presidency of a university with 17 different faculties, I have become more aware of the fact that, as these social institutions are working in the late twentieth century, they have become factories for the production of persons of ever more sharply defined special characteristics that are diplomaed, licensed, and certified further to demarcate them culturally from other subspecies of *Homo sapiens*. Though some other groups may approach them no other group exceeds physicians in undergoing for so long an intense, rigorous, uniform, formal educational hazing, which in turn causes them to be so completely separated from other human beings as indicated by title—the label of doctor—and uniform—the white coat with the stethoscope a further visible badge of office. I ask only that you take note of the risk any person would run in this situation, of being subtly equipped by the process to which you have been exposed with stereotyped answers and guildlike behaviors which you may not have thought through carefully or consciously adopted yourselves.

I am sure that you recognize the frequency in medical writing and discussion with which approving references are made to "hard science," and disparaging references to "soft science" and worse yet, "anecdote"—this despite the importance of case histories in medical practice and the affirmation that it is finally an individual patient that is the object of your care. Let me share with you an experience of some years ago that was for me enlightening as to the nature of scientific investigation: When I became Dean of Arts and Sciences at the University of Michigan, I found that one of my outrigger administrative responsibilities was to the freshwater biological station at Douglas Lake. Its ties with the university were somewhat troubled at that point, and to find remedies, I felt a need to know more about the work of the station and its personnel. Over a period of time I spent several weeks at the station, going out each morning with a different professor and his students as he led them in collecting specimens and making observations in the field. In the subsequent afternoon I attended the session at the station where the professor lectured on related matters and supervised laboratory work with the specimens. It so happened by accident that in one week I was led with different classes three times to the exact same spot, an area hardly more than 100 square feet beside a country road. A creek flowed through the middle of the square before passing under a wooden bridge on the road. The portion of the square nearest the road widened out into a little meadow on both sides of the stream, which then gave way to a stand of deciduous trees that arched over the stream, creating a kind of tunnel ambling off into the distance. On one day I accompanied to this spot an ornithologist in search of bird life. On another day I accompanied an ichthyologist who guided his students toward the larvae of lamprey in the sands of the creek bottom. On the third day an entomologist helped his students net insects in the interface between the air and the watery surface of the creek. Through the selective guidance provided by the three scientists the students and I were led to see three different faces of nature. What I actually experienced was the result of close observation isolating from the same setting three completely different aspects of the universe, three scientific abstractions that seemed worlds apart from each other. Much can be gained from this kind of selective close observation; much can also be dismissed, ignored, lost, and indeed, never seen, though obviously present in the situations before the observer.

It is important to note further that the process of observation itself is a complex affair involving the use of different tools. The ornithologist taught his students to listen closely with their ears to identify birds somewhere in the environment by their distinctive calls and, second, to seek with their eyes any birds darting among the leaves. The ichthyologist did not talk about listening. For him the primary tools were his eyes and the feel of his fingers as he grubbed in the sand. Scientific or rational observation can clearly be mightily affected by one's choice of what one is looking for and by the tools of investigation and observation one uses, not all of which are applicable to all problems. Consequences can then flow from what one is looking for and from the applicability of the particular methods of research for the matter under investigation. Just as the scientist may select out of the phenomena before him his chosen category, his favorite subject, he may also develop a kind of veneration for the particular method or tools of research he has found applicable to his chosen field of investigation, a veneration that can make him intolerant of the work of others if they do not use his methods, even though for one reason or another his method may not be applicable to their area of research. There is a tendency among physicians to insist upon one method of reasoning, that of science based upon an objective stance, a reductionist approach based upon abstraction and the use of quantitative analysis, the only way to go, as it were, even when the results sometimes may be of little consequence or when the method is unsuited to finding answers to the matter in hand.

There simply remain important questions for which the scientific methods often applicable in biology are insufficient or inapplicable. The ideological base of medicine is simply too narrow; the old orthodoxy needs a supplement.

The Flexner doctrine is, so to speak, an old testament, one that added much to the competence of physicians by its emphasis on close observation of human biology, particularly of the parts of the human body, as Flexner said, of the tissues and organs. But there is more to the human being than the body and its tissues and organs; there is the whole human being as a functioning entity, as a unit, as a self, and also as a participant in a larger social group as a social animal. Man as an operating, functional unit engages in behavioral patterns that can also be observed and carefully described, both in individual terms and in terms of repetitive cultural patterns. There are psychosocial as well as biological dimensions to *Homo sapiens*. We now have increasing reason to believe that human behavior and interpersonal relations can be influenced by biological entities, by chemical substances, whether produced internally by bodily action—for example, endorphins—or by the ingestion or injection of externally produced chemical substances—for example, LSD or tranquilizers. We also have an increasing awareness that social relationships and behavioral actions of human beings, their life-style, can produce adverse biological impacts upon the human body. I need only refer to the increasing research interest in stress arising in the personal and social life circumstances of the individual and its impact on his biology and disease conditions.

My contention, then, is that Flexner defined too narrowly the knowledge base for medicine by confining attention to biology. He left out the psychosocial dimension and the establishment within the curriculum of a base of knowledge relevant for it, to accompany the base for biology that he did prescribe. In the course of my experience as a member of the Millis Commission in the first half of the 1960s and, in particular, of our discussions of primary care, I became increasingly concerned by the neglect of this aspect. At a conference at the University of Leyden in 1966 I argued the need for a supplement to the Flexner definition, a new psychosocial testament as an addition of knowledge to the old biological testament prescribed by Flexner. Mind you, I did not engage in an appeal to the human heart of the physician to unleash a flow of loving kindness on patients, to become more of a humanitarian, or to be more humane— though who could be against that? I argued, rather, that the physician should be helped by his medical teaching to expand the range of his rational observations of the patient, that he should be helped to understand the patient not only as a human body but as an operant individual in a social environment, confronting some disease, some dis-ease, some malaise, some crippling. Just as physician teachers have associated themselves with scientists to acquire knowledge about biology relevant to medicine, so should they associate themselves with social scientists and humanists to acquire knowledge about man as a social phenomenon and as an individual.

In this case, as in the case of biology, it is wise to recognize that the basic motivation of the scholars and scientists differs from that of the physician; there are differences in their roles. The former are seeking knowledge for its own sake; the latter are professionals whose purpose is to find and use relevant knowledge for the better diagnosis and therapeutic treatment of their patients. The goal of the former is primarily contemplation; the goal of the latter is primarily action. Though some individuals can navigate comfortably in both roles, some tensions and differences of view often do exist between the disciplinarians and the professionals, but with time a useful symbiotic relationship can be developed between the two parties. Just as useful relationships have developed over time between physicians and basic biological scientists, productive relationships should be possible between physicians and social scientists and humanists.

A physician is carefully taught to listen with a stethoscope to the thumps, gurgles, and sighs that come from the giblets within the bodily cavity of the patient and to identify and interpret these signals, but he is not taught so persistently or systematically to listen to and interpret the sounds which emanate from the throat of the patient in the form of words and their attendant gestures. Anthropology, sociology, and psychology can help equip a physician to identify repetitive, distinctive cultural patterns reflected in the beliefs, expectations, and behavior of patients as participants in various kinds of groups. Though a person may share patterns of behavior, thought, and feelings with other persons, he also exists as a unique individual with a sense of selfhood. The humanistic disciplines, history, philosophy, literature, and the arts, in particular offer insights into man's existence as an individual. It is finally the patient as an individual who must be persuaded to be to some degree a collaborator with his physician if the physician's treatment is to be effective.

It is not enough for the physician to know something of his patient in psychosocial and biological terms. The physician himself is an important participant along with the patient in the diagnostic and therapeutic relationship. He is indeed a part of the cure or the coping with the incurable disabilities of disease. There is much about himself that the physician needs to know for the benefit of both parties in physician–patient relationships, for his own benefit as well as that of his patient. It is in this respect, in the search for himself, that the humanistic studies with their interest in the individual can be helpful to the physician. What they do in essence is provide case histories that enable a person to find himself and to remake himself by a study of comparisons with others and by an analysis of the values that have been chosen by others to guide their actions in various situations. As the physician observes the behavior and values of others and learns more about the various patterns reflected in the lives of others around him, he finds more points of reference for himself as a human being too. As he becomes aware of the thoughts and feelings of others, and finds points of identification with himself as a fellow human being, he may indeed become more sensitive to others. Better informed as to his impact upon others, he may make more of an effort to be understanding; and as he learns to have more empathy for his patient, he may also learn to avoid for himself the hazards of overidentifying with the patient's problems.

These psychosocial and personal matters need to be openly studied and discussed by budding physicians in the course of their medical education. They need to become a part of the medical curriculum. In the 1970s some place was found for nonbiological matters, most commonly in courses labeled behavioral science, offered in the basic science years, less often in so-called humanities courses, which usually focus on critical ethical issues and which sometimes appear as topics within courses in an introduction to clinical medicine. I must confess, however, that my visits to medical schools in recent years have led me to feel that these courses are frequently viewed by students as of peripheral importance in comparison with the real stuff of medicine offered in the basic sciences. This judgment upon the part of students seems to be confirmed and encouraged by the still prevailing large measure of indifference or inattention of clinical professors to these matters. I do not believe that these efforts will assume real significance until a critical mass of clinical professors evidences greater desire to learn more themselves about the psychosocial aspects of their patients so that they can inject these extra dimensions into their own clinical teaching in clerkships and residencies.

I have referred in particular to the need to subject the physician–patient relationship to far more deliberate and planned observations and analyses with the aid of information, perspectives, and methods that could be mined from materials within the social sciences and humanities. There is another problem confronting physicians that deserves attention and for which they have need of knowledge derived from the social sciences and humanities. The delivery of health care in this country is in the hands of what might be regarded as a massive, disorganized, obviously very expensive cottage industry that is still surviving into the late twentieth century. Growing numbers of persons and types of health providers are responsible. Apart from the expense, there are serious problems of discontinuity, jurisdictional disputes, and divided authority. Beyond the physicians, there are obviously other parties with their share of responsibility. Physicians, however, do have a dominant role in influencing the way in which health care is delivered. As captains of the team, they incur a leadership role that means that they are managers of people. Knowledge about people and their social interactions also has its utility in helping physicians play a constructive role in achieving a more effective and efficient delivery of health care.

If the old testament for a bioscience component to medicine is to be supplemented by a new testament for a psychosocial component, there are implications, it seems to me, for possible changes in all three levels of medical education: premedical, undergraduate medical, and postgraduate medical.

To limit my remarks to the premedical phase, I believe it would be desirable to go beyond a recommendation that the college undergraduate have a liberal education, in the sense of an exposure to a modicum of courses distributed among the natural sciences, the social sciences, and the humanities. Such a recommendation might help diminish the tendency of recent years for a high proportion of those admitted to medical schools to take the science courses, to the substantial neglect by many applicants to medical school of experience in the other areas. However, I believe that an attempt should be made to start consultations between medical school and college faculties to discuss courses specifically oriented toward a premedical program. In addition to continuing selected courses in the sciences, I think it would be desirable to plan jointly courses specifically developed to focus on two topics relevant to medicine: to introduce prospective medical students to thinking and learning about physician–patient roles and interaction, and the management of health services.

To turn to the physician–patient relationship, the analysis of the patient aspect could include a study of the impact of ethnic, cultural, and class differences on the sick role and illness behavior, health belief models as they appear in patient populations, and alternative systems of care. The analysis of the physician role could include study of the stresses involved in the care of the sick as they affect the physician and as revealed in historical and literary sources and the physician's need of coping capacity; and students should be made aware of the patient's expectations of the physician.

Health services can be approached from many angles: mode of delivery, cost, participation of and cooperation among different members of the team of health providers, and problems of the management of human beings in institutional groups. I do not for a moment mean to suggest that these matters would be settled once and for all at the premedical level; however, I do suggest that some level of their introduction at the college level would start the process of their legitimization as part of the education of physicians, and they could still be elements within the broader education of undergraduates, whether the students become physicians in time or not.

The very discussion of such matters among faculties could add needed dimensions to the educational background of the faculty members themselves, whether at the college or medical school level. We should not underestimate the importance of providing opportunities for faculty members at all the levels associated with medical education to put themselves through a process of new learning. Though these people may be relatively few in numbers, there exists now a cadre of clinicians, sociologists, anthropologists, psychologists, economists, literary scholars, historians, and philosophers who have been thinking about the psycho-social aspects of health and medical practice and who can share insights with a larger number of interested clinicians.

If such groups were to take seriously the admonitions and injunctions heard in speeches at banquets, and medical school commencements and in the final paragraph of the recent American Association of Medical Colleges overview of medical education, we need not cry, "All hope abandon, ye who enter here." A new testament might be added for the better salvation of patients and—let us not overlook this—the salvation of some of the greatest victims of the present system, physicians and their families.

References

Flexner, A. 1910. Medical Education in the United States and Canada. A report to the Carnegie Foundation for the Advancement of Teaching. Boston: Updyke.

Preface

It is commonly assumed that the delivery of health care is associated only with the identification and alleviation of organic pathology and biological dysfunction. Recent evidence, however, indicates that a significant portion of the practice of primary care physicians has to do with the identification and management of those behavioral factors that contribute either directly or indirectly to the illness behavior of their patients. National health care statistics obtained in both the United States and Canada over the past decade clearly indicate that behavioral factors play a primary role in contributing to the major causes of both mortality and morbidity. It is the purpose of this book to draw the reader's attention to the importance of contributions from the behavioral sciences to a better understanding of the nature of illness behavior and its environmental, social, cultural, and psychological as well as organic determinants.

While medical educators may agree that the behavioral sciences are important in medical education, translating this affirmation into an effective curriculum has proven to be a complex task. Since the late 1960s behavioral sciences at the University of Washington School of Medicine have been taught in terms of their direct applicability to the practice of the primary care physician, with the "behavioral system" providing the point of integration for a general organ system approach.

Our approach to the field has been tightly linked to the burgeoning literature of empirical studies which demonstrate the complex, inter-dependent, and multifactorial nature of the determining mechanisms in illness. We view this model within the context of both historical and cross-cultural perspectives of healing in medical practice, reviewing each of the major parameters of the model so as to examine the neurophysiological correlates of symptom manifestation and cognition underlying patient perception and physicians' decision making, the impact of sociocultural variables on the beliefs of patients and physicians and on symptom presentation and diagnosis, comparisons and contrasts between ethnomedicine and Western biomedicine and the professional healing role within each context, the complex role of operant learning processes in illness and health-seeking behavior, the relation between stress and illness in the field of behavioral medicine and the role of biofeedback, and operant approaches to health care and health maintenance. Finally, we review with the student major problems of primary health care, such as chronic pain, addictive behaviors, hypertension, affective disorders, and cancer. In doing so we illustrate the contributory roles of behavioral determinants in interaction with environmental and biological factors.

Out of our curricular efforts at the University of Washington School of Medicine there emerged a unique series of relations between basic science and the clinical faculty. This faculty is drawn from a wide range of specialty areas, including biomedical history, neurosurgery, physiology and biophysics, anthropology, rehabilitation medicine, pediatrics, family medicine, internal medicine, sociology, psychology, psychiatry, and epidemiology. In the majority of our course meetings topics are presented by M.D. and Ph.D. faculty pairs who are able to demonstrate as well as describe the integration of behavioral sciences within clinical medicine. The response to the course has been especially favorable, as evidenced by the interest and performance of the students and the enthusiasm and involvement of both students and faculty in course evolution.

Out of our efforts there also emerged a course syllabus that rapidly expanded in popularity, not only within the course but also among faculty and students outside the course and the School of Medicine. It was the urging of these many supportive colleagues that led to the expansion of this initially modest course syllabus into the present work. All of the contributing authors are participating faculty within the course and contribute actively to the teaching program at the University of Washington School of Medicine.

We do not presume that this represents the definitive statement regarding the role of the behavioral sciences in medicine. Indeed, one of the fundamental tenets of the group is that the field is rapidly expanding and that there are many substantive areas within the relevant research literature that remain to be tapped and brought to the attention of students, trainees, and practitioners throughout the health care professions.

Although this book has been designed primarily in response to the curricular needs of medical students in their basic science years, the material is directly applicable and especially suitable for training programs at the graduate level within any of the health care professions.

For those of us who have had the pleasure of participating in the unique and rewarding experience of exploring and examining the diverse ways in which a knowledge of the behavioral sciences contributed to our effectiveness as health care professionals, this book represents an especially significant event. We hope that those who read it will come to share in the excitement of that search and exploration.

John E. Carr, Ph.D.

Harold A. Dengerink, Ph.D.

Contributors

George N. Aagaard, M.D.
Professor of Medicine and Pharmacology, Division of Clinical Pharmacology, University of Washington School of Medicine, Seattle, Washington

Cornelis B. Bakker, M.D.
Professor and Chairman, Department of Psychiatry, Peoria School of Medicine, Peoria, Illinois

Robin Beck, M.D.
Clinical Assistant Professor, Department of Family Medicine, University of Washington School of Medicine, Seattle, Washington

Joseph Becker, Ph.D.
Professor, Department of Psychiatry and Behavioral Sciences, University of Washington School of Medicine, Seattle, Washington

Charles Bodemer, Ph.D.
Professor and Chairman, Department of Biomedical History, University of Washington School of Medicine, Seattle, Washington

Thomas A. Brigham, Ph. D.
Professor, Department of Psychology, Washington State University, Pullman, Washington

Albert S. Carlin, Ph.D.
Associate Professor, Department of Psychiatry and Behavioral Sciences, University of Washington School of Medicine, Seattle, Washington

John E. Carr, Ph.D.
Professor and Acting Chairman, Department of Psychiatry and Behavioral Sciences, University of Washington School of Medicine, Seattle, Washington

John A. Chiles, M.D.
Associate Professor, Department of Psychiatry and Behavioral Sciences, University of
Washington School of Medicine, Seattle, Washington

Harold A. Dengerink, Ph.D.
Professor and Director of Clinical Training, Department of Psychology, Washington State
University, Pullman, Washington; Clinical Professor, Department of Psychiatry and
Behavioral Sciences, University of Washington School of Medicine, Seattle, Washington

Peter Fehrenbach, Ph.D.
Post Doctoral Fellow, Department of Psychiatry and Behavioral Sciences, University of
Washington School of Medicine, Seattle, Washington

Wilbert E. Fordyce, Ph.D.
Professor, Department of Rehabilitation Medicine, University of Washington School of
Medicine, Seattle, Washington

Dean Funabiki, Ph.D.
Assistant Professor, Department of Psychology, Washington State University, Pullman,
Washington

Wayne Katon, M.D.
Assistant Professor, Department of Psychiatry and Behavioral Sciences, University of
Washington School of Medicine, Seattle, Washington

Arthur Kleinman, M.D.
Professor and Head, Division of Cultural Psychiatry, and Adjunct Professor of
Anthropology, Harvard University, Cambridge, Massachusetts

Ruth E. Little, Sc.D.
Director, Alcohol and Drug Abuse Institute, University of Washington School of Medicine,
Seattle, Washington

John D. Loeser, M.D.
Professor, Department of Neurological Surgery, University of Washington School of
Medicine, Seattle, Washington

Roland D. Maiuro, Ph.D.
Assistant Professor, Department of Psychiatry and Behavioral Sciences, University of
Washington School of Medicine, Seattle, Washington

Peter E. Maxim, Ph. D.
Associate Professor, Department of Psychiatry and Behavioral Sciences, University of
Washington School of Medicine, Seattle, Washington

George A. Ojemann, M.D.
Professor, Department of Neurological Surgery, University of Washington School of
Medicine, Seattle, Washington

Burton V. Reifler, M.D., M.P.H.
Associate Professor, Department of Psychiatry and Behavioral Sciences, University of
Washington School of Medicine, Seattle, Washington

Gary Rosen, M.D.
Clinical Assistant Professor, Department of Family Medicine, University of Washington
School of Medicine, Seattle, Washington

Gabriel Smilkstein, M.D.
Professor, Department of Family Medicine, University of Washington School of Medicine,
Seattle, Washington

James W. Smith, M.D.
Medical Director, Schick-Shadels Hospital, Seattle, Washington; Clinical Associate
Professor, Psychiatry and Behavioral Sciences, University of Washington School of
Medicine, Seattle, Washington

Orville A. Smith, Ph.D.
Professor of Physiology and Biophysics, Director of Regional Primate Center, University of
Washington School of Medicine, Seattle, Washington

Jeffrey C. Steger, Ph.D.
Department of Behavioral Science, Providence Hospital, Everett, Washington

Eric Trupin, Ph.D.
Associate Professor, Department of Psychiatry and Behavioral Sciences, University of
Washington School of Medicine, Seattle, Washington

Peter P. Vitaliano, Ph.D.
Associate Professor, Department of Psychiatry and Behavioral Sciences, University of
Washington School of Medicine, Seattle, Washington

Nicholas G. Ward, M.D.
Associate Professor, Department of Psychiatry and Behavioral Sciences, University of
Washington School of Medicine, Seattle, Washington

William M. Womack, M.D.
Associate Professor, Department of Psychiatry and Behavioral Sciences, University of
Washington School of Medicine, Seattle, Washington

Suzanne Wu, Ph.D.
Instructor, Department of Psychiatry and Behavioral Sciences, University of Washington
School of Medicine, Seattle, Washington

I

BEHAVIORAL SCIENCE MODELS AND RESEARCH IN HEALTH CARE

1

The Behavioral Sciences in Medicine:
Introduction and Overview

John E. Carr, Ph.D.* and Harold A. Dengerink, Ph.D.†

It has been said that George Bernard Shaw, the brilliant author and essayist, was adamant in his refusal to accept the explanation of bacterial contagion as a cause of tuberculosis. The prevailing medical evidence suggested that Shaw was wrong, since tuberculosis only occurs in the presence of bacteria; however, the medical explanation, while correct, was flawed in that it was overly narrow in perspective. Since the bacterium can be present without the exposed individual contracting tuberculosis, the presence of the pathogen alone is insufficient to account for the disease. Rather, one must take into account the conditions of the host, that is, those factors that determine receptivity or resilience. Thus we come to a consideration of the impact of environmental, genetic, social, and economic factors in determining the response of the organism to disease.

Have subsequent scientific findings supported Shaw's perspective? Initially the evidence was only suggestive. In the case of tuberculosis there was a steady decline in cases prior to the identification of the pathogen and long before the discovery of specific antibiotics effective against the disease. These changes were presumed to be associated with changes in hygienic conditions and in the health-seeking behavior of the public at the time. Patients were isolated in large sanatoriums, frequently in dry climates. Entire families moved to arid parts of the country and the patient was freed of financial and family obligations. Public experience with "consumption," as tuberculosis was frequently called, lead to earlier

*Professor and Acting Chairman, Department of Psychiatry and Behavioral Sciences, University of Washington School of Medicine, Seattle, Washington.
† Professor and Director of Clinical Training, Department of Psychology, Washington State University, Pullman, Washington.

recognition of the symptoms and the seeking of medical attention earlier in the course of the disease.

More compelling evidence of the relation between host characteristics and disease phenomena was provided in a Canadian government report entitled "A New Perspective on the Health of Canadians" (Lalonde, 1974). The document presented convincing evidence that Canadians were no longer dying of smallpox or intestinal obstructions, but were dying of tumors, hypertension-related disease, cardiovascular disease, alcoholism, accidents, suicides, and gunshot wounds, each of which was dependent upon a range of environmental, genetic, cultural, dietary, and social causes. According to this same report, the principal contributing elements of death and disease among Canadians were (1) inadequacies in the existing health care system, (2) behavioral factors or unhealthy life-styles, (3) environmental hazards, and (4) human biological factors.

Nor were these observations limited to Canadians. In 1979 the Surgeon General of the United States released an astounding report entitled "Healthy People" (U.S. Department of Health, Education, and Welfare, 1979) that stated that for the ten leading causes of death in the United States (cardiovascular disease, cancer, etc.) 50% of the mortality could be traced to unhealthy life-styles or behavioral factors (exposure to stress, excessive eating, cigarette smoking, alcohol consumption, etc.). An additional 20% could be traced to environmental factors such as food additives, airborne asbestos particles, and so on. Another 20% could be traced to biological factors and 10% could be related to inadequacies in health care. The Surgeon General's report specifically stated that "environmental factors and factors in individual behavior appear to be the prime causes of most forms of cancer."

Since 1979 the evidence has continued to mount. One recent study (McEvoy and Land, 1981) compared the mortality rates of Missouri residents who avoid caffeine, nicotine, and alcohol and generally lead conservative lives with those for other Missouri residents. Members of the group evidenced mortality rates that were 26% lower than those for other Missouri residents. Similar results have been reported from other studies that compared the mortality rates for groups who adhere to more healthy life-styles with mortality rates for the population as a whole.

This emerging recognition of the importance of behavioral factors in determining U.S. mortality led the Surgeon General to recommend a reexamination of priorities in American health care and medical education. That report specifically recommended that health care professionals should focus their attention on changing patient (or potential patient) behaviors that are responsible for deviations in health in the population.

Is there any reason to believe that attention to these factors has had and will have any significant impact on the mortality rate? The available evidence is reassuring. Numerous governmental and professional programs have been launched to inform the public and to change disease-related and health-seeking behaviors. Media campaigns and physician-distributed pamphlets have informed the public of cancer warning signs. Television talk shows, public service announcements, and newspaper articles have cautioned women to have regular pelvic examinations and have taught them self-examination procedures for the early detection of breast cancer. The myths of venereal disease and the dangers of various substances from illicit drugs to prescription medications have been described on every commercial television station. Patients have been exhorted by television and movie stars to take their hypertension medications and to not expect a prescription from every physician visit.

Such efforts in the early 1960s were followed by a decline in the role of heart disease and in the associated risk factors. In the same time period, European statistics indicated no change in health-seeking behavior, no reduction in risk factors, and no reduction in mortality rates (U.S. Department of Health, Education, and Welfare, 1979). It would thus appear that only when the educational and exhortation effects resulted in specifically changed behavior was there any significant impact upon health.

One is tempted to conclude that massive informational programs are required, but large-scale media campaigns have severe limitations. Significant change for many persons may require changes in the practices and attitudes of individual physicians as well. The Surgeon General's report captured the dilemma of the health care professions by noting that even people who did not modify their behavior "continued to note that they would be more likely to change their behaviors if their physician strongly recommended such changes. Yet health professionals often find themselves too pressed by duties related to diagnosis and treatment to capture the opportunity they have to influence behavior and therefore the health of their patients."

The problem for the physician, however, goes beyond the pressures of the examining room schedule. It includes the manner in which health care professionals conceptualize disease and illness. Traditionally, medicine has relied upon a scientific base that is primarily biological in nature. This scientific knowledge base fails to include many of the elements that the foregoing discussion has emphasized as being important. In contrast, Engel has proposed a "new medical model" that advocates attention to the interaction of biological, psychological, social, cultural, and environmental events in the determination of both disease and illness (Engel, 1977). Throughout this book health care is viewed in terms of the interaction of all these various factors. Taking as our point of departure an organ system approach, the "behavioral system" is viewed as the point of integration among all the organ systems. The rationale for this view is based upon two compelling pieces of evidence: (1) the demonstrated importance of behavioral factors in affecting illness behavior and (2) the observation that the medium of interaction between the patient and the physician is behavioral. This last point is exemplified by the physician's diagnostic evaluation, which is based in part on the behavioral manifestation (symptoms) of organ system dysfunction, and the physician's prescriptive recommendations that result in behavioral change on the part of the patient.

It is the purpose of this book, therefore, to address itself to two objectives: (1) to demonstrate to the student the importance of the broad range of nonbiological factors in health care that we will subsume under the general rubric of "behavioral" and which will include environmental, sociocultural, and psychological factors, and (2) to demonstrate the manner in which these interact with biological factors and with each other in determining the impact of disease-producing conditions on the response of the patient and subsequent illness behavior. We will attempt this demonstration by both detailing some major concepts and exemplifying them within the context of a review of selected examples of major clinical conditions that comprise the day-to-day practice of the primary care physician.

Historical Considerations

From a historical perspective, what accounts for the efficacy of the healing arts down through the ages? In part we may attribute their success to the serendipitous discoveries of natural curative substances utilized by healers throughout the world over thousands of years. Equally important has been the sensitivity, perhaps not always with awareness, of physician–priest– healers to those principles of behavior that affect an individual's responsiveness to disease and to healing procedures. We may note that the unity of mind and body was a common feature of the underlying belief system of many ancient healing arts, and it was the sensitivity of the ancient physician–healer to this relation and his or her ability to utilize it for healing purposes that distinguished successful treatment down through the ages.

Historical events and changing philosophical issues have had an impact on the development of our current attitudes and practices with regard to the delivery of health care. We shall consider the hypothesis that the emergence of Cartesian dualism gave rise to events culminating in medical science focusing on the biological bases of health and disease on the one hand and the development of a unique medical specialty, psychiatry, devoted to the treatment of the "diseases of the mind" on the other. These historical considerations raise an important question. If the concept of Cartesian dualism had not emerged and had medicine evolved on a philosophical basis of mind–body unity, what would have been the impact on current medical concepts and practice?

Several interesting possibilities suggest themselves; for example, would medical care be still further developed in the marriage of the biological with the behavioral and social? And does our increasing interest in the relation between the behavioral and the biological and the recent holistic health movement represent a return to these early universalist concepts? Perhaps it is no accident that at a time when these philosophical issues are reemerging there is renewed interest in comprehensive health care, the emergence of a "new" field, family medicine, and renewed interest in the incorporation of behavioral principals in the training of primary care physicians.

Many scholars of medical history have traced the emphasis upon biologically oriented medicine to the Flexner report of 1910. While the practice of American medicine prior to that time was primarily homeopathic in orientation, the Flexner report had a profound impact on medical education and essentially led to the monopolistic control by allopathic medicine of the educational institutions in the field. Clearly, the Flexner report emerged at a critical time and may well have been the precipitating event to complete the mind–body schism and establish biologically oriented medicine as the predominant orientation.

The concepts we shall consider are neither innovative nor modern, but have roots that reach far into the past. Ancient Chinese medical texts speak of a relation between good health and one's life-style. More than 2300 years ago Hippocrates argued that the physician must consider the whole person in order to diagnose and treat properly, and that social, environmental, and psychological changes influence well-being. Many non-Western healing systems have emphasized the concept of homeostasis in health and have taken a homeopathic approach to medicine, that is, one that facilitates the body's defensive systems against illness, as opposed to allopathic medicine, which involves the introduction of foreign agents to eliminate disease. The ancient Greeks possessed the sophistication to appreciate that both concepts were needed. Healing arts were associated with the god Aesculapius and his two daughters: Panacea, concerned with the development of medications for the sick, and Hygieia, concerned with wise living and healthy behavior.

The concept of mind–body unity did not totally disappear with Descartes. A popular nineteenth century home medical reference, *The American Family Physician* (King, 1860), contained the following quotation: "There is a direct and intimate sympathy existing between the mind and the body. So powerful is this that any disturbance of the one produces a disturbing influence upon the other; hence, it becomes necessary not only that the condition of the body be properly attended to but also what is of equal import, the conditions of the mind." In discussing the reciprocal action between the mind and body, the author reminded the reader the optimal states of mind and physique require challenge and exercise, but neither too much nor too little, since both can be deleterious to health. His description of these conditions anticipates our current concepts of health maintenance and attention to such factors as temperature, cleanliness, diet, fresh air, exercise, and other preventative health care measures.

While behavioral medicine is generally regarded as a recent development, it is interesting to note that there are historical precedents that predate it by a half century. A case in point is the unique and successful treatment program developed by Joseph Pratt in 1905 for the treatment of tuberculosis patients (Harris and Lightner, 1978). Confronted by the conflict between the life-style of his indigent and working class tuberculosis patients in Boston and the treatment of choice (extended bed rest, fresh air, and drinking large amounts of milk), Pratt was challenged to develop a treatment regimen designed to increase the motivation of these tuberculosis sufferers .

Patients were given directions and plans for building outdoor rest areas attached to their houses or tenements. They were also instructed in the keeping of a log book in which they recorded their weight, food intake, pulse, temperature, and other details on a daily basis. The record system was utilized to provide patients with regular feedback on their progress in combating symptoms and was also used in an externally managed reinforcement program where praise and social approval were given patients for increases in targeted behavior, such as time spent in bed, weight gain, and so forth.

The final feature in Pratt's therapeutic program was a system of rewarding patient compliance. Pratt treated his patients in groups of 15–20, which he called "classes." Patients were routinely visited at home by a social worker or nurse who would monitor their progress and make whatever minor modifications in the program that were necessary. If the patient had complied with the treatment program and achieved certain specified goals, then he or she would be allowed to attend a weekly group meeting of the class. Thus the privilege of class attendance was used to reinforce patient compliance. The patients with the best behavioral record were given social reinforcement during class and modeled their positive health behavior to others.

Pratt was able to obtain therapeutic results that were extraordinary, considering his population and the current medical technology. In 1927 he reported a 15-year follow-up of his first tuberculosis class, showing 72% of his patients returned to full work. By contrast, conventional, more expensive sanatorium treatment achieved rates 10–20% lower than Pratt's method.

Though predating the emergence of behavioral medicine by a half century, Pratt faced the same clinical problems faced by health care professionals today, for example, hypertension, diabetes, tuberculosis, etc. His ingenuous treatment approach was significant in that it included applications of operant conditioning and social learning theories to problems of behavior management currently utilized in "modern" behavioral medicine practice.

The Biological–Behavioral Interface

Whereas philosophers are concerned with the mind–body relationship, neurologists and neurosurgeons are more likely to insist that, from an organ systems standpoint, the brain is the organ of the mind. Therefore our concern should be with brain–behavior relations. Since our overall purpose is to look at the complex relations that exist between the biological and the behavioral, a logical starting point is a review of the basic concepts of brain–behavior relations, their impact on health care in general, and the problems they pose for the primary care physician in particular. We attempt to introduce the reader to some of the fundamental concepts of brain structure and function, and elucidate the complex relationships between brain specificity and manifest behaviors (e.g., spatial perception, emotion, and memory). It should be remembered that the brain does not function independently of its external environment and that while the brain itself affects the manifest behavior of an individual, it is in turn affected by factors in the environment, resulting in a complex of interdependent relations.

We are aware that there is substantial individual variability in the patterns of lateralization and intrahemispheric localization of brain functions, and that these individual patterns are as variable as personalities or faces. Such individuality is a function not only of genetic determinants, but also of environmental influences that impact upon the developing brain during critical periods. Thus environmental and hereditary influences begin to blur when one attempts to specify the ultimate causality of behavior. The net effect, however, is that each individual possesses a highly idiosyncratic "computer" uniquely programmed in response to an individualistic set of environmental and genetic circumstances. It is not surprising, therefore,that we manifest unique responses to perception, the processing of information, and emotion, and that the complex integration of these behaviors yields a highly distinctive personality. Thus the unique behaviors and experiences of an individual result in idiosyncratic functioning of the central nervous system. This idiosyncratic functioning then operates to perpetuate the unique behavior patterns that contributed to its formation in the first place.

Recent developments in neurobiology suggest that our search for links between behavior and the nervous system may indeed take us into the realm of molecular structure and cellular mechanisms (Davis, 1980).

Investigations into the physical basis of conscious learning appear to involve altered functioning in existing synapses, as well as the formation of new synapses; but Davis cautions us against overoptimism. Consciousness, like many forms of human behavior, is remarkably complex and may require "some as yet unknown concept—not a return to mind–body dualism, but a set of rules for intercellular information flow as novel as molecular information storage was a few decades ago" (Davis, 1980, p. 87).

The biological–behavioral interface is also evident in the complex biochemical functions that relate to behavior. For example, morphinelike biochemical substances, called endorphins, have been shown to be produced within the body itself and to have the ability to ease pain and induce a feeling of euphoria. These substances are produced by the brain, the pituitary gland, and other tissues in response to both physical and psychological stresses (Davis, 1980). Although the mechanisms are not fully understood, it is clear that the endorphins seem to play a particularly useful role in enabling the individual to deal successfully with psychological stress.

Stress triggers "fight or flight" responses, increasing blood pressure, heart rate, metabolism, and other physical functions to mobilize the body for action. However, this reaction can be dangerous to one's health if it is produced constantly by situations that call for nonphysical responses, that is, psychological stress. Not infrequently vascular diseases, ulcers, and other physical disorders are caused or aggravated by such an appropriate reaction. Endorphins appear to counter these adrenaline-triggered over-reactions by slowing respiration, lowering blood pressure, and calming motor activity throughout the body. Thus the release of endorphins in response to stress seems to have an adaptive value.

While physicians and medical researchers have long believed the immune system to be independent of psychological factors or other brain-related influences, recent research suggests a close, relatively unexplored relation between the immune system and the central nervous system. We have known for years that psychological factors can affect physical health and it seemed only logical that they should have some impact on the immune system. In 1870 Pasteur predicted that one could affect cures of diseases not only by killing the cause but by also bolstering the body's defenses against the invading pathogens. Pasteur indicated that biochemical, physiological, and emotional attitudes all affect the course and outcome of infectious diseases, and that resistance to disease was a function of nutrition, rest, general fitness, and peace of mind. An example is to be found in diabetes, where vulnerability to viral and fungal infections is increased as the result of metabolic abnormalities that activate pathogens lying dormant in the body.

Thus stress appears to be a critical variable in the equation relating behavioral events and illness. Chicken pox and herpes simplex viruses can be latent for years, then, under stress, multiply and cause disease. Some viruses invade the host body and develop within certain cells, but growth is impeded due to chemical processes in the cell. This blocking action of the body's natural defenses can be enhanced or, under conditions of stress, be significantly reduced, resulting in vulnerability to disease.

Recent researchers have investigated the efficacy of a treatment technique called cell-mediated immunity (CMI), in which the body is injected with certain microorganisms that promote the development of scavenger blood cells, which in turn attack a variety of pathogens in the bloodstream (Herberman, 1982).

Another example of the body's natural defenses is the substance interferon, a protein that is diffused throughout body fluids and which serves to protect healthy cells against viral infections. It stimulates the host cell to produce a nucleic acid (RNA), which in turn directs the synthesis of protein that interferes with viral reproduction. Recent research suggests that it may play a role in combating certain forms of cancer, hepatitis, and respiratory disorders (Stewart, 1981). Yet another avenue involves the activation of the endocrine system to alter hormonal levels in the blood, resulting in conditions such as vasodilation or constriction, which may have an effect on pathogen growth and the inflammatory response of the vascular system to infection. It would appear that in addition to being a brilliant author and essayist George Bernard Shaw was also a prophet.

Gender Role and Sex Differences

The relations between behavioral and biological phenomena extend far beyond the molecular and cellular level. The complexity of biobehavioral interrelations are no more clearly illustrated than in the study of the impact of gender differences upon illness and health care. There are major differences between the genders in morbidity and mortality rates with certain diseases. At almost all ages males have higher death rates and are more frequently afflicted with chronic diseases associated with considerable reductions in longevity. As Verbrugge (1980) and Kessler et al. (1981) indicated, there are gender differences in rates of disability, help seeking, and utilization of services, and evidence to suggest that these differences are primarily associated with behavioral rather than biological factors. Other researchers have indicated that there are gender differences in susceptibility to hypertension, with a somewhat greater association for women than men between a family history of hypertension and development of hypertension. Furthermore, there appears to be a greater likelihood that females with a history of hypertension will develop greater cardiovascular reactivity than males with a family history of hypertension. Again, while constitutional factors appear to play a greater role in influencing blood pressure in women than in men, reported gender differences in coping strategies and coping effectiveness may be the result of behavioral factors, for example, environmental or sociocultural influences. Interpersonal relations are often influenced by the prescribed or assumed social roles of the participants. Among the various roles, none is more ubiquitous than those referred to as gender roles. These roles also pervade the examining room and influence the behavior of both the patient and the physician, affecting decisions to medicate, hospitalize, and so forth. Thus consideration of gender and biological sex differences introduces a complicated variable into the myriad of other variables the physican must take into consideration if he or she is to deliver efficacious health care.

Culture and Communication

We move progressively further from biological mechanisms to consideration of the role played by social and cultural variables in determining illness and health-seeking behavior. No set of variables has received more attention in recent years than have cultural factors in influencing not only disease but culturally determined responses to disease. The physician must deal not simply with the pathogenic process of disease but also with the impact of the disease on the patient's life and social network.

Costas et al. (1981) provided an excellent example of the complex nature of this problem in their study of the association of skin color to coronary heart disease risk factors in 4000 urban Puerto Rican males. The authors found that skin color showed a small but statistically significant association with coronary heart disease risk factors, but also pointed out that skin color also tended to be associated with lower socioeconomic status based on income, education, and occupation. Hence it is unclear as to whether the association with skin color represented genetic or environmental influences. Another example has been provided by Palgi (1981), who found hemoglobin levels of Asian Jewish women to be lower than in their European counterparts, but was unable to determine whether the findings reflected genetic and/or socioeconomic differences, such as living conditions, health services, and food supplies to which individuals have access.

We shall consider the complex communication problems posed for the physician by differences in cultural background between the doctor and the patient. Ethnic backgrounds may represent not only potential differences in language but also far more significant differences in beliefs about illnesses, prevention, and health care imbedded in cultural tradition.

In many cultures, our own included, the language of the body is used to describe in metaphor the impact of life's stresses and strains on the individual. Beyond such obvious examples as, "My boss is a pain in the neck," it is the phenomenon of somatization that represents the initial impact point in the doctor–patient relationship. It is where all the variables of the biopsychosocial approach come to bear, since symptomatic description is subject to all the psychological, psychosocial, and biological factors we have discussed up to this point.

The issue of communication is considered further in the context of communication research and the doctor–patient relationship. The health care professions have given little attention to the potential of this enormous body of research not only for explaining the mechanisms that operate within the doctor–patient relationship, but also for improving the relationship and the efficacy of the eventual treatment outcome. A relevant review of communications research offers convincing explanations for some of the dilemmas of medicine, such as the placebo effect and problems of patient compliance.

Evaluation in a Family Context

We shall attempt to bring together the major conceptual issues discussed earlier and demonstrate how they might be utilized in the clinical assessment of a patient's health care problems. The conceptual points are admittedly complex, and any attempt to comprehend how biomedical and psychosocial issues may be blended to enhance health care should be rightly viewed as a major challenge for the physician. Three approaches are suggested to identify and organize relevant clinical data within the context of a biopsychosocial system of health care. An attempt is made to show that through their integration the practicing physician may benefit immensely from a comprehensive behavioral analysis of a patient's health problem, leading to an equally comprehensive health care plan.

Central to each of these approaches is the assumption that the patient functions within the context of family and community and that the impact of the illness on these social systems, together with the supportive resources provided by them, must be accurately assessed and appropriately utilized by the physician if the eventual treatment outcome is to be successful.

Coping and Support

In a landmark interdisciplinary study of health, Vaillant (1979) followed 204 college males in the next four decades of their lives and found a strong relation between emotional adjustment and physical health. Vaillant concluded that anxiety, depression and emotional distress appeared to produce profound effects in host susceptibility to a variety of diseases. "Stress does not kill us so much as ingenious adaptations to stress (call it good mental health or mature coping mechanisms) facilitate our survival."

In a nine-year study of 4725 adult mortality cases between the ages of 30 and 69, Berkman and Symes (1979) found that the risk of death was 2.8 times greater in women and 2.3 times greater in men with the fewest social ties. These findings were consistent for ischemic heart disease, cancer, cardiovascular disease, and circulatory disease.

We drew upon the implications of these and numerous related studies to conclude that the presence of life stress predicts increased psychological and physical morbidity, but that individual differences in resiliency and coping mechanisms, together with social ties, mitigate the pathological effects of stress-produced illness. Thus medical intervention, to be successful, must rely not simply upon the carrying out of mortal combat between the physician and the disease (with the patient as the unwitting and passive battleground) but, rather, on an alliance between the physician and the patient in which the physician provides support and appropriate resources to facilitate the patient's own defenses and coping mechanisms.

The Patient Experience

A brilliant and moving statement of the importance of the relationship between the doctor and the patient has been provided by Norman Cousins, author of the best-selling *Anatomy of an Illness*. Perhaps it required the eloquence of a "literary man," not a "medical man," to focus our attention on the importance of what Cousins has come to term "the engineering of hope." Cousins, founder and former editor of the *Saturday Review*, insists that a physician who does not give much weight to the consideration of behavioral factors in the conduct of his job is in fact only doing half a job. In what is now considered a classic article, required in many medical school courses on the behavioral sciences (*New England Journal of Medicine*, December 1976), Cousins describes the healing of his own potentially fatal collagen disease and the unique partnership between himself and his physician friend Dr. William Hitzig. Cousins insists that the patient, not the doctor, is the healer, and that the doctor's job is to activate the healing mechanism.

It would be erroneous to assume that Cousins' experience was unique or atypical. Similar cases may be observed on an almost daily basis in any physicians' office or clinic throughout the world. They stand in stark contrast to the arrogance and sterility not infrequently encountered in even major medical centers and eloquently, if not disturbingly, reported by one of medicine's own, Dr. Harold Lear, a urologist and surgeon. In the book *Heart Sounds*, Martha Wineman Lear describes her husband's five-year ordeal and the incredible "bungling and callousness" to which he was subjected by trained medical staff. These personal accounts of the patient experience should be read by every physician, practicing or in training.

Stress and Illness

An understanding of the current hypotheses concerning the psychophysiology of stress enables us to begin to appreciate biological mechanisms that bridge the interactions between environmental conditions and behavioral responses (Glass, 1977). We will consider models such as Selye's general adaptation syndrome, which attempts to explain in more detailed fashion the specific series of processes by which the individual organism responds to differential stimulus conditions. Furthermore, we begin to appreciate the illness states that evolve and develop when such adaptation processes begin to break down. The interaction between psychological and physiological variables is explored within the context of the type A personality and these and other characteristics that put individuals at risk for particular types of diseases are reviewed. At the same time, the reader is cautioned against concluding that psychological or personality factors are "causes" of disease states. Rather, as Vaillant has indicated, these factors describe coping skills within individuals that make them especially resistant to the deleterious effects of stress.

Major Health Care Problems

With an overall appreciation of the nature of the relation between stress and illness, we can consider a specific clinical condition that relates directly to stress and which represents a major illness and cause of death in the United States. In reviewing the epidemiology and possible etiology of hypertension, we clearly see the relevance of behavioral and environmental factors in the production of this illness, one that yields measurable changes in vital functions of the body and which, if uncorrected, will result in death. In describing the clinical phenomena, its etiological characteristics, and primary modes of treatment, we may also address the question, What is the mechanism of biobehavioral interaction in hypertension? Three prevailing hypotheses are considered, each based on the current state of knowledge of the physiological, biochemical, and brain–behavior relations known to be related to changes in the hypertensive condition.

An especially important development in the application of behavioral science to medicine has been the rapidly advancing field of behavioral medicine, which evolved in large part from research on operant conditioning techniques applied specifically to the acquisition of illness and health-seeking behaviors. A review of basic principles illustrates the remarkable breadth of application from early research on respondent and operant conditioning to the conceptual issue of self-control and the procedures by which physicians may assist patients in changing their own behavior.

The impact of these behavioral techniques provides a backdrop for a discussion of biofeedback, a treatment technique widely used for various psychophysiological disorders. Biofeedback techniques, like many other behaviorally based techniques, are logical consequences of our increased understanding of the unique "feedback loop" information-processing systems that enable individuals to respond adaptably to incoming stimuli and day-to-day situations. Our appreciation of the role played by learning principles in these processes enables us to develop homeopathic treatment techniques that facilitate and enhance the organism's natural resources in dealing with impinging stress. Several cases of biofeedback treatment of headache disorders are presented in this book to illustrate the utility of the procedure.

The equipment is far less sophisticated but the problems all too familiar when considering the behavioral problems seen in pediatric practice. The behavioral sciences have made an especially unique contribution to the management of problems of pediatric practice commonly encountered by the primary care physician. The techniques, especially designed to provide the practitioner with effective intervention tools, are suitably adapted to the time constraints and heavy patient demands of a busy practice, yet due consideration is given to the frequent dilemmas faced by the practitioner when confronted by the exceptionally difficult or complex case. In our discussion we attempt to provide some insight into how one determines the limits to which these techniques can be pushed and what alternative treatment modalities and expertise may be available to the practitioner.

One of the major problems of modern health care is the treatment of the chronic patient. By differentiating between acute and chronic pain, we are able to meaningfully review the role that environmental and behavioral factors play in influencing pain behavior. Our attention is especially focused on the significance of understanding the essential role played by operant conditioning factors in the acquisition of pain behavior. Given this knowledge, the physician can effectively intervene through the utilization of these same principles in effecting significant reductions in pain behavior and increased health-seeking behavior. In counterpoint to this consideration of behavior factors, the relative effectiveness of other treatment techniques, such as neurosurgical and pharmacological approaches, is reviewed and appropriate utilization of these techniques, as well as both their medical and behavioral risks, are considered. The health care professional should be especially attentive to how ignorance of the role of behavioral factors can unwittingly precipitate medication abuse.

A major portion of this book is devoted to a review of the general area of affective conditions, such as anxiety and depression, and the problems they represent, especially to the practicing primary care physician. It would be erroneous to assume that these problems lie only within the domain of the psychiatrist or that they are rarely seen in primary care. On the contrary, affective disorders are probably the most commonly seen illness conditions in medical practice. Affective states are complex behavioral phenomena that reflect internal physiological conditions, external environmental conditions, and cognitive perceptions of both, with the latter influenced by past sociocultural experiences. All of these combine to determine our emotional states as well as our perceptions and our labeling of them.

It is important to note that those areas of the brain that regulate autonomic functions (and therefore the maintenance of the organism's internal environment) overlap with those areas that regulate emotion. This situation appears to occur at both the cortical and subcortical levels. Thus we are provided with a physiological mechanism by which to explain the common correlation of affective states and illness conditions, for example, psychophysiological and psychosomatic disorders, and our understanding of the relation between stress and illness becomes clearer. In our review of the two most common families of affective states, depression and anxiety, we consider their epidemiology and the complex system of biobehavioral variables that determine them. The major problem faced by the practicing physician is how to determine whether a condition is secondary to another illness or represents a primary disorder. As previously discussed, the complexities of biobehavioral relations do not make this an easy task, and more often than not the physician may be confronted with a situation where the answer to these questions will never become clear. The old adage, "a little knowledge is a dangerous thing," is no more aptly applied in the field of medicine than it is to the treatment of affective disorders by the primary care physician. Quantities of antianxiety and antidepressive drugs, prescribed indiscriminantly and often inappropriately, constitute a problem of major proportion that can only be meaningfully addressed by far greater attention to the treatment of these conditions in the training of primary care physicians.

In a subsequent chapter we shall consider the complex field of drug abuse and especially the issue of medication misuse (by physicians as well as patients). It is important to realize that a knowledge of behavioral principles is as essential to an understanding of drug abuse as is a knowledge of pharmacology—and often more useful when attempting to understand the complex determinants of addictive behavior. We shall review the common families of misused medications and their psychological as well as physiological characteristics. In pointing out that the most dangerously addictive drugs are often the most easily accessible, we are reminded of the risk the physician runs in contributing to, as well as solving, the drug abuse problems of patients.

We shall also consider an equally complex and related problem—

alcohol abuse. The epidemiology of alcoholism describes a highly prevalent medical problem, commonly seen by family physicians, with physiological, psychological, behavioral, and sociocultural determinants. It is commonly associated with stress, depression, and anxiety, and is not infrequently correlated with other illnesses. It provides us with yet another excellent example of the complex interaction between biobehavioral variables.

Finally, we shall consider a problem that is relatively unique as a primary health care area yet quite commonplace from the standpoint of patient and physician experience. The problems of the elderly in medical practice are no longer the ignored domain of a quarter of a century ago but represent an area of increasing importance in health care because of increased longevity as the average age of our population increases and medical science is confronted with new frontiers.

In many respects, the problems of the elderly represent the logical, as well as chronological, culmination of those complex biobehavioral interactions we have traced through so many other examples. In no other arena of health care are the influences of sociocultural variables, environment, biological dysfunction, and psychological function seen in such bold relief.

Origin of This Book

This book is the result of several years of development, beginning with a decision on the part of the faculty at the University of Washington School of Medicine to reorganize the first-year basic science course. In doing so, the dean of curriculum solicited opinions from a variety of physicians, asking what information should be included in the course and what educational goals should be achieved. These physicians, who had been trained in the biomedical tradition but who had practiced, conducted research, and taught for several years, responded in detail. First, they asked that the course be in addition to and separate from consideration of traditional psychopathology topics. Second, they requested that the students understand the role of behavior in patient-caused deviations in health. Third, they requested that students acquire the skills to change patient behavior insofar as these could promote better health. Fourth, they asked that students learn to evaluate the role of patient behavior as it influenced physician decision making in diagnoses and treatment. Finally, they asked that students learn the pitfalls of physicians influencing patient behavior in unanticipated and undesirable ways.

As the course progressed, both behavioral scientists and physician–educators participated in the definition of course objectives and the selection of course materials. These individuals have participated in numerous grueling evaluations of the course content and format. In addition, many students have over the past several years provided valuable feedback that has helped to shape both the content and conduct of the course. The contributors to this volume represent the major contributors to this course. Thus the concepts, information, and procedures they have presented represent the integrated efforts of numerous persons, including both basic scientists and clinicians. The approach, we believe, is unique in that it is not simply an attempt by behavioral scientists to exhort physicians to change their ways, nor is it a review of basic behavioral sciences literature that lacks immediate relevance to medicine; rather, it is an integration of behavioral science principles with biological/physiological principles for the purpose of improved primary care medicine. It typifies the new biopsychosocial model and represents the result of a true conceptual and working partnership between medicine and the behavioral sciences.

References

Berkman, L., and S. Symes. 1979. Social networks, host resistance and mortality: A nine-year follow-up of Alameda County residents. American Journal of Epidemiology 109:186–204.

Costas, R., M. Garcia-Palmieri, P. Sorlie, and E. Hertymark. 1981. Coronary heart disease risk factors in men with light and dark skin in Puerto Rico. American Journal of Public Health 71:614–619.

Cousins, N. 1979. Anatomy of an Illness as Perceived by the Patient. New York: Norton.

Davis, B. 1980. Frontiers of the biological sciences. Science 209:78–89.

Dubos, R. 1978. Bolstering the body against disease. Human Nature (August):68–72.

Engel, G. 1977. The need for a new medical model: A challenge for biomedicine. Science 196:129–136.

Glass, D. 1977. Stress Behavior Patterns, and Coronary Disease. American Scientist 65:177–187.

Harris, B., and J. Lightner. 1978. Behavioral Management of Medical Compliance: Its Role in the History of Group Psychotherapy. Paper presented at 50th Annual Meeting of the Midwestern Psychological Association, Chicago.

Herberman, D. 1982. Natural killer cells. Hospital Practice 17:93–103.

Kessler, R., R. Brown, and C. Broman. 1981. Sex differences in psychiatric help-seeking: Evidence from four large scale surveys. Journal of Health and Social Behavior 22:49–64.

King, J. 1860. The new American family physician. Indianapolis: Robert Douglass.

Lalonde, M. 1974. A New Perspective on the Health of Canadians. Ottawa: Ministry of National Health and Welfare.

Lear, M. 1980. Heart Sounds. New York: Simon and Schuster.

McEvoy, L., and G. Land. 1981. Lifestyle and death patterns of the Missouri RLDS Church members. American Journal of Public Health 71:1350–1357.

Palgi, A. 1981. Ethnic differences in hemoglobin distribution of Asian and European Jewish women in Israel, both pregnant and nonpregnant. American Journal of Public Health 71:847–851.

Stewart, W. 1981. Clinical status of the interferons: Will their promise be kept? Hospital Practice 16:97–105.

U.S. Department of Health, Education and Welfare, Public Health Service. 1979. Healthy People: The Surgeon General's Report on Health Promotion and Disease Prevention. Washington, DC: U.S. Government Printing Office DHEW (PHS) Publication No. 79-55071.

Vaillant, G. 1979. Natural history of male psychologic health: Effects of mental health on physical health. New England Journal of Medicine 301:1249–1254.

Verbrugge, L. 1980. Sex differences in complaints and diagnoses. Journal of Behavioral Medicine 3:327–355.

2

Behavioral Research in Health Care

Harold A. Dengerink, Ph.D.* and Cornelis B. Bakker, M.D.†

Historically the relation between behavioral sciences and medicine has generally been one of mutual neglect. Although the early histories of psychology and medicine were the same (persons such as Hippocrates were important to both), medicine has largely developed independently of psychology and other behavioral sciences. As the biological bases of disease became apparent, medical sciences pursued these bases and provided the medical professions with major innovations for improving health. The behavioral sciences continued to develop in other directions and overlapped with medical sciences only insofar as the two were concerned with mental retardation and some abnormal behaviors.

After this long period of mutual indifference, the behavioral sciences are bursting into the medical scene with great vigor and have succeeded in just a few years in establishing the basic structure of a new discipline, behavioral medicine. Observing this phenomenon, one must wonder about the source of this vigor and whether this is only a new fad of passing interest or an essential building block in the growing structure of medicine.

A review of some basic facts that bear on health and illness in modern society leads unavoidably to the conclusion that behavioral medicine is a logical and necessary response to some major issues in health care. First, while the medical professions have made major improvements in health care, the most promising remaining frontiers involve behavioral rather than strictly biological factors. If the medical profession is to provide major

*Professor and Director of Clinical Training, Department of Psychology, Washington State University, Pullman, Washington.

† Professor and Chairman, Department of Psychiatry, Peoria School of Medicine, Peoria, Illinois.

advances in the health of developed countries, then it must foster changes in an individual's behavior patterns, including personal habits, life-style, and coping skills. Second, the medical profession must address the behavioral factors that influence persons to avail themselves of or comply with medical interventions. In doing so, the medical profession must recognize that it does not operate in a vacuum but, rather, overlaps with and has a reciprocal relation with other sociopsychological systems. The day-to-day practice of medicine is influenced by a variety of behavioral phenomena, and medical intervention itself (including nonintervention) may have important social and behavioral consequences.

What Has Led to the Emergence of Behavioral Medicine?

There are two basic reasons why behavioral medicine is emerging. First of all, the behavioral sciences themselves have sufficiently matured to be able to provide practical assistance. Medical psychology, as it was previously taught in medical schools, tended to provide interesting insights to human existence and may have led to a deepening appreciation of the patient's plight; but while this may have improved the physician's interviewing style and his relation with the patient, it did not provide him with tools that were helpful in either curing or preventing illness. Such practical assistance and some specific techniques developed by behavioral sciences are a major focus of this volume.

The second and equally important reason for the late emergence of behavioral medicine can be derived from Table 1. Table 1 shows that up until 1950 there has been an enormous growth in effectiveness of the battle against mortality. Year after year, the death toll of various diseases was effectively reduced. However, beginning in the 1950s, the mortality tables show less and less improvement. This slowdown has occurred in spite of a rapid expansion in medical expenditures. In fact, we are now confronted with a situation where, at tremendous cost, little or no progress is made in mortality reduction. The reasons for this are obvious. The major causes of our increased longevity are related to our ability to cope with microorganisms by means of hygiene, disinfection, immunization, and antibiotics, as well as to the general improvement of the living situation in terms of nutrition, shelter, and availability of medical care.

The enormous successes of medicine themselves focused all attention on concepts and efforts that thus far had proven to be effective. When in the 1950s this payoff began to be less and less spectacular, we responded in typical human fashion, doing more of the same thing and doing the same thing better. This strategy is still called for in many developing parts of the world where adequate health care remains unavailable. In more developed parts of the world, however, doing more of the same has led to only minor improvements. In 1967 the Canadian Ministry of Health

Table 1. Changes in Life Expectancy (1900–1970)[a]

		Change from previous years	Percentage of change
1900	47.3		
1916	50.0	+2.7	5.7
1920	54.1	+4.1	8.2
1930	59.7	+5.6	10.4
1940	62.9	+3.2	5.4 (Depression)
1950	68.2	+6.7	10.7
1960	69.7	+1.5	2.2
1970	70.9	+1.2	1.7

[a]Data courtesy of the Center for National Health Statistics.

conducted a long-range study of that country's health (LaLonde, 1974). That study found that despite major advances in medical techniques and the availability of health care through socialized medicine, mortality rates failed to further improve for Canadians.

Equally characteristic of the human way of problem solving was the gradual, although reluctant, recognition that the current direction of efforts was approaching the limits of its potential and that a new conceptualization of health and disease was needed. This state of affairs fostered a perspective on the determinants of mortality as well as morbidity, from which behavioral medicine has begun to emerge. In the following, we will exemplify the observations made as a result of this shift in focus and the possibilities created by this new medical discipline. A closer look at the U.S. mortality tables will serve as a starting point.

Causes of Death

Tables of life expectancy are statistics derived from composites of a total population (see Table 2). It is obvious that life expectancy is reduced most significantly by individuals who die young. The most dramatic improvements in life expectancy statistics, therefore, were more indicative of the reduction of infant mortality (due to perinatal care and elimination of childhood infectious diseases) than of an actual longer life-span of those who had reached adulthood. Following this initial impressive result and partially overlapping with it was the gradual elimination of major infectious diseases, poor work and living conditions, and so forth, as was already mentioned above. What we are left with now is a rather stable rate of mortality. The impact of any improvement in medical care on life expectancy can be computed by multiplying the number of people affected with the potential number of years gained. For example, assuming an average additional life expectancy of 50 years, a 50% reduction in car

Table 2. Leading Causes of Death in the United States in 1977[a]

All ages		Ages 1–14		Ages 15–34	
Male	Female	Male	Female	Male	Female
Heart diseases 396,431	Heart diseases 322,294	Accidents 6,275	Accidents 3,327	Accidents 31,881	Accidents 8,331
Cancer 210,459	Cancer 176,227	Cancer 1,407	Cancer 957	Suicide 8,826	Cancer 3,454
Cerebrovascular diseases 77,351	Cerebrovascular diseases 104,583	Congenital anomalies 902	Congenital anomalies 840	Homicide 8,358	Suicide 2,566
Accidents 71,935	Accidents 31,267	Homicide 421	Homicide 345	Cancer 4,015	Homicide 2,269
Pneumonia, influenza 27,618	Pneumonia, influenza 23,575	Pneumonia, influenza 382	Pneumonia, influenza 336	Heart diseases 2,608	Heart diseases 1,234
Suicide 21,109	Diabetes 19,357	Heart diseases 280	Heart diseases 260	Cirrhosis of liver 927	Cirrhosis of liver 470
Cirrhosis of liver 20,167	Arteriosclerosis 17,106	Meningitis 181	Cystic fibrosis 135	Cerebrovascular diseases 774	Pneumonia, influenza 467
Homicide 15,355	Cirrhosis of liver 10,681	Suicide 160	Cerebrovascular diseases 121	Pneumonia, influenza 722	Congenital anomalies 440
Diabetes 13,632	Diseases of infancy 9,953	Cerebrovascular diseases 153	Cerebral palsy 116	Congenital anomalies 638	Cerebrovascular diseases 412
Diseases of infancy 13,448	Suicide 7,572	Cerebral palsy 123	Meningitis 113	Epilepsy 387	Diabetes 303

	Ages 35–54		Ages 55–74		Ages 75 and over	
	Male	Female	Male	Female	Male	Female
	Heart diseases 43,592	Cancer 27,972	Heart diseases 191,458	Heart diseases 99,105	Heart diseases 157,986	Heart diseases 107,990
	Cancer 26,646	Heart diseases 13,338	Cancer 117,884	Cancer 87,555	Cancer 60,417	Cerebrovascular diseases 73,663
	Accidents 13,660	Cerebrovascular diseases 4,759	Cerebrovascular disease 28,585	Cerebrovascular disease 25,531	Cerebrovascular disease, 43,064	Cancer 56,222
	Cirrhosis of liver 7,607	Accidents 4,634	Accidents 12,424	Diabetes 8,316	Pneumonia, influenza 15,028	Pneumonia, influenza 16,310
	Suicide 5,612	Cirrhosis of liver 3,892	Cirrhosis of liver 10,205	Accidents 6,322	Arteriosclerosis 8,725	Arteriosclerosis 14,949
	Cerebrovascular diseases 4,679	Suicide 2,760	Pneumonia, influenza 8,425	Cirrhosis of liver 5,264	Accidents, 6,944	Diabetes 9,257
	Homicide 4,532	Diabetes 1,435	Emphysema 7,040	Pneumonia, influenza 4,566	Emphysema 4,887	Accidents 8,142
	Pneumonia, influenza 2,083	Pneumonia, influenza 1,178	Diabetes 6,840	Emphysema 2,175	Diabetes 4,731	Hernia and intestinal obstruction 1,985
	Diabetes 1,687	Homicide 1,142	Suicide 5,034	Arteriosclerosis 2,058	Nephritis 1,918	Hypertension 1,818
	Emphysema 630	Nephritis 438	Arteriosclerosis 2,711	Suicide 1,848	Hypertension 1,471	Nephritis 1,744

[a] Adapted from Silverberg (1980).

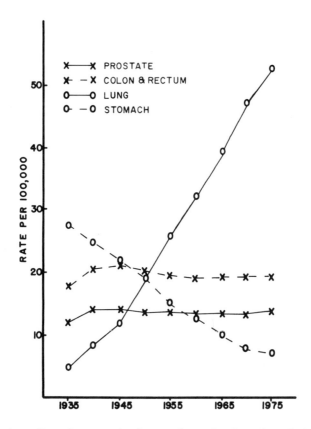

Figure 1. Age-adjusted cancer death rates for males for selected sites. Adapted from Silverberg (1980).

accidents would add approximately 23,000 × 50 = 1,150,000 man-years to the U.S. male population. In contrast, a 50% reduction in heart disease in males over age 65 (assuming an average additional life expectancy of 7 years) would yield only 135,000 × 7 = 945,000 man-years. As it is claimed that 50% of the car accidents are related to alcohol, one can readily recognize the impact of, for instance, more effective measures to control drunk driving as compared with the application of surgical procedures to improve the blood supply to the heart muscle. In any case, it is clear that violence—including accidents, homicide, and suicide—is the greatest problem bearing on mortality in the age group under 35.

Beginning at age 35, the statistics reflect the increasing impact of habit patterns that must be present for a long time before they begin to significantly affect health. Table 2 shows that after age 34, cancer and heart disease replace accidents as the major causes of death. An enormous effort

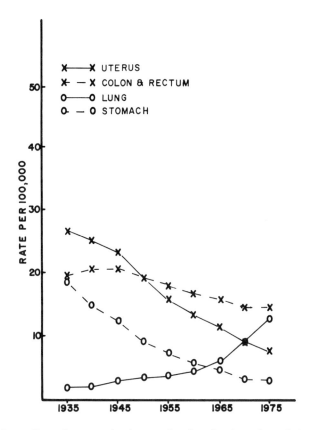

Figure 2. Age-adjusted cancer death rates for females for selected sites. Adapted from Silverberg (1980).

is being made to reduce their impact. The result of this effort relative to cancer is shown in Figs. 1 and 2, which represent a composite graph of the trends in cancer deaths from 1935 to 1975. These graphs provide an interesting and compelling picture. First of all, most types of cancer have maintained a stable relative death rate in spite of all of our efforts to push it back. The only consistent decline is in stomach cancer. As it is well known that the treatment of stomach cancer is one of the least successful of all cancer treatments, it must be clear that the reduction is not due to the fact that an effective treatment of stomach cancer has been found but, rather, is the result of a lower incidence. It may well be that the strenuous efforts of the Food and Drug Administration to eliminate carcinogenic substances from our food supply is having the intended results. Changes in habit patterns may also play a role. It has been noted that in countries where people eat or drink things that are very hot there is a high incidence of

Table 3. Person-Years Lost due to Cancer

Male		Female	
Site	Person-years lost	Site	Person-years lost
Lung	695,083	Breast	569,167
Colon	190,054	Colon	261,703
Lymphoma	182,613	Lung	197,047
Leukemia	178,362	Ovary	187,197
Prostate	151,024	Cervix, uterus	158,894
Pancreas	128,168	Leukemia	156,882
Stomach	123,747	Lymphoma	152,977
Brain	111,124	Pancreas	107,355

cancer of the stomach (Japan, 43.8 out of 100,000 population, versus the United States, 6.6 out of 100,000 population; World Health Statistics Annual, 1977–1978).

The most obviously impressive aspect of Figs. 1 and 2 is the line indicating the mortality rate of lung cancer. The tremendous rise over the past 40 years in the incidence of lung cancer has now made it the leading cause of death due to cancer in males, and, as Fig. 2 shows, females are steadily catching up. The shape of the curves indicates that as yet there is no reason to anticipate a reduction in the relative rise of lung cancer deaths, and for the females we must foresee that lung cancer will become the leading cause of cancer death in the near future. The actual impact of lung cancer becomes even more apparent if one examines Table 3, which exemplifies the impact of cancer death in terms of person-years lost and which shows that in males lung cancer alone accounts for as many person-years lost as the next four major types of cancer combined.

The relation of lung cancer to smoking is, of course, so well known that it need not be belabored at this point. It does indicate, however, that improved mortality may depend upon efforts to reduce smoking rather than upon medical interventions that are applied after the cancer has developed.

The importance of personal habits is also illustrated by the effects of consuming alcohol. Liver cirrhosis becomes the fifth leading cause of death in males between 35 and 54. The same abuse, however, has a far greater impact when one considers the number of homicides, suicides, and accidents that are alcohol related. Indeed, alcohol abuse contributes to a substantial increase in the probability of dying from all causes at all ages. The interaction of alcohol with other factors has been most clearly

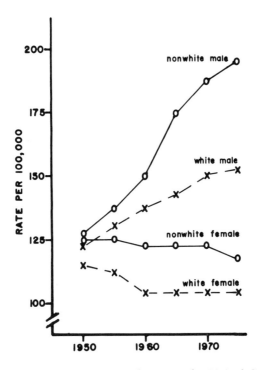

Figure 3. Cancer death rates by sex and race in the United States 1950–1977. Adapted from Silverberg (1980).

demonstrated in a study by Rothman and Keller (1972) that shows that the occurrence of oral cancer is correlated with both smoking as well as drinking, but that the combination of smoking and alcohol does not increase the risk linearly but, rather, exponentially. Thus someone who smokes more than 40 cigarettes and drinks 1½ oz. of alcohol per day has more than 15 times the incidence of oral cancer than the non-smoker who does not drink. Impressive as these types of statistics may be, they do not reflect the far more devastating impact of alcohol in certain target populations. For instance, alcoholism is extremely prevalent and may account for as much as 35% of all mortality among Alaskan natives (Kraus and Buffler, 1979).

This type of interaction between sociocultural factors and health is also demonstrated by Fig. 3, which shows the difference in cancer death rates by sex and race, when compared with Fig. 4, which reflects the smoking habits of these groups. We could be in a better position for reducing the

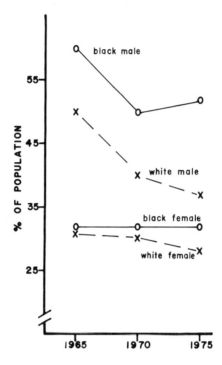

Figure 4. Estimated percentage of cigarette smokers in black and white American populations. Adapted from Silverberg (1980).

cancer mortality if we knew more about the determinants of smoking incidence in these populations.

The leading cause of death for both genders over the age of 54 is cardiovascular disease. Although all the factors that bear on the incidence of cardiovascular disease are by no means known, a number of correlations are apparent. Such correlations are especially important because of the fact that it is nearly impossible as yet to do anything of medical significance once the vascular degeneration has proceeded far enough to produce symptoms. Factors associated with cardiovascular disease include smoking habits, high-fat diets, hypertension, and stress. Both cardiovascular disease and hypertension are affected by obesity and salt intake (personal habits). The high-sodium diets in China may be associated with that country's prevalence of hypertension, and obesity may play a similar role in the United States. The importance of weight control is exemplified by the Framingham study, (Kannel & Gordon, 1979) which followed 5209 people from 1948 until the present. This study indicates that a weight loss of 12 lb is followed by a systolic pressure drop of 26 mmHg; a loss of 18 lb results in a drop of 57 mg of cholesterol per 100 ml of blood. A 10% increase in weight appears to increase the probability of having a coronary by 30% and a 10% loss in weight may reduce one's chance of coronary thrombosis by 20%. Again, specific habit patterns appear to have a major impact on the individual's health, ultimately affecting the individual's life expectancy.

A particularly intriguing issue is the extent to which cardiovascular disease is related to social circumstances and personal life-style, not including the already apparent importance of overeating, lack of exercise, and smoking. Friedman and Rosenman (1974) gathered impressive support for the hypothesis that the incidence of coronary occlusion is particularly high in individuals with a characteristic behavior pattern that they labeled as type A behavior. This behavior pattern includes being engaged in an excessive, chronic struggle to obtain more and more from the environment against resistance, but without loss of hope. Such individuals are forever fighting against the constraints of time. They are highly competitive people, very busy, always short of time, never giving up. This impresses as a life-style characterized by a high level of stress (Glass, 1977).

Stress can probably best be defined as the emotional and physiological reaction (including increased physiological arousal) to an overwhelming environmental challenge. The type A personality would then characterize people who, by virtue of their habit patterns, abilities to cope, and objectives in life, are likely to experience a great deal of stress. This notion is supported by the observation that truly successful, competitive individuals, such as executives who establish a secure position at the top, have a lower rather than a higher incidence of heart disease.

It is important to recognize that life-style and behavioral patterns are not merely a function of the personality characteristics that typify a person. They are also a function of the sociocultural environment in which the individual lives and the specific response patterns of the people with whom he or she interacts. This—as will be demonstrated later—is of great importance if one seeks to facilitate changes in these behavior patterns. If the observations of Friedman and Rosenman are borne out, then it is obvious that a change in life-style ranging from learning how to relax to acquiring skills to better cope with the competition may play an important role in the prevention of coronary disease (see Roskies, 1980).

Determinants of Morbidity

While the incidence and causes of mortality may reflect the health of a society, they are far from complete. Morbidity tables provide additional information. If health is defined as the effective functioning of an individual in all respects, then morbidity can be understood as a significant reduction in levels of functioning. Unfortunately, good morbidity statistics are hard to come by; there are a variety of reasons for this. First of all, morbidity is not an all-or-none affair. Individuals can be partially incapacitated all of the time and completely incapacitated during other periods. It is easiest to measure morbidity in terms of the ability to perform a job. Although this is of importance, it certainly does not tell the whole story. The impact on personal well-being as well as on the functioning of the family and wider community must be taken into account, as must the economic impact of the cost of medical care for the chronically ill. In terms of economics, chronic illness is, of course, far more expensive than death. Being able to keep the paraplegic alive or maintaining individuals with nonfunctioning kidneys on renal dialysis has significant consequences economically, socially, and psychologically for the individuals involved. Although comprehensive and adequate statistics are lacking, there is sufficient information available to identify some of the major determinants of morbidity.

An important example is chronic back pain and the suffering and reduced functioning that results from it. The pain can vary widely in location, but in our society the most frequent kinds and the ones associated with the most impressive morbidity are low back pain, neck pain, and headaches. In terms of economics, it has been estimated that chronic low back pain may cost the United States as much as $50 billion a year, both in disability payments and medical expenses. A total of 60% of both men and women at some time in their life suffer low back pain severe enough to warrant medical attention. It accounts for a loss of 1.4 work days per year for every employee in the United States and in other western European nations. It is also the most common basis for awarding compensation payments. In short, this complaint represents the single most costly medical condition, but it has no impact whatever on the mortality tables. While the onset of low back pain is ordinarily associated with some types of trauma, its maintenance and the degree of disability is hardly affected by the application of medical techniques. Aside from a smaller number of rare physical causes for back pain (such as spondylitis, tumors, and congenital defects), there is, in the majority of cases, no adequate and sufficient structural explanation of the suffering of the patients. It is interesting to observe relative to this condition how physicians are often inclined to keep on doing what they do best, even if it has no relevance to the condition they are treating. Rockey et al. (1978) observed that x-ray examinations had no effect on either diagnosis or treatment in cases of low back pain. Nevertheless, the practice of taking these pictures is continued, costing million of dollars and subjecting patients to radiation (back radiation is the major contributor to gonadal irradiation, which may result in a significant increase in lethal mutations in the population gene pool). An even more dramatic demonstration of such unfortunate behavior by the physicians and a major contributor to morbidity is provided by surgery for low back pain. Such operations continue to be carried out in spite of the fact that statistics show that such interventions do not improve the individual's functioning more than conservative treatment, unless there is a well-defined neurological defect.

In Chapter 16 Loeser and Fordyce demonstrate that the suffering of pain is dependent on the behavior that the individual engages in as a consequence, the so-called pain behavior. This behavior, which keeps the suffering alive, is maintained by the responses of the environment to the suffering individual. The environment in this case includes the relatives and the work situation, as well as the physician. In recognition of this fact, pain clinics have sprung up in most major medical centers and the first rather hesitant steps have been taken to combat the problem by means of behavioral intervention rather than with the aid of the scalpel or the pill.

Behavioral Science and Medical Practice

The foregoing material indicated that physical health depends to a major extent upon the recreational, consumatory, and other behaviors of the persons concerned. It further indicates that social policies regarding activities such as driving, alcohol consumption, food processing, and so forth, may have more to do with future improvements in national health than advances in the biological and medical sciences. It also indicates that the medical profession may have to incorporate procedures from the behavioral sciences to improve its effectivenesss as a health care system.

During recent years there have been increasing indications that behavior interventions are the treatments of choice for a variety of medical or medically related problems. One of the prime examples of such problems is enuresis. Barring a small percentage of cases in which bed-wetting is secondary to some physical disorder, biological interventions are less useful than behavioral ones. In one study, a simple conditioning procedure was proven effective in eliminating enuresis in approximately 80% of the cases. Sleep-lightening medication was less effective (23%) and resulted in more frequent relapses (Forrester et al., 1964).

Another example is that of hyperactivity. Although stimulant medication may be at least temporarily helpful for such children, this medication may be differentially helpful for different aspects of the problem. Low doses of stimulant medication may facilitate a hyperactive child's performance on cognitive or school-related tasks without influencing the child's social behavior; higher doses may improve social behavior but not performance on school tasks (Sprague and Sleator, 1977). As Pelham (1978) noted, it may be necessary to combine biological interventions for cognitive performance with behavioral interventions for social behavior.

The emerging importance of the behavioral sciences in medical practice stems not only from an analysis of mortality and morbidity tables or from the apparent success of some behavioral interventions. The need for behavioral sciences is also apparent when one considers the complexities of patient behaviors and physician–patient interactions that center around the shared problem of improving the patient's health. Patients play a far greater role in the initiation and execution of medical interventions than would be apparent if one considered medical practice only from the perspective of the biological sciences. Furthermore, the interaction between physician and patient can markedly influence the decision making and the overt behavior of both the physician and patient as these relate to medical care.

Patient Initiation of Medical Care

Most medical care begins with some behavior on the part of the potential patient. The patient perceives a pain or altered bodily state and then labels the symptoms as normal, temporary, insignificant, or as something that requires medical attention. The simple perception of pain or altered bodily states may vary markedly from person to person and from situation to situation, with such variation being in part cultural. Persons from certain socioethnic backgrounds are more likely to report pain from the same physical stimuli than are persons with other heritages (Tursky, 1974). Individuals who are experiencing other sensations may be relatively insensitive to acute bodily changes. Accordingly, persons who experience chronic pain may be less likely than others to recognize some new ache. Persons intensely involved in some other activity such as a sporting event may be less sensitive to pain than they would otherwise. These variations may also depend on the emotional state of the person. Depressed persons, for example, may be more sensitive to altered bodily states than the average person and thus seek medical care at a higher rate than their physical conditions would warrant. Similarly, persons who have recently experienced stressful life events may be more sensitive than they would otherwise.

Once recognized or attended to, the altered bodily conditions or symptoms must be labeled as ones requiring medical attention before one is likely to seek such attention. Thus the process of labeling one's physical symptoms and responding to these labels can have some major medical implications. Clearly, whether one labels a thoracic discomfort as indigestion or as a cardiovascular dysfunction will determine the likelihood of seeking medical attention. The sophistication and complexity of biological and medical sciences often precludes the average individual from having sufficient knowledge to adequately assess many symptoms and their medical implications. As a result, naive individuals will rely upon whatever information or information sources they do have, whether accurate or not. Other information such as alterations in diet or exercise may be taken into account and lead a person to attribute symptoms to these activities. The similarity of one's ailments to those of some other family member or friend may contribute to one's labeling of symptoms. The reactions of other family members to one's suffering may also contribute to viewing one's symptoms as medically irrelevant or as requiring professional attention. Finally, one's belief in folklore such as "growing pains," the "curse" of womanhood, and so on, will contribute to one's labeling of symptoms. The processes of perceiving and labeling one's own aches and pains are extremely complex and often occur without the physician being able to influence them directly. Furthermore, the lack of public sophistication in the medical sciences may result in some discrepancies between the patient's and the physician's evaluations of the same symptoms.

Once one does determine that symptoms require some attention, the potential patient is likely to seek nonprofessional advice first, from friends, the spouse, parents, persons known to have similar problems, and so on. The physician is seldom the first link in the chain of medical attention and may be several links removed. Furthermore, once that decision is made, it is not always acted upon. There are several possible reasons why people may not seek treatment even when it appears warranted.

Acting upon such a judgment will depend in part upon one's expectations concerning the efficacy of medical intervention. Even if one believes that the condition is quite serious, seeking medical attention is less likely if one expects that such attention will have little or no advantageous effect. Furthermore, expectations concerning the degree to which the physician's interventions will be painful, degrading, and so on, may interfere with seeking treatment. Individuals who expect that the medical intervention may interfere with other aspects of their lives (taking time off work, etc.) may choose to tolerate the symptoms rather than seek remediation. Such expectations may arise from a number of sources, including previous experience and cultural or religious beliefs. Seeking medical advice may also require several different behaviors on the part of the potential patient. One must call for an appointment, rearrange other commitments, arrange for a sitter, find transportation, and often then wait in a physician's office. These behaviors require varying amounts of effort and for some persons, relative to some symptoms, the effort may outweigh the expected benefit.

These points suggest that patients, rather than the medical community, contribute in large measure to the initiation of medical care. The information upon which and the proceses by which one decides to seek medical care may be very different for the population as a whole or for the average patient than for the physician. The traditional disease model of health care focuses on biological processes, disorders, and cures; patients, on the other hand, will interpret illness within contexts that are far broader, including the emotional, social, and informational contexts often not attended to within the basic biological model. Effective medical care then requires that the medical professions and individual practitioners provide more information for the general public and evaluate disease processes within the broader illness contexts.

Evaluating Patient's Problems

In addition to relying on the patient to initiate the health care process, the physician must depend in part on information provided by the patient in order to diagnose the problem, monitor the effectiveness of the treatment, and so forth. The patient's descriptions of bodily functions, of alterations in pain, and of adherence to medical regimes, and so on, form an important part of the information needed by the physician. Still these self-reports may be grossly inaccurate. When a patient reports that he took some medication that was prescribed, he may mean once a day while it was prescribed for four times a day. He may also fail to mention some other medications he is taking. If a patient with back pain reports that he has complied with the prescription for 5 days of complete bed rest, he may mean exactly that; or he may mean that he spend an extra 4 hours a day in bed. A parent's description of a child's eating habits and defecation schedule may lead to the decision that a case of appendicitis is only a case of the flu. A patient's report of the amount of coffee she drinks may lead to the conclusion that she requires a prescription for tranquilizers when all she needs is to reduce her caffeine consumption. Obviously a patient's self-reports can make a major difference in the kind of treatment that he or she receives.

There are several factors that may contribute to this kind of inaccuracy. First, the general public's ignorance of medical science may preclude the patient's attention to a variety of relevant phenomena. Being unaware that aspirin may cause gastrointestinal discomfort may lead some persons to not report such self-medication when seeking assistance for stomach ailments, although they would report it if seeking assistance for headaches; that is, patients will edit the kind of information they volunteer and such editing may be based upon misinformation. Second, patients often lack the habits of monitoring and attending, which are required for accurate information. Many parents may not be aware of their child's elimination habits. Few persons who have not attempted to lose weight have practiced monitoring their calorie intake. When asked to retrospectively provide such information, their reports may be mere guesses. A third possible factor may involve some motivated distortions on the part of the patient. Physicians are generally regarded as prime examples of society's authority figures. As a general rule people will do their best to have a "good" appearance in the eyes of those they consider to be authority figures. As a result they may minimize their faults, such as smoking, or overstate their compliance with recommendations.

Misinformation may be most appropriately considered as failures in communication to which both parties may contribute. Patients obviously contribute to such miscommunications, but so do physicians. The physician may contribute by appearing (accurately or inaccurately) to be uninterested in some items of the patient's report, by failing to explain the importance of certain procedures or information, by appearing hurried and so forth. Such appearances may lead a patient to mistakenly edit information in ways that result in incomplete or inaccurate medical decisions.

Physicians may contribute to miscommunication in other ways as well. The process of medical decision making is complex and not always traceable to the diagnostically relevant medical information. Rather, such decisions require attending to the context in which the information is acquired as well as to the information itself. Thus complaints of pain from a patient who is generally regarded as stoic may be considered differently from similar complaints on the part of another patient. Perez (unpublished dissertation, 1981) concluded that an obstetrician's choice of analgesics during delivery depends upon just such reasoning. He reported that the potency of the analgesics prescribed increases with the amount of information seeking in which these patients engage; that is, the more questions these patients ask about the nature of the delivery process, the pain they will experience, and so forth, the more potent will be the medication the physicians prescribe. Greater information seeking by the patient apparently leads the physician to conclude that the patient will be in more pain.

Perez concluded, however, that this relation between medication potency and information seeking seemed to be the case only for those patients who were judged to be reasonably stoic. If the physician had originally characterized the patient as being one who was overly sensitive and complaining, then greater information seeking by the patient was related to less potent analgesics. In these latter cases the greater information seeking apparently confirmed the physician's original assumption that the patient was excessively sensitive and complaining.

The physicians relied upon nonverbal and contextual information in making medical decisions. It is not clear that the physicians' original classifications of patients were accurate or that greater information seeking indicates greater pain. What is clear is that the physicians' medical decisions varied with the patients' behavior and their labeling or classification of a patient was based upon their interactions with that patient.

Patient Execution of Medical Procedures

The patient not only initiates medical care and provides the physician with much of the information that is necessary for making medical decisions, but also carries out most of the medical interventions. Patients administer the medications prescribed, carry out exercise programs, relax, stop smoking, curtail alcohol or food consumption, increase fluid intake, and so on. The patient is clearly the physician's most important potential ally.

Despite an implicit assumption that patients can or will follow such medical orders, there is increasing evidence that they do not. A review by Stimson (1974) indicates that as many as 72% of the patients do not take or administer medications as prescribed. The National Heart, Lung, and Blood Institute (NHLBI) estimates that 50% of hypertensive patients do not take their medications. This latter figure does not include patients who take medications inappropriately, in conjunction with other medications, at the wrong time, in improper doses, and so on.

The potential causes of noncompliance are numerous. Although it is often assumed that patients will understand and remember instruction, it is apparent that they often do not. Instructing patients to take medications or to follow other, even more complex procedures may be situations that have a particularly high potential for miscommunication. In a 1977 study sponsored by the NHLBI (National Institutes of Health, 1977) 60% of the hypertensive patients who had inappropriately stopped taking medication claimed they did so because they understood their physician to have instructed them to stop. Statements such as, "Your blood pressure is responding to the medication," were taken to mean that the treatment was no longer needed.

Johnson and Brown (1969) compared several means of influencing parents to modify their children's behavior and reported that verbal instructions were the least effective of those evaluated. This finding is especially sobering, since physicians rely primarily upon verbal instructions to influence their patients' self-medication behaviors. When one considers that a 15-minute office visit must include an examination, an explanation, and instructions, it is not surprising that patients may misunderstand. These misunderstandings are exacerbated by the patients' lack of fundamental medical knowledge. Few patients have reason to be aware of why some medications should be taken between meals or why antibiotics should be taken even after the symptoms have disappeared.

Another reason for noncompliance may relate to a person's perceived need for relief; that is, willingness to comply may depend upon the amount of pain or discomfort a person is experiencing. Persons who are experiencing severe pain will likely take all the medication prescribed and perhaps more; but a person with hypertension may not experience any discomfort as a result of the elevated blood pressure. Obese patients may experience some social discomfort but no physical symptoms they are able to detect. The patient who smokes may not be able to associate any physical problems with his habit. These patients may have very little immediate reason, therefore, to change their behavior. As a general rule, the more delay there is between a person's behavior and the resulting benefits, or the less apparent these benefits, the less likely the patient is to engage in that behavior. Similarly, the greater the delay between a behavior and the resulting aversive consequences, the less likely the patient is to avoid that behavior.

Compliance with instructions may also depend on the cost or effort of complying. The NHLBI study noted earlier indicatd that 2% of non-complying hypertensives stopped taking medications because of cost. Arthritis patients who are instructed to exercise may find it overly painful and disregard the instructions. The importance of effort in compliance is illustrated in a study cited by Stimson (1974). In that study 67% of the patients who were instructed to take iron tablets three times a day defaulted. Only 25% of those instructed to take an equal amount, but only once a day, failed to do so. Similarly, parents instructed to give their child medication every 6 hours may find that such instructions are difficult to follow if their son goes to camp or trades lunches (pills included) with a school friend. A mother of three young children may find it impossible to get a complete week of bed rest. The immediate "cost" of complying with medical recommendations may seem greater than the more long-term "cost" of not doing so.

A fourth and final reason for noncompliance is that patients will sometimes simply forget. In fact this may be the most frequent reason for noncompliance. Fully informed and well-intentioned patients may thus fail to take hypertensive medications because the disorder has very few symptoms to remind them and they have little else to remind them of the need to take such medications. Persons who have been faithfully taking antibiotics may discontinue when the symptoms disappear. Patients confined to wheelchairs may be asked to lift themselves up on the arms of their chairs periodically to prevent the development of skin ulcers. Paraplegics in particular may be likely to forget this simple task because they lack the physical sensations to remind them of the need.

Physician–Patient Interaction

Traditional medical interventions have resulted in major advances in physical health. In order to appropriately apply these procedures, however, the physician must rely upon information from and communication with patients whose orientations may not be based largely upon the biological sciences. Furthermore, the disease processes and the biological interventions occur within contexts that may have little immediate relevance for either that disease process or the medical intervention. The interpretation of the disease process by the potential patient, however, will depend to a considerable extent upon the context in which the disease process occurs. The efficacy of many medical interventions will also depend upon the interaction of those interventions with the context in which they are applied. Medical interventions that intrude upon other aspects of the person's life than just the disease processes are less likely to be carried out by the patient. Those medical interventions that can be supported by other aspects of the person's life, such as supportive family members or a structured environment which assists patients with memory and execution of the procedures, are more likely to be carried out. Medical interventions that improve other aspects of a person's life, social inter-actions, employment, recreation, and so on, are most likely going to be executed by the patient.

Effective medical care may depend considerably on the degree to which physicians and other medical professionals are able to view medical treatment as an effort shared with the patient. It will also depend upon the physician's ability to promote the patient's efforts toward the common goal through information, negotiation, and two-way communication. Doing so will require that the physician assess the social or behavioral context in which the disease process occurs, determine the meaning of the disease for the patient and the degree to which the disease influences other aspects of the person's life, anticipate the intrusive possibilities of the medical intervention, and take steps to avoid failures in the execution of treatment.

This chapter implies that medical professionals are accountable for medical care beyond accurate diagnosis and appropriate prescription. Indeed, Ware et al. (1977) indicated that there is a broad trend "toward holding those who control and provide essential services more account-able to their consumers in ways other than the ones that commonly operate in the marketplace (Ware et al., 1977, p. 1). They concluded that in medicine the ultimate measure of quality care is its effectiveness in promoting physical health and patient satisifaction. Patient judgments of quality care and satisfaction do not center most often on the technical aspects of medical care; rather, the most frequent dimension of patient judgment involves the degree of "humanness" or "caring" evidenced by the medical professionals (Ware et al., 1977). Even when considering the technical quality of care, which includes skill in diagnosis and treatment, patient assessments include the ability of the physician to "clearly explain what is expected of their patients" (Ware et al., 1977, p. 5).

References

Forrester, R. M., Z. Stein, and M. W. Susser. 1964. A trial conditioning therapy in nocturnal enuresis. Developmental Medicine and Child Neurology 6:158–166.

Friedman, M., and Rosenman, R. H. 1974. Type A: Your Behavior and Your Heart. New York: Knopf.

Garfinkel, L., C. E. Poindexter, and B. S. Silverberg. 1980. Cancer in black Americans. Ca. A Cancer Journal for Clinicians 30:39–44.

Glass, D. C. 1977. Stress, behavior patterns, and coronary disease. American Scientist 65:177–187.

Johnson, S. M., and R. A. Brown. 1969. Producing behavior change in parents of disturbed children. Journal of Child Psychology and Psychiatry 10:107–121.

Kanfer, F. H., L. E. Cox, J. M. Greiner, and P. Karoly. 1974. Contracts, demand characteristics, and self-control. Journal of Personality and Social Psychology 30:605–619.

Kannel, W. B., and Gordon, T. 1979. Physiological and medical concomitants of obesity: The Framington study. In G. A. Bray (ed.) Obesity in America. Washington DC: U.S. Goverment Printing Office, DHEW Publ. No. (NIH) 79-359, pp. 125–163.

Kleinman, A., L. Eisenberg, and B. Good. 1977. Culture, illness, and core: Clinical lessons from anthropological and cross-cultural research. Unpublished manuscript, University of Washington, Seattle, Washington.

Kraus, R. F., and P. A. Buffler. 1979. Sociocultural stress and the American native in Alaska: An analysis of changing patterns of psychiatric illness and alcohol abuse among Alaskan natives. Culture, Medicine, and Psychiatry 3:111–151.

Lalonde, M. 1974. A New Perspective on the Health of Canadians: A Working Document. Ottowa, Canada: Ministry of Health and Welfare.

Martin, S., S. Johnson, S. Johensson, and G. Wahl. 1976. The comparability of behavioral data in laboratory and natural settings. In E. Nash, L. Hammerlynck, and L. Handy, eds.: Behavior Modification and Families. New York: Brunner/Mazell.

National Institutes of Health. RFP NHLBI-1977-20.

Pelham, W. E. 1978. Behavior therapy with hyperactive children. Symposium on behavior therapy. Psychiatric Clinics of North America.

Perez, R. 1982. Psychosocial factors affecting prepartum anxiety and delivery processes in a sample of Hispanic women. Unpublished doctoral dissertation, University of California at Los Angeles.

Pomerleau, O., F. Bass, and V. Crown. 1975. Role of behavior modification in preventative medicine. New England Journal of Medicine 292:1277–1282.

Rockey, P. H., R. K. Tompkins, R. W. Wood, and B. W. Wolcott. 1978. Usefulness of x-ray examinations of patients with back pain. Journal of Family Practice 7:455–465.

Roskies, E. 1980. Considerations in developing a treatment program for the coronary-prone (Type A) behavior pattern. In P. O. Davidson and S. M. Davidson, eds.: Behavioral Medicine: Changing Health Lifestyles. New York: Brunner/Mazell.

Rothman, K., and A. Keller. 1972. Effect of joint exposure to alcohol and tobacco on risk of cancer and pharynx. Journal of Chronic Diseases, 25:711–716.

Silverberg, B. S. 1980. Cancer statistics, 1980. Ca. A Cancer Journal for Clinicians. 30:23–38.

Sommer, R., and F. D. Becker. 1969. Territorial defense and the good neighbor. Journal of Personality and Social Psychology 11:85–92.

Sprague, R. L., and E. K. Sleator. 1977. Methylphenidate in hyperactive children: Differences in dose effects on learning and social behavior. Science 198:1274.

Stimson, G. V. 1974. Obeying doctor's orders. A view from the other side. Social Science and Medicine 8:97–104.

Tursky, B. 1974. Physical, physiological and psychological factors that affect pain reaction to electric shock. Psychophysiology 11:95–112.

Ware, J. E., A. Davies-Avery, and A. L. Stewart. 1977. The measurement and meaning of patient satisfaction: A review of the literature. Unpublished manuscript, Southern Illinois University, Carbondale, Illinois.

World Health Statistics Annual. 1981. Geneva, World Health Organization.

3

The Interpretation and Treatment of Pathological Behavior in Historical Perspective

Charles Bodemer, Ph.D.*

Primitive Cultures

It is appropriate to begin a historical review of concepts of pathology with a consideration of conditions in primitive or preliterate societies. This permits identification of factors that enter into the interpretation of disease which in turn underlie therapeutic procedures and general attitudes toward the sick. It is assumed that the world view and derived medical practices in primitive cultures resemble most closely those developed early in human history and in the earliest stages in the development of Western civilization.

A world view represents an interpretive scheme according to which people measure the universe, themselves, and the natural phenomena that surround and intrude into their lives. Three clear elements enter into a world view: the human; the natural, that ensemble of nonhuman entities ranging from stones and plants to celestial bodies; and the supernatural, or that which is considered divine. The perceived relation of these three elements in a formulated world view determines the configuration of medicine and the nature of healing practices appearing within a particular society or civilization.

Characteristic of the world view developed within primitive societies, as well as the archaic civilizations of Mesopotamia and Egypt, is the lack of a sharp distinction between the human, the natural, and the supernatural. In the absence of a clear demarcation of these three elements, the human, natural, and supernatural realms are equally real. This interpretive setting

*Professor and Chairman, Department of Biomedical History, University of Washington School of Medicine, Seattle, Washington.

makes logical the supernatural causation of natural events. Hence in primitive and early literate cultures, natural and supernatural explanations have the same degree of validity. It is possible, then, to explain a natural event by strictly natural processes, and it is equally possible to explain an event in terms of the supernatural. This has great relevance to ideas of disease causation.

Within the framework of the primitive world view it is generally assumed that the flesh is heir to certain problems and accidental injuries. Disorders of this variety, which are considered ordinary, receive naturalistic explanations. The explanation of serious and/or dramatic illness, however, most often involves invocation of supernatural agencies, operating either directly or indirectly in causation of the disease. A supernatural causation is especially likely to be assumed when the disease presents a dramatic aspect. In general, acute disease of sudden onset is considered to result from the intrusion of a foreign object into the sick person's body. Thus a suddenly developed fever and a serious acute illness may be explained in several ways, both supernatural in orientation. The fever or the illness may be attributed to the presence of an object somehow implanted into the sick person's body. The object may be, among other items, a pebble, a stick, or a bone fragment. The object itself is less important than the entity responsible for its intrusion into the body, which may be a demon, a god, or a sorcerer.

The most typical representation of the idea of disease causation through object intrusion is an arrow shot into a person's body by an external agent. The image of the arrow as a disease agent of supernatural origin is prominent in medical history. It appears early in the Western tradition in Homer's *Iliad*, when Apollo at the behest of his priest, Chryses, causes an epidemic among the Greek troops besieging Troy. Chryses prayed to Apollo, "Let your arrow make the Danaans pay for my tears shed," and an angered Apollo

came as night comes down and knelt then apart and opposite the ships and let go an arrow. Terrible was the clash that rose from the bow of silver. First he went after the mules and the circling hounds, then let go a tearing arrow against the men themselves and struck them. The corpse fires burned everywhere and did not stop burning. Nine days up and down the host ranged the god's arrows. (Lattimore, 1951)

The pestilence continued until Chryses prayed to Apollo to desist. Apollo is thus both the source and cure of the disease, the direct cause of which is the god's arrow. The arrow as a disease-causing agent appears later in Western history in various places, such as the mechanism of disorders caused by the elf shot described in the ninth century Anglo-

Saxon *Lacnunga* as "spirits of evil" that roam the land, (Grattan and Singer, 1952) and it is the *Hexenschuss* of German tradition.

The idea of object intrusion also appears in concepts of disease causation as a demon or supernatural entity that enters the body directly and causes the disease. The supernatural agency itself is the cause of the disease, and so long as it is lodged in the body the disease state will continue. Elimination of the supernatural entity and the disease it causes requires some sort of direct action on the entity itself. Illnesses of all kinds are frequently explained on the basis of possession by evil spirits, and this is especially true of the disorders with behavioral manifestations.

Chronic diseases, particularly those involving progressive deterioration, generally receive a supernatural explanation in primitive medicine. They are most often ascribed to soul loss, whereby it is assumed that in some way the individual's soul has been captured and/or separated from the body, and as a consequence the person withers away and may die unless the soul is freed and/or restored to the body.

It is obvious that the interpretive scheme of primitive medicine is magical and religious in orientation, and thus it requires magicoreligious therapeutic procedures. Accordingly, primitive healers are of a composite type, priest–physicians, who operate within a magicoreligious conceptual framework and deal with supernatural forces primarily through incantations, prayers, charms, and amulets, supplementing the various magico-religious rituals with empirical remedies. The priest–physician functions at the junction of the human, the natural, and the supernatural, mediating between the sick person and transcendental agencies.

The priest–physician may exorcise individuals suffering from demoniacal possession, although this may also be approached surgically through trepanation. The latter, one of the earliest and most widespread surgical procedures known, has been and is practiced throughout the world as a means of permitting egress of a possessing demon through openings made in the skull. The idea of possession and the practices of exorcism and trepanation are especially important in considerations of psychopathology. Quite often in the history of Western civilization behavioral disorders have been attributed to divine or demoniacal possession, and appropriate procedures have been employed in attempts at therapy.

In the primitive situation magicoreligious explanations account for disorders today likely to be distinguished as psychological. The primitive medical approach, it should be emphasized, generally does not make the distinction between somatic and psychological illnesses, and a disease state, regardless of its manifestations and the presumed etiology, is dealt with as a single entity. Thus behavioral disorders are explained and treated in the same way as the more obviously physical disabilities. Confession and suggestion are important elements in therapy, and the activities of the healer involve much ritual religion and magic for its presumed efficacy. Moreover, a great deal of ritual and ceremony associated with the healing process is designed for its psychological effect upon the patient and others in the kinship or social group. The healing ritual is one in which the healer and the patient share, and it is based in their common world view. Thus many of the activities of the medicine man or shaman are designed to focus the patient's attention on his activities and to impress the patient and the group with his special powers to deal with the supernatural and to engender, as much as possible, optimistic expectations. The healing procedure often involves members of the family or social unit and frequently approaches what is today known as group therapy.

In a primitive culture, disease quite often acquires moral significance, and violation of a taboo, for example, may be considered as the precipitating cause of disease. Thus much of the priest–physician's ritual, including use of the social group, may be directed toward detection of moral transgressions by the sick person or by members of that person's kinship group. This allows identification of the depth of the offense, the offended deity or deities, and selection of the appropriate therapeutic regimen, which not infrequently involves forms of penance.

Primitive medicine reveals certain universal characteristics surrounding the activities of the healer, the relationship of the healer to the sick person, and the nature of the healing transaction. An effective relationship requires a shared world view and a belief in the special abilities of the healer to deal with the causes of disease. Thus the medicine man, shaman, or priest–physician in primitive and archaic civilizations is assumed to possess a special understanding of and a favored relation with super-natural agencies related to disease causation. The healer's ability to mediate between the sick person and these supernatural entities gives him a special authority in that culture, and, since disease is usually given moral significance, the healer becomes a powerful arbiter of morals and a powerful regulating force of social orthodoxy. Therapy normally has a moral component, involving the expiation of guilt and restoration of the patient and, perhaps, the kinship group into the moral and social order. To enhance his image and reinforce his authority the healer necessarily relies upon various devices in order to become an object of awe, thereby augmenting the suggestive component in the therapeutic regimen. The healer, then, tends to rely upon the psychological element involved in recovery from illness, and the healing art in general has a well-defined psychotherapeutic aspect, whatever the disease or its presumed etiology. The shaman with a drum, the medicine man with a rattle, and the modern physician with a white coat all rely upon symbols that declare special status and powers and which grant these special privileges and the medical authority that affect the nature of the healing art.

Antiquity

Mesopotamia and Egypt

Medicine appearing in the earliest, archaic stages of development of Western civilization corresponds quite closely to what has previously been described as primitive medicine. Both the Mesopotamian and Egyptian medical ideas and practices were suffused with magic and, especially, religion. The Babylonians conceived of a tightly structured, morally ordered universe. Their world view gave special importance to the supernatural and included innumerable demons and gods. The human was at the mercy of these transcendental beings and sought to maintain a harmonious relationship with them through morally correct behavior and appropriate prayers and sacrifices. Egyptians also postulated the existence of a large pantheon of gods capable of affecting human lives. Both Babylonians and Egyptians made use of amulets, charms and fetishes to offset evil supernatural forces. Egyptian jewelry is to a large extent a testament to preventive medical practices.

In the presence of illness the priest–physician acted through prayers, incantations, and other magicoreligious means to mediate between the gods and the sick person in order to restore health and reintegrate that person into the moral and social order. As in the case of primitive medicine, the distinction between the natural and the supernatural realms was obscure, physical and psychological disorders were not sharply delimited, and psychopathological conditions were most frequently ascribed to spirit intrusion or demoniacal possession.

Greece

The first substantial departure from the magicoreligious interpretation of disease occurred in ancient Greece around the fifth century B.C., in the teaching of Hippocrates and the Coan school of medicine. There was a coeval form of medicine, apparently dating from the pre-Homeric era, that centered upon the Asclepieia, those temples dedicated to the god of medicine, Aesculapius. There priest–physicians followed healing procedures that were clearly of magical and religious character. Hippocratic medicine, however, was a reflection of totally different intellectual impulses, impulses more rational than religious, more philosophical than theistic.

During the sixth and fifth centuries B.C. Greece gave birth to a great burst of creative philosophical inquiry. The thrust of this inquiry was an attempt to *understand* the universe and its mode of action, to place things and events external to the human being within the grasp of human reason, and to substitute comprehension for wonder and awe. The pre-Socratic philosophers tended to remove the gods from nature and make it more impersonal than it had been in the Bronze Age cosmologies. Thus they attempted to define the nature of the universe, its material basis, and the nature of change. They were generally monists, designating a single substance capable of changing physical states as the basis of material reality. Thales, for example, suggested that all material bodies had their origin in water, and Anaximenes designated air as the basis of being, the physical nature of bodies reflecting its varying states of condensation and rarefaction. Eventually, Empedocles argued that all material bodies in the universe were composed of four primary elements—air, earth, fire, and water—and this doctrine endured for many centuries thereafter.

Hippocratic medicine attempted a naturalistic explanation of disease, and Hippocratic medical theory was essentially a composite of various pre-Socratic philosophical speculations. It included the Empedoclean doctrine of the four primary elements as the basis of material being. However, the Hippocratic physiological scheme did not depend directly upon the primary elements but, instead, upon four humors or fluids related to those elements and possessing the same qualities. Thus the humor phlegm, with the qualities of cold and wet, was related to water; blood, hot and wet, was related to air; yellow bile, hot and dry, was related to fire, and the humor black bile, cold and dry, was related to the element earth.

Hippocratic theory combined with the Empedoclean doctrine of the four primary elements the concept of *harmonia*, a contribution of the Pythagorean school. According to the Pythagoreans, reality lay in number rather than in any physical element; they proposed that the mathematical relations between elements were more important than the elements themselves. *Harmonia* was the result of optional numerical relations and accounted for the orderly function of the universe and the general order of things. Thus when the mathematical relations of the spheres containing the celestial bodies was like that encountered in the musical scale, *harmonia* prevailed and the perfect order of the cosmos gave rise to the "music of the spheres." The Hippocratics adopted the idea of *harmonia*, positing that health was a condition in which the four humors existed within a given body in a state of appropriate proportions, or *harmonia*, and disease was the disturbance of this *harmonia* through imbalance of the humors, either through excesses or depletions. Treatment therefore aimed at restoration of the normal harmonious relation existing between the humors of the body.

The Hippocratic doctrine of the four humors supplied the basis of medical theory and practice for more than a thousand years (see Fig. 1). It supplied also a lasting variety of psychological theory. According to this theory, the proportional relations of humors existing in an individual are quite specific and one humor is dominant. Individual temperaments can thus be attributed to the normal predominance of one humor. Hence the

49

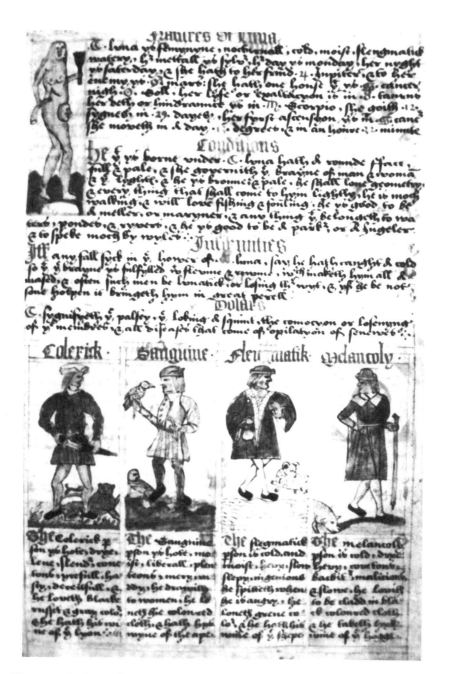

Figure 1. A sixteenth-century English medicoastrological manuscript depicting men of different humors, with a discussion of character types.

sanguine personality is derived from the dominance of the humor blood, the phlegmatic temperament from the dominance of phlegm, the choleric temperament from yellow bile, and the melancholic personality from the normal dominance of the humor black bile.

Thus psychological theory evolved out of the Hippocratic humoral doctrine. A humoral imbalance in a specific individual was pathological and accounted not only for physical ailments but behavioral abnormalities as well. An excess of black bile, for example, caused the psycho-pathological state of melancholia. The Hippocratic physician approached this psychological disorder in the same way as any somatic disease without psychiatric symptomatology, relying upon the healing powers of nature, diet, and perhaps bleeding to redress the humoral imbalance, probably the administration of hellebore as a cathartic, and rest and quiet. The physician did not consider any specifically "emotional" etiology to a psycho-pathological condition: Although he might treat and think about a mental disturbance, his interest in the details of the disturbance itself went only as far as they were part of the clinical picture of the disease as a whole. A psychopathological condition such as melancholia, for example, was thought to have a clear physical cause and a definite relation with other diseases of the black bile. This was thoroughly consistent with the naturalistic orientation of Hippocratic medicine, the fundamental premise that all diseases have a natural origin and a natural cure, and the perception of the disease as a state involving the entire organism.

Thus the people of ancient Greece were not overly concerned with those individuals who demonstrated grossly abnormal behavior patterns; and, if they were not a threat to other individuals, they were generally allowed to roam. In those cases where the individuals were disabled, it was the responsibility of the family to provide for their care. In the event there was no family or it was unable to care for the severely disordered person, he became a ward of the state and, if necessary, confined in the jail. There is some evidence that such incarcerated madmen were used as scapegoats or as essential sacrificial elements in various fertility rites, but generally, especially during the later periods of Greek antiquity, the mentally deranged were not necessarily singled out for abuse or harsh treatment.

Rome

The psychologically disordered were not treated much differently in ancient Greece and Rome. As in Greece, there were no institutions devoted exclusively to the mentally ill in Rome. Their care was entrusted to the family, and the state assumed responsibility only in the last resort. The Romans did not demonstrate great concern for those suffering from behavioral disorders, except as it affected property rights. The Romans were the first to deal with the question of competence in law, because they had a very well-developed and complex legal system, much of it related to property relationships and inheritance rights. They were the first to deal with the legal question of competence. Thus the Romans developed a set of procedures according to which an individual could be deprived of his property on the basis of mental incompetence. Interestingly, the decision regarding the property holder's sanity was made by a jurist, rather than a physician, although on occasion the latter might be consulted.

This relative lack of distinction between the physical and the psychological reflected the influence of Greek thought on Roman medicine. Greek medicine, along with much of Greek culture, was transplanted to Rome, and the best of Roman medicine, exemplified in the writings of the second-century physician, Galen, was naturalistic and based in Hippocratic theory and practices. The medical interpretation of psychological states, then, generally conformed to those of earlier Greek physicians. Most Roman physicians did not write specifically on the subject of psychopathology and its management, although some medical writers, particularly patricians, like Cicero, who were physicians but who did not practice medicine for gain, did consider the subject. These writers recommended a humane pattern of treatment for those manifesting psychological disorders, suggesting that the patients be housed in pleasant, clean, and well-lighted rooms. They recommended quiet and cheerful conditions, and the opportunity for diversion and creative activities as a means of enhancing recovery from mental as well as all disorders.

The Medieval Period

Galen synthesized the naturalistic medical knowledge of Greco-Roman antiquity. The future, however, lay not in the growth and refinement of naturalistic medicine, but with Hippocratic and Galenic theories and practice suffused with religious and astrological elements. Christianity was the major force that lay behind this development. It was operating in Galen's time, and the environment it created then and especially after the collapse of Rome led to different interpretations of disease and distinctly different perceptions of psychological states.

A characteristic of imperial Rome between the first and third centuries was widespread anxiety and a sense of guilt. The old value systems were in decay and an inordinate variety of religions and philosophies competed for the people's attention and loyalty. This environment of anxiety, guilt, and moral pluralism engendered a general wave of religiosity and superstition and a corresponding interpretation of health and disease. The naturalistic explanation of physical and psychological disorders began to recede in the presence of a revived interest in the supernatural. This development received great impetus from the rise, growth, and eventual dominance of Christianity.

Early Christianity was a religion of healing: the New Testament abounds with accounts of the healing powers and miraculous cures of Jesus Christ. Consistent with this emphasis the sick and their care acquired a special importance in Christian thought. Christianity removed the sinful connotation from disease transmitted in the Judaic tradition, and early Christian writers placed a positive value on sickness, declaring it an avenue toward grace through suffering. Consequently, the sick person was favored and enjoyed privileged status in the Christian community. Thus it early became a Christian duty to care for the sick. The covenant loyalty lies at the base of Christian ethics, and the medical covenant is one of the most profound. From the outset it conditioned attitudes toward the sick, the practice of medicine, and the development of institutions.

As Christianity became an increasingly powerful and finally the dominant cultural force in Western civilization, the world view placed increasing emphasis upon the supernatural. This was reflected in ideas of disease causation and healing. During the early centuries of the Christian era belief in the intercession of saints in healing took root, and thereafter people prayed to specific saints for protection or relief from disease. Incantations, conjurations, and prayers reappeared as a part of medical therapy, comprising an important part of medieval medicine. Simultaneously, the interpretations of psychological disorders underwent profound transformation, eventually leading to the establishment of psychopathology as a condition clearly distinct from physiopathology.

The basis for the separation of mental and physical diseases lay in the fourth-century writings of Saint Augustine, which were, in turn, influenced by earlier ideas regarding the relation between the soul and the body. In treatises that shaped Western thought for centuries, Augustine equated the intellect with the soul. Thus disturbances of the rational faculty were disturbances of the soul, an immaterial entity totally distinct from the grossly material body. Disorders of the soul were, accordingly, the concern of the Church and priests, rather than of medicine and physicians. The restriction of medicine to the diagnosis and treatment of somatic disorders profoundly affected the progress of medical psychology, the configuration of medicine, and the interpretation and treatment of behavioral disorders.

Christian beliefs and practices basal to medieval civilization generally favored humane care of the sick. Certain beliefs, however, had a destructive effect upon the understanding of and attitudes toward illness. The Devil has a long history, antedating Christianity. As a consequence of various factors, demonology and Satan entered Christian theology during the late Roman period. At first largely a theological entity, by the ninth century Satan was hypostatized as evil, having at his command a host of malevolent transcendental agents.

Belief in the Devil and his powers rose to great prominence in the medieval and early modern periods. As the European social scene changed, especially after the twelfth-century Renaissance, there was a certain amount of unrest and social and religious unorthodoxy. During the late medieval period this disrupted considerably the stability of the social and political order and consitituted a threat to the authority of the Church. The Devil, whose reality was a widely accepted belief, provided a ready explanation for all forms of disturbances, natural as well as social, political, and religious. Thus a fifteenth-century papal bull attributed to Satan and witches operating in the northern provinces of Europe events ranging from crop failures and hailstorms to infertility in women and impotence in men (see Fig. 2). Most importantly, witchcraft was defined as heresy, and the Church, in concert with the secular arm of society, undertook to identify and eliminate witches, the agents of Satan. This started a witchcraft hysteria that was especially pronounced during the late medieval and early modern periods and which did not abate until the end of the eighteenth century.

The belief in witchcraft and satanic or demoniacal possession led to the identification and persecution of many individuals suffering from various forms of psychological as well as physical conditions, and it served to reinforce the exclusion from medicine of the consideration of behavioral disorders. Indeed, it was during the early modern period that physicians were legally restricted to treating bodily ailments only. The lot of the mentally ill was now especially hard: Many were identified as witches and tortured and executed as heretics in the grasp of the Devil.

During the medieval period public authorities took only limited responsibility for the mentally deranged. Mentally or emotionally disturbed members of the community were left at liberty so long as they caused no public disturbance. Custody of the mentally ill generally rested with their relatives and friends; only those considered too dangerous to keep at home, or with no one to care for them or who were socially disturbing were dealt with by communal authorities.

Acutely disturbed, agitated patients were admitted to general hospitals in some places. Some institutions had either separate rooms or a separate facility for such patients. The insane who were native to other communities were frequently expelled and returned to the town from which they had come. In an attempt to avoid the burden of caring for the emotionally disturbed, authorities commonly drove them out of the community, allowing them freely to roam the countryside. Frequently the mentally ill in a community were handed over to boatmen. Thus during the late medieval period and Renaissance the "ship of fools" appeared in reality as

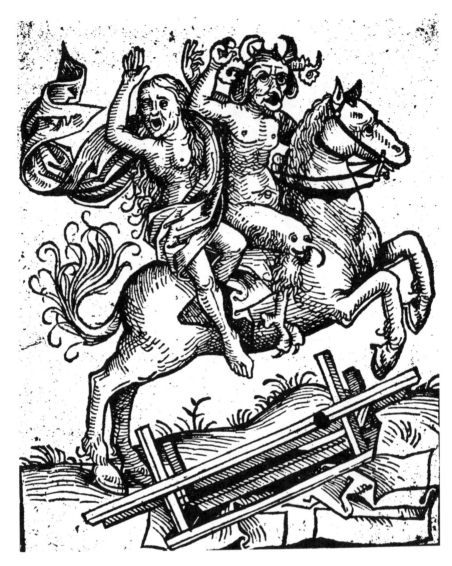

Figure 2. A witch and the Devil illustrated in the Nuremberg Chronicle of 1493.

well as literature. The numerous waterways forming the trade routes of the continent were employed to transport the mentally deranged and abnormal away from communities along the routes. The ship of fools may have provided a symbolic cleansing and purification; it certainly made it possible for communities to remove from their midst those individuals considered undesirable for behavioral reasons.

The Sixteenth and Seventeenth Centuries

The most recent roots of modern civilization are located in the Renaissance of the fifteenth and sixteenth centuries (see Fig. 3). This was a period of discovery and exploration: There was new appreciation of Greco-Roman antiquity; there were new lands and a new economy based in capitalism. Most importantly, it was a time during which new value was placed on the cosmos and the human being. It was the first step away from the medieval world view toward that of the twentieth century, and it laid the groundwork for the growth of the natural sciences.

The motive for scientific study began to change during the Renaissance from that of demonstrating through nature the wisdom of God in the creation and the manifestations of divine order toward that of improving the human condition through mastery of nature. The perceived new dignity of man created a new interest in the nature of man, engendering a burst of study aimed at analyzing the structure of the human body and inquiry into the workings of human reason and the nature of emotions. Thus the first major and original treatise devoted to human mental operations after Augustine appeared during the sixteenth century, and it introduced the term *psychology*. Human psychology thenceforth became an increasingly popular subject of study; the number of treatises devoted to psychiatric matters rose from about 6 during the fifteenth century to over 250 during the sixteenth century.

The scientific revolution of the seventeenth century firmly established the world view in which the human and the natural were in the ascendant. Nature was desacralized, and during the next two centuries the supernatural was gradually displaced. Eventually the human component of the world view came to outweigh the supernatural and the natural. The scientific method, stressing observation, quantification, and experiment, was clearly developed during the seventeenth century, and, although it would be several centuries before it assumed its modern form, the "new learning" underlaid numerous investigations into the nervous system and the basis of behavior.

During the seventeenth century Thomas Willis and others began to analyze the structure of the brain and the significance of various anatomical parts in explanation of behavior. In a more philosophical vein, René Descartes developed a system for studying physiological processes according to the rules governing mathematics and physics, proposing that the organism is essentially a machine, operating in the same way as a mechanical clock. Descartes was the first to develop the concept of the neural reflex and to apply it in explanation of behavior. Thus he argued that mechanical agitation of the nerve fibers transmitted along the nerves to the brain and thence to the muscles explains apparently purposeful behavior without necessary recourse to any principle or agent other than matter and motion. The rational faculty, according to Descartes, is the chief

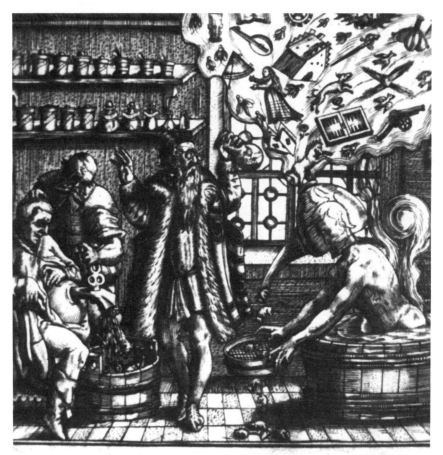

RTE MEA CEREBRVM NISI SIT SAPIENTIATOTVM

Figure 3. A sixteenth-century Flemish woodcut showing mad thoughts being removed from an insane man through distillation.

characteristic distinguishing the human being from other animal–machines. This mechanistic view combined with the general intellectual currents to condition the view of medicine toward psychopathology and the treatment of the mentally ill during the seventeenth century, or the Age of Reason.

The seventeenth century witnessed the emergence of strong national states, absolute monarchs ruling by divine right, and a mercantilistic economy. A work ethic developed that placed a special value upon contributions to the national welfare and condemned idleness, beggary, and vagrancy. The desire to suppress these nonproductive behaviors led

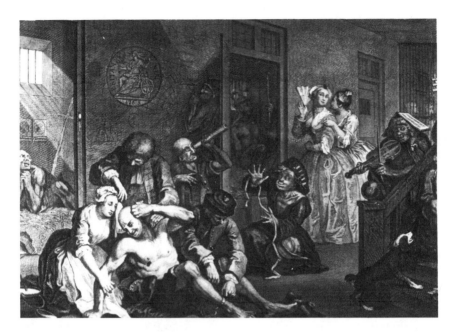

Figure 4. Print by Hogarth illustrating the famous insane asylum Bedlam, including two fashionable visitors.

to the development of workhouses and general hospitals. Confinement became a prime characteristic of the early modern period and it extended to those displaying socially unacceptable behavior. Thus criminals and prostitutes, for example, were confined, and with them in the general hospital were placed epileptics, the mentally retarded, the mentally disabled, and, not uncommonly, the rebellious teenager.

Rationality was the touchstone of normal behavior during the Age of Reason. Irrationality was madness, and it could be demonstrated in failure to observe the strict rules governing social behavior as well as in more dramatic psychopathological states. The emphasis upon reason as the distinctly human characteristic and the equation of irrationality and madness encouraged evaluation of the irrational person as something less than truly human. The harsh and inhumane treatment of the confined psychopaths typical of the early modern period is consonant with this general attitude, and it also explains recreational visits of the fashionable to hospitals like Bedlam to view the antics of the inmates, as shown in Fig. 4.

The great confinement of the seventeenth century firmly established the lasting practice of creating and maintaining a separate life space for the socially unacceptable. In time the criminals and others were separated from the psychologically disturbed and specific institutions were dedicated exclusively to confinement of those demonstrating conditions perceived as psychopathological. Institutions developed primarily for moral, social, and economic reasons thus became hospitals for the insane. There was, however, no change in the conditions under which they were kept. This awaited the end of the eighteenth century and the endeavors of Philippe Pinel as a model of Enlightenment thought.

The Eighteenth Century

Pinel was appointed director of Bicêtre and Salpêtrière, the large institutions in the Paris environs devoted to confinement of the mentally deranged. He demonstrated the spirit of the new era by developing a therapeutic program free of physical restraints and abuse (see Fig. 5). His "moral treatment" derived from the eighteenth century sensationalist psychology of Locke and Condillac. According to sensationalist theory, sensory impressions provide the basis of brain function; ideas and emotions thus relate to external stimuli. The basis of Pinel's moral treatment was the regulation of sensory stimuli so as to reduce the psychologically disturbing stimuli and substitute in their stead an environ-

Figure 5. An engraving showing Philippe Pinel unchaining the insane.

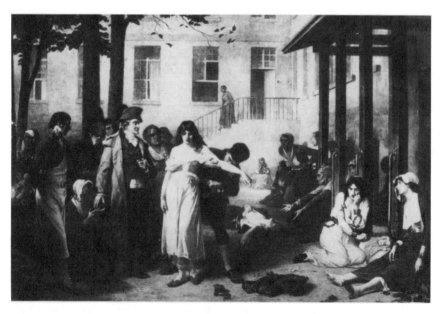

ment modeled after the existing social order. It was believed that this regimen would restore the disturbed person's rational faculties and normal behavior. Pinel's moral treatment was designed to demonstrate to patients that their behavior was inappropriate to the normal behavior prevailing outside the walls of the institution. Establishing as the norm behavior based on middle-class French morality and maintaining conditions conducive to calming the agitation of the nervous system, Pinel attempted, often utilizing other inmates, to have patients recognize the incongruity of their behavior and subsequently adapt it to the established standard.

Bicêtre and Salpêtrière housed an enormous number of inmates. The Quaker Retreat at York in England, on the other hand, dealt with a relatively small number of inmates. There Samuel Tuke dealt with patients in a generally humanitarian manner, without restraints, using guilt as a means of altering maladaptive behavior. The standard established was that of Quaker morality, and, since the Retreat was intended for members of that faith, the pyschotherapeutic program was aimed at restoring behavior appropriate to the standards of that religion. Like Pinel, Tuke reveals the final flowering of the humanitarian and libertarian impulses of the Enlightenment. The institutions with which Pinel and Tuke were associated form the foundations of the asylum movement of the nineteenth century, and Pinel, especially, was a powerful influence in the numerous asylums that were developed with great enthusiasm and a spirit of optimism.

The Nineteenth Century

The Asylum

During the nineteenth century there was a mounting concern with nervous disease and insanity. It was generally accepted that insanity was a price of the progress of civilization. This was especially true in the United States, where competition and the drive to succeed were recognized as dangerously stressful. Blighted ambition and failure, it was believed, were clearly precipitating causes for nervous exhaustion and insanity. The interpretation of insanity as the obverse of civilization did not, however, necessarily elicit an attitude of wretched hopelessness, for Americans during the age of Jackson believed in the ability to correct both social and individual ills through institutions. Thus the penitentiary was developed to reform criminals and restore them to society as productive, conforming citizens, and the asylum was developed to reform and restore the insane.

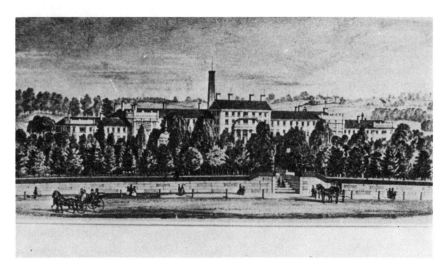

Figure 6. The Worcester State Hospital for the Insane around 1855. The structure was typical of the ideal asylum of the nineteenth century.

The Jacksonian ideal was a well-ordered asylum, in which that order began with its architectural design (see Fig. 6). In the design of the American asylum, architecture acquired a clear moral purpose. Operating according to a theoretical stance based on an amalgam of Pinel's moral treatment, American faith in the formative powers of the environment, and a belief in the curability of insanity, the asylum of the Jacksonian era carefully ordered and strictly regulated the daily routine of the inmates, confident that this would result in their eventual return to society as normal individuals. The asylums had a medical and therapeutic orientation. The use of restraints was unusual; occupational therapy was not. There is some evidence that the early asylum movement achieved some success in the treatment of the insane. This was not, however, destined to be the beginning of a powerful and continuing upward thrust in the management of mental illness. Indeed, it was to be little more than a brief moment of light and hope introducing a longer period of darkness and despair.

Various factors account for the change in orientation of asylums from therapy to custodial care. Among the social and economic factors were the Civil War, massive immigrations, and the rising cost of maintaining increasingly overcrowded institutions. The earlier asylum, with a regimen appropriate to a relatively small patient population, was incapable of meeting the new demands, and eventually most therapeutic efforts were buried by the weight of numbers and inadequate funding. This development was also encouraged by a change in medical thought.

Neurology and Neuropsychiatry

During the nineteenth century medicine escaped metaphysics and adopted the methods and techniques proven so successful in the physical sciences. Great advances were made in basic biomedical science. In this period the cell theory was formulated and the animal experiment was established as an avenue to physiological knowledge. By the third quarter of the century experimental medicine was a reality. Analysis of the nervous system progressed steadily throughout the century, the bulk of investigations revealing a relation of localized structure and function. This changed the interpretation of psychopathology. Neurological and psychiatric disorders alike were explained on a physiological basis. Psychological causes were not excluded totally, but abnormal behavior was generally linked to abnormal function of localized anatomical entities. Insanity was thus considered to be a symptom complex of anomalous states of the brain.

The triumph of the somatic outlook in neurology created a pessimistic attitude toward psychiatric illness. Little could be done to treat abnormal brain structures or lesions. Consequently, even as asylums began to turn away from moral treatment for essentially nonmedical reasons, advanced medical thought supported the idea of the incurability of insanity. The nonphysical therapeutic orientation of institutions, already attenuated, entered into decline and at the century's end asylums were custodial institutions where restraints were common, occupational therapy absent, and attempts at treatment as ineffectual as they were miserable.

Neurology developed as a special branch of medicine during the nineteenth century, and clinical psychiatry emerged as a part of neurology. The treatment of disturbances of the psyche once again became the province of medicine. The somatic approach to psychiatric illness reached its zenith in the writings of Emil Kraepelin at the century's end. His classification scheme of psychiatric diseases represents the clear definition of modern psychiatry as a medical discipline theoretically free of poetic and moralistic attitudes. The concept of localization of mental diseases and their symptoms and the assumption of physical causes operative in disturbed mental states dominated psychiatric thought in Kraepelin's time, and this general organic approach continues as a powerful aspect of contemporary psychiatry.

Dynamic Psychiatry

During the same period that neurology and neuropsychiatry were taking form, the foundations of dynamic psychiatry were being established. Dynamic psychiatry has broad and diverse origins. In part it is rooted in neurology and clinical psychiatry, in part in the outgrowths of Mesmer's

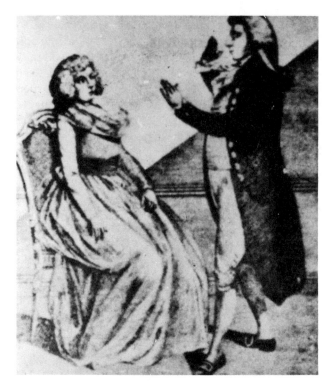

Figure 7. Anton Mesmer's "magnetizing" procedure.

eighteenth-century concept of animal magnetism, and in part in various manifestations of that broad cultural movement termed Romanticism.

Toward the end of the eighteenth century Franz Mesmer proclaimed his discovery of a rarefied fluid that bathed the entire universe, penetrating and surrounding all bodies. He extolled the application to medicine of this primeval agent of nature. Sickness, Mesmer maintained, resulted from an obstacle to the flow of the fluid through the body, which was analogous to a magnet. Individuals could control and reinforce the fluid's action by "mesmerizing" or massaging the body's poles, thereby overcoming the obstacle and inducing a "crisis," often in the form of epileptiform convulsions, to restore health (see Fig. 7). In this way Mesmer cured people of diseases ranging from blindness to ennui produced by an overactive spleen.

Everything in Mesmer's clinic was designed to induce a crisis in the patient. Not all crises took a violent form: Some developed into deep sleeps. Some of these sleeps provided communication with dead or distant spirits, who sent messages by way of the fluid directly to the somnambulist's internal sixth sense, which was ordinarily receptive to what would later be called extrasensory perceptions. This feature of mesmerism was to have an eventual impact upon the development of psychiatric thought.

Accused of charlatanism and rebuffed by a royal commission, Mesmer retired from public life. Nonetheless, mesmerism had extensive therapeutic successes to its credit, and it did not depart with its creator. Instead, it diffused throughout France, Germany, Great Britain, and the United States, where it was especially important in the development of Christian Science.

Early in the nineteenth century some realized that the sleeplike states that often occurred in the course of mesmeric treatment were the result of psychological rather than magnetic forces. The idea was more widely accepted after the mid-nineteenth century when Braid introduced the terms *hypnosis* and *suggestion* in explaining the phenomenon. And now neurology, which had at first served to strengthen somaticist trends in psychiatry, produced pioneers in psychogenic research.

"Neurasthenia" was a major concern of late nineteenth-century medicine. It was a condition believed to result from an organic weakness of the nervous system. "Nervousness," a catalog of complaints later to be defined as neurotic, functional, or psychosomatic, became fashionable in psychopathology. Thus during the last decades of the century Jean-Martin Charcot, physician-in-charge at the Salpêtrière, turned his attention to a functional neurosis, hysteria, eventually utilizing hypnosis in his investigations, as illustrated in Fig. 8. Hypnosis, until then despised and neglected in academic circles, became a legitimate if not stylish field of study and treatment because of its use by the greatest living neurologist and the most influential physician in France. The numerous studies in hysteria and hypnosis that followed Charcot's investigations resulted in new facts, the formulation of new theories, and undoubted therapeutic successes. These, whatever their basis, tended to mitigate the apathy and hopelessness that had spread throughout neuropsychiatry.

Charcot's approach was not a therapeutic one. The modern approach to psychotherapy sprang mainly from the work of Hippolyte-Marie Bernheim, professor of medicine at Nancy. Originally of frankly somatic orientation, Bernheim, following the lead of his predecessor, Ambrose-August Liébault, turned his attention to psychological methods of healing, using hypnosis and suggestion as a means both to treat and investigate the neuroses. He argued that suggestion, not the sleep, was the essential element in treatment with hypnosis. His experiments indicted that the results achieved by means of hypnosis could almost all be obtained by means of suggestions made in the waking state or by autosuggestion. Bernheim's experiments with posthypnotic suggestion seemed to him to prove the existence of latent memories and produce interesting and quite

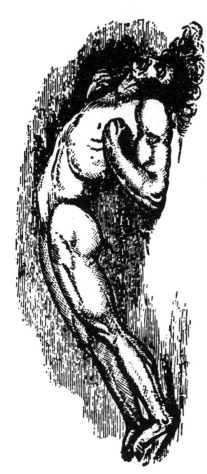

Figure 8. Opisthotonos, illustrated in *Iconographie photographique de la Salpêtrière,* one aspect of hysteria studied by Charcot.

unrealistic explanations of behavior on the part of the patients. These would later be termed "rationalizations."

The full significance of Bernheim's observations was realized later, when, as a result of the great interest aroused by his and Charcot's investigations, hypnosis was studied experimentally and used therapeutically by many outstanding neurologists and psychiatrists. For example, the neurologist Pierre Janet, who became professor of psychiatry at the Collège de France, used hypnosis in his studies of various forms of neurotic behavior, encountering the phenomenon of the split personality. He extended Charcot's theory that the hysteric has a weakness in the nervous system to embrace the concept that this constitutional weakness contributes to a lack of psychic cohesiveness, which results in aspects of the consciousness becoming split off and resultant hysterical and dissociative phenomena. The split or double personality thus represents behavior of the individual caused by those processes that become separated from the consciousness. Janet's research into hypnosis revealed that traumatic memories forgotten by the patient could produce neurotic symptoms. He found that such memories could be discovered through hypnosis and that making them conscious could lead to cure. This would later be called the cathartic method of treatment.

Psychotherapeutic and psychogenic ideas were clearly abroad in the 1880s. They were reinforced by powerful currents of philosophical and social thought emphasizing the irrational, the amoral, and the aggressive drives and the self-deceptive nature of human beings. The ideas of Arthur Schopenhauer, Karl Marx, and Friedrich Nietsche especially conditioned the environment in which dynamic psychiatry took its origins. All that was lacking in psychiatry was the grand synthesis. This was the accomplishment of Sigmund Freud, undoubtedly the most renowned of all psychotherapists and psychogeneticists of the late nineteenth century. Freud molded the ideas that emanated from France into the form in which they became an international movement and provided the base for the development of twentieth-century dynamic psychiatry in its diverse manifestations.

Originally an extreme somaticist, Freud was always convinced that ultimately all psychological illnesses are attributable to neurological processes. But neuroanatomical and neurophysiological research had yielded no positive results for the psychiatry of the neuroses and functional psychoses, and thus he resolved to confine his work first of all to the purely psychological level. Disappointed with the then fashionable electrotherapy, he turned to hypnosis, collaborating at the outset with Josef Breuer. Like Janet, Breuer had observed that during hypnosis hysterical patients could recall traumatic experiences and that the reproduction of psychic events repressed at the time had a therapeutic effect. He and Freud later reported this as the cathartic method.

Freud eventually abandoned hypnosis as a psychotherapeutic technique and used other methods of recalling forgotten memories, developing the free association technique and dream analysis as avenues to the unconscious and clarifying the full role of repression in neurosis. Freud developed an elaborate deterministic theory of psychological function, locating unconscious processes at the base of psychopathological phenomena. Symptoms were interpreted as substitute gratifications and the therapeutic task was to uncover repressions and resolve them by conscious decisions. The basic tenet of this psychoanalytical method was that to achieve a cure it is necessary for the patient to relive past events and gain insight into the meaning of those events. The removal of inner conflicts thus underlies the elimination of maladaptive behavior.

Thus Freud's synthesis represents the culmination of various diverse currents in nineteenth-century thought, and provides the foundation of twentieth-century dynamic psychiatry in all its aspects. The general concepts and outlook resident in late nineteenth-century dynamic psychiatry have in turn directly or indirectly affected subsequent biomedical views regarding psychiatric conditions and have extended into the intellectual fabric of twentieth-century society.

There have been many developments and advances in the understanding of behavioral factors in health care and especially the treatment of the mentally ill during the twentieth century. Knowledge is still incomplete, however, and methods of treatment are still in the process of evolution. It is well to remember the long history of ideas in medicine and the development of treatments and institutions dedicated to those suffering psychological as well as physical ailments, especially remaining cognizant of the nonmedical factors that have operated in this regard throughout the history of Western civilization. It is possible to gain insight into the roots of contemporary ideas and practices and better judge the manner in which medical knowledge progresses. A historical perspective permits some satisfaction about the progress in the understanding and treatment of illness in general; it also serves as a reminder of the limitations and imperfections of the manner in which contemporary medicine and society cope with the problem of mental illness in particular.

References

Grattan, J. H. G., and C. Singer 1952. Anglo-Saxon Magic and Medicine. London and New York: Oxford U. Press, p. 155.

Lattimore, R. (Trans.) 1951. The Iliad of Homer, Chicago and London: University of Chicago Press, p. 60.

4

Brain–Behavior Relations and the Delivery of Health Care

George A. Ojemann, M.D.*

Many human brain functions can be viewed as responses to internal or external environmental changes. Brain responses to changes in an individual's internal environment are largely directed toward providing uniformity and homeostasis. These responses utilize mechanisms of negative feedback to regulate respiration, heart rate, blood pressure, and salt and water metabolism and modulate pituitary hormone output. The reactions to the external environment generated by the brain make up that individual's behavior. These reactions include a group of "subconscious" involuntary or reflex responses, most of which are present at many phylogenetic levels and early in human development, and a group of more complex "conscious," "voluntary," or "higher" functions, such as language, that are largely unique to man and appear later during human development. In this chapter we will consider how alterations in brain function modify reactions to the internal or external environments. These changes are involved in many significant health care problems, ranging from hypertension to the major psychoses. But, in addition, the way in which individual patients' and physicians' brains react to the environment colors every interpersonal interaction; this touches on every aspect of health care.

Despite the great expansion in the neurosciences in the last decades, knowledge of human brain function lags behind many other areas of biology. Indeed, quite fundamental issues are still controversial. One such issue is the extent to which brain responses to the environment are learned from previous contacts with the external environment, and how much is

*Professor, Department of Neurological Surgery, University of Washington School of Medicine, Seattle, Washington.

"wired in," an innate property of that individual's brain "machinery." There is general agreement that some functions are "wired in"; examples include the homeostatic mechanisms to regulate the internal environment, the reflex responses to noxious stimuli, the sleep–wake and other circadian (24-hour) cycles, and the sexual drives that appear at puberty. Most would also agree that there are innate brain mechanisms for some "higher functions" as well, such as an innate mechanism for the acquisition and generation of a language. Presumably the nature of these innate properties of the brain is largely genetically determined, perhaps modified by any early acquired damage. On the other hand, some brain responses are clearly learned. The exact length of circadian cycles, for example, can be altered to some extent by changing the environmental periods of light and dark. The higher functions in particular are clearly molded by the environment. The particular language(s) one acquires is certainly environmentally determined. There is no innate brain mechanism for English, only, at most, one for acquisition of some type of language. The extent to which innate brain mechanisms or learning contribute to the behavioral repertory of an individual is particularly controversial in the area of emotional responses. Studies of animal behavior suggest innate patterns of emotional responses, but the extent of these innate responses in human emotionality is unknown.

This issue of the role of innate and environmental factors in brain functions is now further complicated by the recent identification of the phenomenon of "critical periods." In this phenomenon, the presence or absence of certain environmental experiences at one critical stage of development determines the kinds of connections made by nerve cells. Thus the nature of the brain machinery subsequently available is modified by the environmental experiences during that particular developmental period. The role of innate brain machinery or subsequent environmental experiences, then, remains one of many unresolved issues in human brain function.

This chapter focuses on how alterations in brain function impact on the individual's response to the environment. However, present knowledge does not provide a comprehensive understanding of the brain mechanisms that underlie these reactions to the environment, particularly those involving the uniquely human higher functions, for an understanding of these processes is dependent on observations made in man. Even the simplest of these higher functions, language, has no suitable animal model. Study of the behavioral changes after spontaneous brain damage in man, such as strokes, focal seizure disorders, or surgical excisions of local areas of brain, is the source for most of these observations. The relation between brain function and behavior is established by identifying the areas of the brain that are consistently damaged when a behavior is altered.

However, these studies are limited by several problems. One is identifying exactly where the brain is damaged. The extent of gross pathological changes after a stroke is generally smaller than the changes thought to represent damaged brain on the diagnostic study known as a computerized tomographic (CT) scan, and this in turn seems to be much smaller than the extent of the metabolic derangements as measured by the new technique of positron emission tomography (PET). The area that should be related to the behavioral deficit is not always clear.

A second problem is that the behavioral deficit following brain injury is not static but changes over time, generally with some recovery of function. The way in which this recovery occurs is not known. Some of it probably represents a gradual return of function in neuronal circuits that were damaged but not destroyed; but some recovery takes a year or more. This probably represents reorganization in the brain circuits that are used for a particular function. Recovery of function then depends not only on the extent of the lesion, but also on the status of the remainder of the brain, which can be influenced by such factors as age or previous injury. Commonly this problem is dealt with by assessing the changes in behavior long after the brain injury, but then, of course, the pattern of change represents the sum of the effects of the initial damage and the recovery process.

Small electric currents applied to local areas of the human brain often have a disruptive effect on higher functions, acting like temporary reversible lesions. This technique, sometimes called electrical stimulation mapping, is of great value for identifying discrete localization but is applicable only to selected patient populations, those who are appropriate candidates for neurosurgical operations under local anesthesia. Some of the conditions for which these operations are done may also alter brain organization so that findings with this technique may not always reflect brain organization in the "normal" population.

Another technique for establishing relations between human brain function and behavior is to identify where neurons are working during a particular behavior. Working neurons locally increase the blood flow; this can be detected in a number of ways, most often by techniques using inhalation or intravascular injection of radioactive xenon tracers. A major limitation with these techniques is that they show where neurons are working, but not what they are doing. Inhibitory neurons work just as hard as excitatory neurons, though with very different functional implications.

Selected issues in the relation of the brain to behavior can also be addressed by innovative environmental manipulations, such as in tests to determine lateralization of functions to one cerebral hemisphere. These tests depend on introducing simultaneously competing stimuli into either ear or either visual half field, with the stimulus going to the side of the brain concerned with that function preferentially processed. This technique can be used to assess lateralization of function in normal subjects, but the magnitude of these effects is often quite small and variable. Also, some of the results obtained with these techniques are in conflict with those derived from most other techniques for looking at lateralization of human higher functions.

Because of these technical limitations, the data base on brain mechanisms that underlie human higher functions is surprisingly small. Nevertheless, this field has been subject to a great deal of theorizing. As a result, factual underpinnings for many theories are often slim. A critical attitude toward all theoretical frameworks for human brain organization is warranted, with particular questions about the nature of the data on which the theory is based. In view of this, this chapter presents a series of examples of the way in which altered brain function impacts on the environmental responses related to health care, rather than attempting a coherent theory.

This discussion assumes some knowledge of human neuroanatomy and neurophysiology. If, in the vagaries of curricular organization this material has not been presented, reference is also made to portions of a brief illustrated paperback on brain function intended for the general public, *Inside the Brain* (Calvin and Ojemann, 1980), which will provide the needed nontechnical background in neuroanatomy and neurophysiology. That volume also is a source for further reference to more comprehensive review articles and original work on each topic.

Motor Systems

The human brain demonstrates a substantial degree of localization of function; neuronal systems represented in different areas are commonly involved in different functions. Thus focal brain damage in different areas usually has different behavioral consequences. Some examples are relatively simple and not at all controversial (Calvin and Ojemann, 1980, pp. 1–7). Damage to lateral portions of the motor cortex or the efferent pathways through the internal capsule produces a motor paralysis of the opposite face and upper extremity, a paralysis that is most dense in the distal hand and lower face. Damage outside this area does *not* produce such a paralysis. The potential impact of this deficit on the patient's behavior is obvious. Clearly there is a group of motor functions, especially those involving the opposite hand, that the patient could perform before the brain damage and not after. The way the patient will cope with this deficit will be a function of the innate and learned behavioral responses of the remaining uninjured brain and the reaction of the external environment to the deficit.

If small electric currents are applied to the motor cortex, a pattern of highly discrete functional localization becomes evident. Movements in the larynx are often evoked by stimulation of the motor cortex just above the sylvian fissure, with a progression of effects as the electrode is moved upward a few millimeters at a time: movements of the tongue next, then the lips, then the remainder of the face, followed by the individual digits and the arm. As the electrode passes on to the medial face of the hemisphere, leg movements are evoked. This pattern is called a "homunculus." It seems to be relatively uniform from person to person, and the pattern it illustrates, different discrete brain areas involved in different functions, also seems to be a general one, not only in the motor cortex, but also in the remainder of the brain.

Language

The effects of damage to the motor system are symmetric, that is, damage on the right side alters left body function in the same way that damage on the left side alters function on the right. But damage in certain areas of cortex on the left hemisphere is associated with deficits in language that are not seen in most patients with similarly placed right brain lesions. This is the phenomenon of functional lateralization known as language "dominance."Such asymmetrically localized functions seem to be unique to man (Calvin and Ojemann, 1980, pp. 67–74).

There is some individual variability in the lateralization of language. Nearly all right-handed individuals are left brain dominant for language, but only about 70% of left handers have this pattern of dominance. The remaining left handers are about equally divided between those who seem to have language represented bilaterally, in each cerebral hemisphere, and those who are right brain dominant for language. The bilateral pattern is probably familial. There is some evidence that this arrangement is less than optimal, for the expressive language disorder stuttering seems particularly likely to occur in the presence of bilateral language representation. Language lateralization seems to be slightly greater in males than females as well.

Language lateralization has been associated with a number of asymmetries in the anatomy of the cerebral hemispheres. The most notable of these asymmetries is the size of a cortical area known as the planum temporale, that portion of the superior temporal lobe that lies buried in the sylvian fissure, extending posteriorly from the primary auditory cortex in Heschl's gyrus. This area is smaller on the left than on the right in about the same proportion of brains as there are people who are *not* left brain dominant for language. However, the role of this area of the cortex in language is unknown. This anatomical asymmetry has been identified in the fetus, suggesting that lateralization of language is genetically determined, and this asymmetry too seems to be slightly less marked in females than in males.

However, lateralization of language is not totally fixed until about age 5. If there is a major insult to left brain, particularly in the frontal or parietal lobe prior to age 5, language function may then develop in the homologous areas of right brain. However, recent evidence suggests that this language is not entirely normal. There is a congenital anomaly of the cerebral blood vessels called Sturge–Weber syndrome that is sometimes lateralized to one cerebral hemisphere. Removal of that hemisphere in infancy has been indicated to prevent later damage to the good hemisphere by seizures induced by the abnormal blood vessels. Usable language develops in these patients, regardless of which hemisphere is removed in infancy. But those who had the left hemisphere removed have deficits in language, compared to those who had the right hemisphere removed. These patients are relatively quiet individuals who use spoken language infrequently and have a limited range of grammatical expression. The brain then seems to have intrinsic mechanisms that lead to language lateralization, but these mechanisms remain plastic until about age 5. This plasticity, however, is not complete. Failure to develop the usual intrinsic mechanisms leads to less than optimal language function and rather surprisingly, learning and producing the full range of language's grammar seem to depend especially on intrinsic mechanisms.

Damage within different parts of the perisylvian cortex of the left brain of adults has been associated with different language deficits (Calvin and Ojemann, 1980, pp. 19–29). Damage in the posterior frontal lobe has been generally associated with a language deficit in which the patient is nonfluent, that is, produces relatively few words. Most language consists of nouns or noun–verb pairs and there is a poverty of grammar; words or phrases are frequently repeated (perseveration). Language understanding is relatively preserved. These patients may speak with single words, indeed, occasionally with only one word, but they are not mute. For example, the patient of Paul Broca's in whom this picture was first related to frontal lobe function over a century ago could only say "tan-tan". This type of language disturbance is then often called Broca's aphasia or motor or expressive aphasia.

Damage in the posterior temporal portion of the language area is more commonly associated with a language deficit where speech production is relatively intact but language understanding seems to be highly defective. Speech is fluent and grammar intact, but the individual words frequently do not make sense; they are neologisms, nonsense words, jargon, or paraphasias, that is, words that are close but inaccurate approximations of the correct sound or meaning. This type of aphasia is often called sensory or receptive aphasia or Wernicke's aphasia (after the neurologist who described it in the 1870s).

More recent studies using electrical stimulation mapping techniques have demonstrated discrete localization of a number of language-related functions in the general region of the perisylvian cortex (Calvin and Ojemann, 1980, pp. 29–31 and 35–41). Such different language-related functions as naming, reading, and short-term verbal memory are frequently altered in response to electrical stimulation of different though nearby areas of the cortex in a particular patient. Indeed, naming of the same information in two different languages may be altered by stimulating different cortical sites. What determines the location of cortical sites involved in a particular language task is presently unknown. One model suggests that a subcortical, perhaps thalamic switching mechanism selects the cortical sites appropriate to the task. In the adult, these sites seem to be quite stable for a given language function over hours to months. Whether they change over longer periods is unknown. There is a suggestion that larger areas of the language cortex are involved in more difficult language tasks (Ojemann and Whitaker, 1978b). Perhaps as facility in a particular language function is acquired, less and less brain is primarily functional, as crucial to the task. In this model, then, the exact areas of brain functioning during a particular task are a function of the underlying neuronal organization, the task, and previous experience with the task.

These studies have also suggested a somewhat different model of the general organization of the language cortex. In this model, the posterior area of the inferior frontal gyrus is still concerned with the motor speech output, but in the remainder of the frontal language areas and in the superior temporal and parietal areas there is a system in which language understanding and speech motor production share a common cortex. This is surrounded by areas of cortex related to short-term verbal memory. In this model, specialized language functions, such as grammar or word finding are related to sites at the interface between the cortical system common to language production and understanding and the surrounding memory system, both frontally, parietally, and temporally. This is one of a number of pieces of evidence that supports the view that language, including language understanding, utilizes areas of the brain whose original functions were related to motor control and motor learning.

Gross defects in the language system have an enormous impact on behavior. The inability to verbally express one's thoughts, as in a motor aphasia, even though much evidence suggests that the thoughts are still there as "inner speech," is a devastating problem; nor is this deficit always easily recognized. It is not at all uncommon to see patients with aphasias whose defects were thought only to represent a nonspecific confusion. Patients with deficits in language production regularly have considerable insight into the presence of the defect and are greatly distressed by it, while patients with deficits in language understanding seem to have less insight into their disability.

It is the milder defects in the development of the language system that have the greatest impact on health care, however. Developmental dyslexia, one of the significant problems in language education, is in many cases a genetically determined, male sex-linked delay in maturation of portions of the dominant language cortex. Indeed, there is evidence that in some individuals with this problem, the anatomical organization of language cortex may be defective, presumably also on a genetic basis (Galaburda and Kemper, 1979).

Further evidence that the individual patterns of organization of language cortex are sometimes related to overall verbal function is presented below in the discussion of individual variability in cortical localization. Contemporary Western society with its emphasis on education puts a high premium on verbal skills. Thus the quality of brain mechanisms for language, to the extent that they are reflected in this overall verbal ability, have a major impact on each individual's career opportunities and development. Indeed, the system for educating the health care providers is heavily biased toward the selection of individuals with strong verbal performance. Such skills are not present in perhaps the majority of individuals seeking access to health care systems. Thus people with rather different brain mechanisms are likely to be found in the health care provider or recipient roles.

Memory

Injury to a number of brain areas alters recent memory (Calvin and Ojemann, 1980, pp. 55–67). Of these, damage to portions of the medial temporal lobe, particularly the hippocampus and thalamus, seems especially crucial. Areas of cortex also seem to play a role in recent memory. At all these areas, recent memory deficits are modality specific in man; that is, damage to the left brain tends to interfere with recent memory for verbal material, and damage to the right brain with recent memory for spatial material. Unilateral damage to these structures, however, usually produces only mild recent-memory deficits; but bilateral injury prevents the development of any new recent memories.

This memory deficit does not involve immediate memory, the kind of memory measured by the digit span, nor does it involve long-term memory for material acquired in the distant past. Rather, the deficit involves "post distraction" recent memory. A memory can be retained so long as the patient is not distracted by having to engage in some task involving similar material. But once that occurs, the patient with bilateral hippocampal damage is unable to retain the material. Such memory deficit generally extends in a retrograde manner for several years prior to the injury. Memories developed prior to that are preserved.

This global loss of recent memory is very disabling: Not only can the patient not retain the telephone numbers of friends but, indeed, he cannot remember where he has been or what he has said. But even more devastating is that the development of new long-term memory requires an intact postdistractional short-term memory. Thus the individual with the global memory deficit is unable to form new long-term memories as well, he is left only with those from his distant past.

Bilateral damage to either the hippocampal or thalamic components of the recent memory system can produce this deficit. Bilateral thalamic damage with recent memory loss is usually seen as a sequela of chronic alcoholism and is a condition known as Korsakoff's disease. Bilateral hippocampal damage may occur under a number of conditions. This part of the medial temporal lobe is often damaged in major head injuries—even the head injury associated with normal birth! It is a common site of nerve cell loss in the presenile and senile dementias, such as Alzheimer's disease, and with distortion of the adjacent cerebral ventricles in hydrocephalus. Neurons here are unusually susceptible to hypoxia. It is this unusual vulnerability of the hippocampal neurons that probably accounts for the prominence of recent memory loss in all these conditions and with aging. There is some evidence that neurons in these recent memory circuits use acetylcholine as a transmitter; it has even been suggested (but not proved) that increasing acetycholine metabolism might improve function of these circuits.

At the thalamic level a part of the memory mechanism seems to involve circuits related to specific attention (Calvin and Ojemann, 1980, pp. 50–54). These circuits can be experimentally manipulated in man by electrical stimulation of the ventral lateral thalamus. Activation of these circuits at the time of input of information enhances the likelihood that that information will be later recalled from either recent or more remote memory. Activation of these circuits in left brain alters verbally codable material, and those in right brain have the same effect on spatial material. These alerting circuits, active at the time of input of information, then, seem to modulate the probability of later recall of specific items of information and the availability of previously internalized information to be associated with the incoming material. The activity level of these circuits at the time information is registered would seem to have a major impact on whether this information is remembered or not. One can imagine the consequence of defects in such a system: A mild deficit results in inability to sustain attention on a task, with a reduced learning rate, as in the "minimal learning disability" child; with a more severe deficit, incoming information is ignored and attention is directed only to previous internalized material. A child with this situation might appear very much as being autistic, where the child seems unable to relate to the external environment but, rather, acts as though he is continually "daydreaming," attending only to some internal cues. Deficits in the function of these thalamic alerting circuits seem likely in these conditions but remain to be demonstrated.

Sensory Systems

Damage in the posterior bank of the central sulcus of cortex is associated with deficits in sensation in the contralateral body (Calvin and Ojemann, 1980, pp. 5–9). The deficit is not equal in all sensory modalities, touch and joint sensation are predominantly involved while temperature and pain are relatively preserved. Like the motor cortex, stimulation mapping of the sensory cortex shows discrete homuncular organization, with face and predominantly lip representation just above the sylvian fissure, and extremity representation, predominantly of the hand and especially the thumb, more superiorly. Leg representation is again on the medial face of the hemisphere. The organization of the sensory cortex has been meticulously examined in experimental animals. There it shows a discrete pattern of localization, with individual columns of sensory cortex connected to specific areas in the thalamic sensory nuclei devoted to sensory input from specific parts of the contralateral body.

Damage to the sensory cortex is often associated with a condition called thalamic syndrome (Calvin and Ojemann, 1980, pp. 103–111). These patients have an elevated threshold for touch sensation in all or part of the contralateral body, but once that threshold is exceeded, any sensation is interpreted as extremely disagreeable. The importance of this rather rare syndrome for brain–behavior relations is its indication of the internal mechanisms in the brain for modulating the sensory input that is received at higher centers. Systems to modulate sensory input are present at many levels of the nervous system, from peripheral receptors to the spinal cord, thalamic nuclei, and sensory cortex. Under normal circumstances these modulating circuits have properties that apparently diminish sustained sensory input into the brain and certainly diminish the response to sensory inputs. This effect is commonly encountered; the ongoing touch of one's clothes is not usually detected, though the new touch of a mosquito landing on a sleeve will be. The peripheral touch inputs adapt to the continuing touch sensation and now only respond to the novel touch. Such a system has great utility, preventing massive sensory overload of the central nervous system by irrelevant information, but it also has significant behavioral implications. The model of the pathophysiology of the thalamic syndrome is that when an inadequate amount of sensory input has been received at cortical sensory levels due to damage to the afferent pathways, sensory modulating sites at lower levels are signalled to turn up the gain in the sensory system. What follows seems analogous to what happens to an audio amplifier when gain is continuously turned up. At a certain point even the most melodious music becomes disagreeably loud. In the thalamic syndrome, with the alteration in normal sensory modulation, even the most innocuous touch sensation becomes disagreeable.

A cortical role in interpreting sensory phenomena is also evident in the behavioral pattern seen after damage to portions of the parietal lobes, predominantly in the non-language-dominant hemisphere (Calvin and Ojemann, 1980, pp. 75–80). The deficit after this injury does not involve language, memory, or primary motor or sensory processes, rather, the patient with right parietal lobe damage acts as though the left half of the world were not present. Thus if a group of examiners is standing around this patient's bed, the patient may totally ignore those standing to the left and converse only with those on the right. More subtle forms of this defect can be shown by the phenomenon of "extinction." Although single sensory inputs to either the right or the left side of the body are readily detected, when simultaneous inputs are presented to both right and left body, those on the left side are ignored. In the florid form, this deficit may extend to the patient's own body image. He may not recognize portions of the left side of his own body. If that patient is shown his left arm, he is likely to become very distressed, not understanding what this strange arm is doing in bed with him. This deficit in body image may also extend to the inability to relate his own body to clothing, a phenomenon known as dressing apraxia; the patient is unable to relate his arms and legs to the appropriate sleeves and trouser legs. Nondominant parietal lobe damage is also often associated with deficits in the ability to manipulate objects in space, a phenomenon called constructional apraxia. Associated with this is the inability to read a map and to find one's way from one spot to another, such as from the bed to the bathroom, without using verbal cues.

The lateralization of spatial abilities to the right brain is not just the reverse of the lateralization of verbal abilities to the left brain. Left brain lesions produce language deficits about 13 times as often as right brain lesions, but right brain damage produces dressing apraxias only about 5 times as often as left brain damage, and constructional apraxias only about 2 times as often. Thus there are individuals who have spatial abilities bilaterally represented, but with language strongly lateralized to the left; and conversely, there are individuals with very strong lateralization of spatial abilities to the right brain, with language to the left. Thus there is substantial individual variability in the exact patterns of lateralization of spatial functions.

Some of this individual variability is determined by the individual's sex. Spatial abilities seem to be more strongly lateralized in males than in females. Indeed, a recent study suggests that testosterone must be present in early life for development of spatial skills, including their lateralization (Hier and Crowley, 1982).

There seems to be less of the anatomical asymmetry between right and left hemisphere perisylvian cortex in females than in males as well. Some evidence suggests that in boys with the familial form of developmental dyslexia, the strong lateralization of spatial functions to the right brain, which is commonly a feature of males, is less well developed. One model of the delayed maturation of the language areas in that form of developmental dyslexia suggests that there is competition between language and spatial abilities within the left hemisphere (Whitelson, 1977). The reverse pattern of competition between language and spatial abilities certainly occurs. When language is displaced from the left to the right hemisphere by early left brain injury, spatial functions generally are severely impaired. One cerebral hemisphere generally seems to be unable to handle both spatial and verbal abilities by itself.

Nondominant parietal lobe deficits, including neglect of half of space, distortion of body image, and inability to manipulate objects in space, represent a significant problem in the health care area. Patients with these deficits often do not recognize their own illness (even to the extent of not recognizing one's own arm as paralyzed). In its more minor forms, these patients may not recognize their own limitations. Such deficits greatly color motivation to engage in therapy or rehabilitation programs, or one's judgment of an appropriate behavioral response. Thus a patient with right parietal damage is likely to come to the hospital but then claim nothing is wrong with him and not wish to stay. He is not going to be interested in treatment programs or rehabilitation. Indeed, such patients are most difficult to rehabilitate because of their lack of insight into their disability.

Nondominant parietal lobe deficits are frequently reflected in the patient's drawings. Some of the most dramatic illustrations of these deficits have occurred when damage to this brain area has occurred in professional artists (Gardner, 1976). There is some suggestive evidence that functions of this area of the brain may be particularly important to skills involving artistic ability and spatial manipulation, though what if any structural differences there might be in the brain organization in these areas in individuals with or without visual artistic skills is unknown.

Another example of the brain's ability to manipulate sensory phenomena occurs in one type of seizure discharge that arises in the temporal lobe (Calvin and Ojemann, pp. 85–88). Seizures reflect local hyperactivity of neurons. When seizures arise from these hyperactive neurons in the posterior temporal lobe, the patient frequently reports sensory hallucinations. When the hyperexcitable neurons are very far posterior in the temporal lobe, near the region of the temporal–occipital junction, these hallucinations may take the form of patterned visual phenomena in the contralateral visual field and often geometric patterns of colored lights are reported. When the discharges involve areas more anterior in the posterior temporal lobe, the visual phenomena often include specific visual scenes. These visual events may be quite stereotyped from one seizure to another in a particular patient: a man and his dog walking across the visual field in one patient, a particular bucolic farm scene in another. Such hallucinations are most commonly of visual origin when the seizures arise in the right hemisphere. Seizures arising in the left temporal lobe are more likely to be associated with auditory hallucinations such as hearing a specific song. Seizures arising in more medial portions of the temporal lobe sometimes are associated with olfactory hallucinations, a disagreeable odor being a common report. And even further anteriorly in temporal lobe, the seizure phenomena may be manifested by reports of visual and auditory sensations that represent a specific experience from the patient's earlier life, an experience that is often recalled with all its emotional as well as sensory coloration. All of these phenomena often seem very real to the patient. All are generated by the brain independently of any environmental sensory events. The brain then has the ability to generate sensory phenomena that seem to represent a real view of the world. In some circumstances these are totally detached from sensory phenomena available to other individuals.

There are brain mechanisms, then, at many levels that filter the incoming sensory information. Other mechanisms in nondominant parietal lobes integrate the information passing such a filter into a comprehensive image of the external environment and one's body. Temporal lobe mechanisms seem to add emotional coloration and memory components to these images. Abnormalities in these mechanisms alter the perceptions used to generate overt behavior, obviously with major consequences for the interaction between the patient and his surroundings.

Emotions

The examples of behavioral consequences of specific brain damage discussed to this point are ones on which there are considerable supporting evidence and general agreement; however, the brain mechanisms that underlie certain aspects of human behavior are more controversial. This is particularly true of those behaviors labeled as judgment and emotion (Calvin and Ojemann, 1980, pp. 151–162). Animal studies suggest that damage to certain brain areas alters patterns of behavior in a way that seems to represent changed emotional responsiveness. The most dramatic examples generally involve lesions in the medial or lateral hypothalamus. Lateral hypothalamic lesions will change a quiet, passive cat into one that attacks any stimulus, regardless of how inappropriate; medial hypothalamic lesions tend to make cats placid. The medial hypothalamus also has circuits where electrical stimulation evokes responses such that the animal will continue to provoke stimulation to the total exclusion of other activities, including feeding and sleeping. These responses have been interpreted as pleasurable. These hypothalamic effects have been modeled as representing the raw qualities of rage and pleasure. Occasional cases of damage to the human hypothalamus with similar changes in emotional responsiveness have been reported.

Areas of the cerebral cortex are thought to modulate this raw hypothalamic rage or pleasure. The portions of the cerebral cortex most often
related to this role are the medial faces of each hemisphere, which on
anatomical grounds have been defined as the limbic lobe. Indeed, those
human lesions that seem to produce alterations in emotional responsiveness generally involve injury, commonly bilateral, to the limbic lobe on the
medial face of the frontal or temporal lobes. Bilateral frontal lobe injuries
are often associated with a general decrease in emotional responsiveness,
the patient becoming relatively flat and unconcerned. There is a suggestion that medial temporal injury may be associated with inappropriate
aggressive emotional responses, inappropriate in that they can be
triggered by trivial stimuli.

The hypothalamus, of course, has another group of functions involving
maintenance of the internal environment of the organism. Nuclei in the
base of the third ventricle regulate pituitary hormone secretion, salt and
water balance, appetite, reproductive cycles, heart rate, respiration, blood
pressure, and the sleep–wakefulness cycles. At the level of hypothalamus,
then, the areas of brain that regulate autonomic function and those that
regulate emotion overlap. Indeed, cats with lateral hypothalamic damage
not only show rage but become very emaciated; those with medial damage
are not only placid but obese. The same situation seems to occur at the
cortical level. Those areas of the cortex where one can modulate heart rate,
respiration, or gastric secretions are the same portions of the medial faces
of the frontal and temporal lobes that have been implicated in the
regulation of emotion. This feature of brain anatomy, that is, that common
areas seem to be used for the regulation of both autonomic functions and
emotions is probably the anatomical substrate for that large group of
diseases that are sometimes labeled as psychosomatic. This group
includes, among others, hypertension and gastric ulceration diseases,
where emotional states seem to have a major impact on the evolution of
the condition. It has been suggested that in these diseases, excessive
neuronal activity related to emotion spills over into the autonomic
regulatory activity of the same area. These conditions, then, might be
equally effectively treated by reducing the neural activity related to
emotional excitement or by blocking the peripheral autonomic end organ.
Among the large number of autonomic mechanisms that share common
anatomical substrates at the hypothalamic and cortical levels are those that
control pituitary adrenocortical stimulating hormone release and thus the
basis for the adrenal steroid response to "stress" and other hyperactive
emotional states. Hormonal mechanisms regulating reproductive activity
also overlap with brain areas regulating emotion, providing an anatomical
basis for the role of emotion in infertility.

A number of the symptoms of altered brain function have some features
in common with the symptoms of major psychoses. The hallucinatory

alterations in perceptions of the environment with temporal lobe seizures have some parallels to the altered perception that is part of the thought disorders (schizophrenias). The alterations in emotion associated with medial frontal damage have some parallels with the major affective psychoses, particularly depression. There is a substantial body of evidence, most of which is on the inheritability of the major psychoses, to suggest that they represent biological phenomena in which some type of brain abnormality is present. Indeed, for the affective disorders the biochemical nature of the abnormality is beginning to be defined and seems to involve neural systems that use norepinephrine and serotonin as transmitters; and there are hints that excessive activity of certain neural circuits that use dopamine as a transmitter may occur in some schizophrenias. Nevertheless, behavioral changes that are exactly the same as the major psychoses generally are not produced by brain lesions or evoked by brain stimulation or seizures, and focal abnormalities of brain function have not been reliably identified in the major psychoses. The brain mechanisms that underlie these behavioral disorders, then, remain unknown. Even less is known about altered brain function in the less severe emotional disturbances.

Individual Variability in Brain Mechanisms

While there is a considerable body of evidence that relates deficits in particular functions such as language, recent memory, spatial abilities, and even emotional responsiveness to particular brain areas, it has been considerably harder to show that differences in brain structure and function account for individual behavioral differences; yet there is reason to think that they might. Recent studies of identical twins reared separately have shown some remarkable degrees of behavioral similarity. This would be quite likely if individual behavior depends heavily on brain mechanisms in view of the common genetic basis, but rather unlikely if individual behavior were environmentally determined in view of the very different environments in which some of the twins were raised.

It is tempting to speculate that particular levels of ability may be related to the development of different capacities in various brain systems. The artist, for example, may have a particularly well-developed nondominant parietal lobe, but confirmatory data is not presently available. The one exception to this is in the area of language. One of the striking findings in the studies of electrical stimulation mapping of language processes in the dominant cortex has been the high degree of individual variability in the exact location of language functions from one patient to another (Ojemann and Whitaker, 1978a; Ojemann, 1983). In that data it was possible to correlate some of the patterns of evoked language change with the patient's overall language abilities. Patients who showed evoked language changes from the inferior parietal lobe had statistically significant lower overall verbal abilities than those who did not. This suggests that the development of language processes in this particular anatomical area is concomitant of a less facile verbal system. It may well be that with increasing knowledge of the detailed brain organization of particular functions, similar correlations will be found for other abilities. Then much of the variance in the behavioral responses encountered in the course of health care delivery may well be attributable to the differences in the brain machinery available to that patient.

The Critical Period

It has generally been assumed that the available brain machinery is largely a reflection of the genetic background of the patient, with environmental influences playing only a negative role, that is, in the avoidance of trauma, hypoxia, or other conditions that might damage genetically determined brain systems. A series of recent findings in experimental animals has added another factor to that model of brain development (Calvin and Ojemann, 1980, pp. 113–126) by demonstrating that in some sensory systems certain experiences during early development are necessary for the normal pattern of neural organization to develop. Thus the environmental influences during early life, if sufficiently adverse, seem to alter the structure of the brain that is then available to the individual. Specifically, the cells in certain levels of the visual cortex in various mammals receive varieties of complex inputs that at some levels represent inputs from both eyes. But if one eye is covered during a certain critical period, the inputs to various neurons will no longer show binocular interaction but only represent inputs from one eye or the other. The presence of a binocular visual experience is necessary to generate binocular visual inputs to cells in the visual area of the cortex. Such critical periods have been identified for the visual systems of man as well. Whether they extend to other sensory systems or to more complex functions such as language has not been established, although there are suggestions that critical periods may exist for many abilities. These critical periods all occur relatively early in development, usually in the first few weeks to months of life in animals. In man the critical period for the visual system may extend to 2–3 years of age. Critical periods for language development, if they exist at all, are probably much longer, extending to age 8 or so.

The environmental deficits during the critical periods that give rise to altered neuronal wiring are rather dramatic ones—lack of visual perception in one eye, for example. An ordinary environment presumably would be adequate to avoid such deficits. Whether enriched environments alter brain function remains problematical, though it is known that when neurons in a particular systems are heavily utilized, at least in experimental animals, they become metabolically more active and generate new proteins and larger dendritic trees, allowing for the possibility of a greater number of contacts with other neurons. It may well be that environments that make increasing demands on the brain in particular areas are associated with increased development of the neuronal systems involved in that function.

Summary

This chapter has examined a number of ways in which alterations in brain function impact on behavior and thus the health care system. Damage in various focal areas of the brain has differential effects on behavior, effects that include alterations in motor function, speech, perception of the environment through changes in the sensations that reach the brain, in their interpretation there, or in the brain generating its own sensory patterns independently of environmental inputs, and in emotional response. Brain anatomy provides the basis for a group of diseases where emotions and autonomic functions are linked.

There is considerable individual variability in the exact way the brain is put together, a variability that is expressed as differences in lateralizations of function and in the individual patterns of localization of some functions. In some cases these individual variations can be correlated with overall ability, suggesting that differences in patterns of brain organization may underlie some of the variability in behavior. There is a suggestion that the nature of that brain machinery may not only be a consequence of the individual's genetic background but is perhaps altered by the kinds of experiences encountered during early development.

Behavior represents the response of a particular brain to an environment. Here we have highlighted how changes in the brain alter these responses, factors that the health professional must consider in analyzing the behaviors that result from brain–environment interactions.

References

Calvin, W., and G. Ojemann. 1980. Inside the Brain. New York: New American Library.

Galaburda, A., and T. Kemper. 1979. Cytoarchitectoric abnormalities in developmental dyslexia: A case study. Annals of Neurology 6:94–100.

Gardner, H. 1976. The Shattered Mind. New York: Vantage Press; Chapter 8.

Hier, D., and W. Crowley, Jr. 1982. Spatial ability in androgen-deficient men. New England Journal of Medicine 306:1202–1204.

Ojemann, G. 1983. Brain organization for language from the perspective of electrical stimulation mapping. Behavioral and Brain Sciences 6:189–230.

Ojemann, G., and H. Whitaker. 1978a. Language localization and variability. Brain and Language 6:239–260.

Ojemann, G., and H. Whitaker. 1978b. The bilingual brain. Archives of Neurology 35:409–412.

Whitelson, S. 1977. *In* C. Shagass, S. Gershon, and A. Friedhoff, eds.: Psycho-pathology and Brain Dysfunction. New York: Raven Press; pp. 15–50.

5

Social Science in the Clinic:
Applied Contributions from Anthropology To Medical Teaching and Patient Care*

Gary Rosen, M. D.† and Arthur Kleinman, M. D.‡

Introduction

The purpose of this chapter is to illustrate the utility of clinical approaches derived from anthropology and other social sciences. It is our hope that through a review of certain clinical approaches, using patient examples from our own practices, it will be apparent that these add a necessary dimension to patient care. Together with psychiatric input, they contribute to a more systematic and rigorous assessment of the core psychosocial issues in clinical work and make the clinician a more effective healer.

Many writers have demonstrated the inadequacies of the narrowly defined biomedical model in adequately conceptualizing and managing the life problems that result from the patient and family's experience of serious sickness (how they live through and respond to it) (Engel, 1977; Kleinman et al., 1978; Eisenberg, 1977; Leigh and Reiser, 1980; Good and Good, 1981). We will first review some of the problems upon which this criticism of biomedicine is based and then set out specific concepts and practical strategies from clinical social science that complement the biomedical side of clinical practice by offering clinical knowledge and skills that can address these and related problems.

*Work supported by the National Institute of Mental Health Training Grant No. 15648.

† Clinical Assistant Professor, Department of Family Medicine, University of Washington School of Medicine, Seattle, Washington. Formerly, Senior Fellow in the Clinically Applied Anthropology in Psychiatry and Primary Care Training Program, University of Washington School of Medicine, Seattle, Washington.

‡ Professor, Department of Psychiatry and Behavioral Sciences, University of Washington School of Medicine, Seattle, Washington. Present address: Professor and Head, Division of Cultural Psychiatry, and Adjunct Professor of Anthropology, Harvard University, Cambridge, Massachusetts.

Influence of Social Structure and Culture

Social structure (a society's institutional arrangement of social relationships) and culture (a group's core beliefs and norms) exert a profound
influence on the health status of individuals and their health care
responses (Berkman, 1981; McKinlay, 1981; Waitzkin, 1981; Harwood,
1981; Mishler et al., 1981). Epidemiological and social research has
demonstrated how sickness rates relate to social deprivation (low
socioeconomic class, poverty, broken social networks, widowhood),
gender, migration and refugee status, genetically distinctive populations,
ethnicity, and ecological and sociopolitical determinants (Berkman, 1981;
McKinlay, 1981; Waitzkin, 1981; Harwood, 1981; Mishler et al., 1981;
Kleinman and Hahn, in press). Tay-Sachs disease among Ashkenazi Jews
and sickle cell anemia among blacks are pertinent examples from our own
society, as are low back problems among migrant agricultural workers who
do stoop labor; alcoholism among native Americans; depression in
married women with young children, no job, and a socially confining
relationship; and poor outcome for myocardial infarction among men
without intact and supportive social networks. The recent public concern
with environmental pollutants' effects on health is but one important
indicator of the significance of this relation. That cultural beliefs and
practices also yield epidemiologically and clinically significant effects
worldwide is impressively demonstrated by the case of kuru among the
south Fore people of New Guinea, which resulted from the transmission
of a slow virus producing progressive destruction of the central nervous
system due to ritualized cannibalism (Lindenbaum, 1979). Such beliefs
and practices have also been recognized to influence rates of parasitic and
other infectious diseases.

But social relations and culture have also been shown to influence how
stress is perceived and appraised, coping resources deployed to meet it,
symptoms labeled and experienced, and help sought out (Kleinman,
1980). For example, distinctive ethnic responses to pain among Italian,
Jewish, and Northern European Americans; the predominance of physical
complaints among Chinese, Japanese, and most non-Western depressive
patients; and the fact that pathways to the mental health center among
psychiatric patients differ principally owing to membership in different
ethnic groups all illustrate this pervasive influence (Zborowski, 1952; Zola,
1966; Kleinman and Lin, 1981; Lin et al., 1982). Cultural differences in
belief and behavior have also been shown to strongly determine how
patients from the major ethnic groups in our society experience and cope
with a wide range of serious medical disorders; whether they enter,
comply, and are satisfied with particular medical care delivery systems;
and whether they experience major problems in care because of inadequate clinical communication and conflicts in value orientations with
care givers (Harwood, 1980). Such problems are not limited to ethnic

patients. Noncompliance, dissatisfaction, and inadequate care are ubiquitous problems in health care to which ineffective clinical communication and inadequate therapeutic relationships contribute mightily. It has been estimated that between one-third and two-thirds of primary care patients, more than half of chronic pain patients, and perhaps the great bulk of "problem patients" generally are suffering from psychosocial problems that are usually misdiagnosed and mistreated (Katon et al., 1982). We could cite many other pieces of evidence in support of our contention, but rather than review arid though impressive statistics, we will illustrate our point with dramatic case instances from our own practices that speak to the practical concerns of clinical students.

Case Illustrations

CASE 1
Mr. N. is a 28-year-old Chinese American male with "impotence" referred by his primary care physician for psychiatric evaluation. The patient reports to the psychiatrist nocturnal emissions and several episodes of masturbation with ejaculation. Hence by biomedical definition he is not "impotent," but he is culturally "impotent" in the eyes of his family, since he has never had sexual relations with his wife of 6 months. Assessment by an anthropologist reveals that the patient was forced into the marriage by his family against his strong objections and that the patient strongly dislikes his wife whom he resents for going along with the family pressure and whom he believes is educationally and socially inferior to him. Furthermore, he holds the widespread belief among traditionally oriented Chinese that intercourse leads to loss of "vital essence," which weakens the body's constitution and leads to progressive illness. Hence, besides refraining from intercourse so as not to comply with the forced marriage, he also fears becoming ill if he does so. Such illness, he reasons, will make him "weak" and less able to stand up "strongly" to his authoritarian parents. Finally, by avoiding intercourse he can avoid making his wife pregnant, which would make divorce more difficult, and try to have the marriage annulled. From knowledge of Chinese culture, the anthropologist is able to inform the primary care physician not only about these facts, but also about the tremendously stressful situation the patient's wife and parents are in. Without this knowledge a social problem is converted into a narrow biomedical complaint and the possibilities for intervention are greatly limited.

CASE 2
A 16-year-old with juvenile diabetes previously under excellent control has had several hyperglycemic reactions in quick succession. There is no evidence of infection or other biological reasons for the increasing difficulty his pediatrician faces in helping him manage his diabetes. Finally, the information is elicited that the patient has broken up with a girlfriend who he feels "rejected" him because he is "different" (i.e., must follow a strict diet and take

insulin and hence cannot "eat whatever anyone else" can and go to the quick food stands where his friends "hang out"). When confronted with this information, the patient angrily admits to his frustration over his chronic sickness, which he feels is incompatible with the "normal" life-style of his peers. He further admits that he had purposefully stopped taking his insulin and adhering to his diet over the several days following his breakup with his girlfriend. The patient's noncompliance explains the difficulties in clinical management and points to maladaptive coping, not a biomedical problem, as the chief reason. This common problem is similar to those in the management of many patients with chronic diseases in whom personal and family stress may significantly exacerbate their sickness and undermine their treatment plans.

CASE 3
The patient, an 11-year-old boy, has had a chronic cough for 6 months. He has had several full-scale workups from his primary care physicians, without documentation of a specific organ pathology responsible for the cough; yet, owing to its severity, he has stayed home from school for several months. His mother fears that he has a dangerous, progressive disorder that the doctors cannot diagnose. Because of this fear she keeps the child home from school, in spite of advice from her doctors to the contrary, and pursues specialist after specialist in hope of a biomedical solution. Finally, psychosocial assessment reveals that the patient's mother had gone through a divorce 1 year ago and 6 months before (at the time of onset of her son's cough) had begun living with a boyfriend. The son was fearful that his mother would "run off with him and leave me alone." As a result he has successfully used the sick role associated with a chronic low-grade psychosomatic symptom (cough due to dry throat and associated with anxiety) that he has amplified to become closer to his mother and prevent separation. But this behavior has had substantially negative effects on his school and family life. Again, it is the psychosocial evaluation that is crucial in the identification of the source of the clinical management problem and, again, this evaluation has come late in the course of care after high cost to patient, family, and practitioners.

Conceptual Framework and Clinical Strategies

In response to the kinds of clinical problems we have illustrated with case vignettes, clinically applied anthropological and social science studies support a conceptual distinction between two aspects of sickness: *disease* and *illness* (Kleinman et al., 1978; Eisenberg, 1977; Katon and Kleinman, 1981). Illness is the way sickness is perceived, labeled, experienced, expressed, and coped with by patient *and* family. Illness problems are the day-to-day life problems created for them (and by them) owing to the sickness and its treatment. When patients fall ill, they first experience illness, which is the organization of symptoms and disabilities into a characteristic personal and cultural pattern under the influence of beliefs, norms, and psychodynamic and interpersonal constraints. But when patients bring their illness to doctors, these are reorganized as *disease* within biomedical categories; that is to say, the illness experience is refracted through the lens of biomedical assessment and becomes a defined malfunctioning in biological and/or psychological processes. The disease is often made into an *entity*—a thing, an "it"—by the physician for the patient. ("You are suffering from sinusitis, Mr. Jones!" "The problem is heart failure, Mrs. Smith!" "If I could only get rid of my ulcer, Doctor Williams, *it* burns and hurts and drives me crazy. Can't you cut *it* out?") This is different from the research scientist's understanding, which is usually an *explanation* of dysfunction at different levels of analysis (biochemical, cellular, physiological, behavioral) that he uses as a shorthand for a complex, open-ended, changing understanding of a reality which is always limited in description by our analytical concepts and tools. For the clinician and the patient, however, disease is saturated with value sentiments. It is something "bad," "wrong," "dangerous"; it is the "enemy," a "threat," "loss"; and it comes to represent not just the biomedical perspective on it (which itself is influenced by historical and social forces), but also important values that emerge from the experiences of being ill and of giving care, and which represent both general cultural and specific personal ways of acting in these capacities (as patients or healers). Through this process, everyday meanings, relations, and behaviors that are bound up with who we are become associated with illness behavior and clinical judgment. Hence for the professional football player who becomes paraplegic in an auto accident owing to a severed spinal cord (the disease), the illness includes a tremendous sense of loss of body function, body image, source of income, pride, self-esteem, way of relating to others, and so on. For the primary care physician who fears psychiatric disturbance as something too threatening for him to handle, the detection of substantial psychosocial problems in his patients is not an easy issue to face and may be strictly avoided, much to the detriment of effective patient care.

Illness experience, as we saw in the case examples, feeds back on disease such that illness problems can (and often do) exacerbate disease problems, and vice versa. This interaction between disease and illness is, of course, one of the cornerstones of psychosomatic relations. Through it meaning and social relations come to affect physiology, affect, and behavior. Think of a patient with chronic asthma who develops an anxiety reaction to stress in his family life. That reaction can physiologically precipitate asthmatic attacks and worsen respiratory functions, with concomitant disability. The anxiety that is frequently experienced by patients as an integral part of their reaction to a serious illness suggests just how inseparable illness and disease usually are.

Consider the cardiac patient who after years of stable angina presents with an increased frequency of anginal attacks during periods of marital discord; the anxiety and distress generated by his social relationships raise his catecholamines, leading to elevated blood pressure and pulse, thus precipitating angina. Or consider the young male who has a recurrence of duodenal ulcer disease when he and his wife separate. Psychosocial stress leads to a coping style that indicates increased ethanol, nicotine, and caffeine intake, which results in higher gastric acid levels and ulceration.

In summary, then, the utility of this distinction is fourfold: (1) to underline the crucial part played by psychosocial and cultural processes in all disorders, (2) to pinpoint a concrete focus for therapeutic intervention that complements biological intervention, (3) to emphasize the psycho-somatic and somatopsychic interactions routinely active in sickness and care and avoid clinically and scientificly indefensible distinctions between "real" and "functional" disorders, and (4) to highlight the essential recognition that all sickness understandings are "cultural" in the sense that they systematically construct pictures of sickness based on distinctive belief and value systems, be they scientific, clinical, or lay (commonsense approaches in the mainstream or ethnic populations).

The provacative problem for health care emerging from this analysis is that biomedicine is primarily interested in the recognition and treatment of *disease*, whereas patients and families are primarily interested in *illness problems*, the practical difficulties in living resulting from sickness, and their resolution. Thus the stage is set in routine clinical encounters for substantial differences and even conflicts in orientation that, though they are often tacit and hidden, nonetheless frequently cause miscommuni-cation, troubled relationships, practical problems in day-to-day clinical management, as well as patient dissatisfaction, noncompliance, and inadequate care. Such differences and conflicts may also lead to delay in seeking care and the use (both appropriate and inappropriate) of alternative health care providers. This striking gap between physician and patient "interests" simply cannot be bridged by the biomedical model itself but requires a systematic approach to the psychological, social, and cultural dimensions of practice that can be applied (side by side with the biomedical approach) as part of a comprehensive biopsychosocial ap-proach to diagnosis, clinical decision making, and treatment. Clinical social scientists have developed clinically relevant concepts and management techniques that can be integrated into everyday clinical practice to achieve this desired end (Kleinman, 1980; Katon and Kleinman, 1981). In what follows, we will outline several of these clinically applied social science strategies.

Explanatory Model Framework

This clinical method aims to systematically elicit the patient's view of the illness in his own perspective, words, and belief and value system. Each patient and family maintains a particular explanation of the sickness they experience. This explanatory model (EM) usually includes a lay view of the etiology (why?), onset, pathophysiology (how it works), expected course (what to anticipate), and desired or expected treatment. Patient and family EMs may not be the same and can at times be in conflict. Hence, where feasible, both should be elicited. We can regard the physician's view of the problem as his medical EM, and this too can be systematically assessed. This is to say, the clinician should be self-reflexively aware of his own EM and the liaison psychiatrist consulting on physician–patient or physician–family conflicts should openly elicit the physician's EM. These EMs will change in the course of care for a particular illness episode and will come to include ideas and values concerning the particular treatments provided and received (e.g., expectations and attributions regarding side effects, chronic drug use, rehospitalization, treatment with high-technology instruments, multiple referrals, and care from interdisciplinary therapy teams in place of a single practitioner). Closely related to EMs, though appreciated only over time and as part of a broader assessment of the patient's family and work situations, is the *meaning* the symptoms and illness behavior hold for the patient and key others and their social *function* in the patient's life.

For most symptoms and illness experiences, it is possible to describe particular personal and interpersonal meanings. Threat, loss, and gain are but common illustrations ' of a very wide range of meanings; others include illness as punishment, sin, atonement, retribution, test of will to survive, test of religious faith, opportunity for change and growth, undermining of personal sense of indestructability, premonition of death, inherent weakness (moral as well as physical), and altered identity (e.g., among the severely disabled), to name just a few. Some meanings may be "natural" concomitants of particular illnesses. Hence quadraplegia, in our experience, almost always involves grave loss and immensely altered identity; cancer induces a fearsome cultural as well as personal threat; and chronic pain syndromes often involve major disability suits or potential secondary gain, a gain that cannot be openly admitted because this would contravene the dictates of the sick role that you must *want* to get better. Yet in most instances it is not so much that illness brings with it predictable significance, but it enters the network of meanings that surround the patient and family, where it can be understood only as part of this web of significance. For example, the "black sheep" in a family develops a life-threatening illness and his illness is attributed to his wayward behavior, though it may help reintegrate him into the family; a young wife whose husband has had a series of extramarital affairs becomes disabled and develops a reactive depression owing to her fear that her husband will abandon her for someone more attractive and better able to fit into his lifestyle; a farmer develops severe arthritic pains but denies their significance and refuses to seek help because it is harvest time and he "must work"; or a previously healthy and outdoors-oriented lumberjack receives a relatively minor injury in a logging accident but becomes so disabled with pain that he is unable to get out of his house because of the fulfillment of dependency needs never before sanctioned. These examples also illustrate the social functions that illness may fulfill in a person's life: for example, sanctioning failure, changing jobs, distancing a spouse sexually, making family members feel guilty, manipulating key others toward a desired end, and so forth. The upshot is not to memorize a list of possible illness meanings and functions, but to remember to look for these meanings and to interpret patient and family responses to treatment in light of them. Hence a core clinical task that practitioners must master is the *interpretation* of the personal, social, and cultural significance of illness and patient-hood. Recognizing responsibility for acquiring and honing this skill is, in our experience, a major step toward building clinical competence in the performance of psychosocial interviewing and intervention.

CASE 4

Mr. K. is a 33-year-old male who 4 months prior to his office visit had injured his back on the job. He had been cared for by an orthopedist with rest, narcotic analgesics, and sedatives. He complained of constant low back pain, was unable to work, and was receiving disability payments. Past history revealed a compression fracture of the lumbar vertebrae, a lumbosacral sprain, valium addiction, and depression 10 years earlier while in the army. Review of the symptoms revealed a 3- to 4-month history of sleep disturbance, decreased appetite and libido, constipation, dry mouth, and decreased energy level. Social history revealed that he had been working as an automobile parts manager, a job with which he was quite dissatisfied, feeling it made no use of his art training. He openly stated he would prefer working in the areas of photography or advertising. His EM was elicited and he felt he had injured a disk in his back that could necessitate additional time to loaf. The physician's EM consisted of (1) an acute low back strain, (2) concomitant depression precipitated by unmet career goals, and (3) subacute somatization secondary to the depression. This EM was presented openly to the patient, who was anxious for a multifaceted approach to his problem. In the presentation, emphasis was placed on the acceptability of desiring a job change. Physical therapy was prescribed, nonnarcotic analgesics were gradually substituted for narcotics and sedatives, and an antidepressent was given. Mr. K. rapidly showed improvement, with fewer pain complaints and a lessening of his depressive symptoms. After 3 months of treatment he was off disability, resuming normal daily life activities and beginning to establish himself in the advertising area.

CASE 5

Scott is a 12-year-old white male with an 8-year history of asthma. When first seen, Scott had been followed by a specialty clinic at a children's hospital; his treatment included theophylline, oral steroids, and oral adrenergic agents. At the clinic he had multiple care givers and, in addition to regular clinic visits, he was visiting the emergency room (ER) two to four times monthly for acute asthmatic attacks.

At the first office visit, some history was briefly obtained and a longer visit scheduled. Before that visit, Scott was seen one night at the ER for one of his "typical attacks." At that time he was found to be in minimal distress, easily clearing with a single injection of epinephrine.

At the next visit, in addition to biomedical data, Scott's psychosocial history revealed that his parents had divorced early in his childhood and that his mother had become extremely close to Scott during his chronic illness. She readily admitted that when he started wheezing at night, she feared for his life. Scott openly stated that he enjoyed his ER visits and after thorough questioning admitted he did not always take his medications on time. In fact, a major on-going battle over taking his medications existed at home.

The physician's assessment was that Scott had chronic asthma as a disease, that a biomedical approach had failed in controlling that disease, and that an analysis of his illness could perhaps be of benefit to Scott and his mother.

In this context Scott was viewed as an adolescent in an enmeshed family unit struggling with independence–dependence issues. As a result of this family dysfunction, lack of compliance, utilization of the sick role, and inappropriate use of medical facilities resulted; in addition, the medical care system acted to reinforce this behavior.

This assessment was presented openly to Scott and his mother, who willingly accepted it. A treatment plan was negotiated where Scott assumed more responsibility and independence over the timing and taking of his medications. An inhaler was prescribed to be used by Scott after discussing his condition with his mother. In addition, they both agreed to set aside time each week to do "fun" things together.

Over the ensuing 9 months, Scott had no further ER visits and had successfully been weaned off steroids and oral adrenergics. Both he and his mother reported a marked improvement in their relationship.

Systematic elicitation of EMs, then, as well as assessment of the meaning and function of symptoms and illness behavior provide the practitioner with often crucially important information that influences his therapeutic relationship with patients, their diagnostic workup and treatment recommendations, and the patient's and family's responses to and acceptance of these recommendations.

The EM elicitation should be a formal part of the medical evaluation and can be contracted or expanded as is appropriate for a particular patient

with a particular disorder in a particular circumstance. The EM can be
efficiently elicited by asking the following questions:

1. What do you think has caused your problem?
2. Why do you think it started when it did?
3. What does your illness do to you? (How does it affect your body?)
4. How severe is it? (What course, acute or chronic, will it take?)
5. What kind of treatment do you believe you should receive?
6. What results do you expect from your treatment?
7. What are the chief problems caused by your illness?
8. What do you fear most about your illness?

This set of questions is merely a suggested format and the actual
wording of questions will vary with the patient, the clinical problem, and
the setting. The practitioner must demonstrate warmth, empathy, and
persistence in order to convince patients that their ideas are of genuine
interest and relevance. This process not only provides important data but
also serves to reinforce the physician's concern for the patient and thereby
helps to build a therapeutic relationship.

As a corollary to this process, it is imperative that physicians coherently
formulate their own EMs. Physicians, like patients, are profoundly
influenced by sociocultural factors. Physicians were patients long before
they entered medical training and thus have deeply ingrained beliefs
derived from their own social and cultural backgrounds. Through medical
training, physicians are socialized into the subculture of biomedicine. Thus
physicians' beliefs are derived from a mixture of subcultures and will vary
from practitioner to practitioner. With an understanding of both the
patient and his own EM, the physician can begin to negotiate a diagnostic
and therapeutic approach, a process we will outline further. To be
effective, biomedical explanations must be articulated in a commonsense
idiom accessible to the patient. Where feasible, the practitioner will find
that he can be especially effective in clinical communications if he employs
the concrete terms and images his patients use. This core clinical skill, so
rarely formally taught, correlates with improved compliance and satisfaction (Katon and Kelinman, 1981).

Illness Experience Problems

As we have demonstrated earlier, patients undergo sickness as a life or
illness experience. For patients the difficulties arising from the illness,
illness experience problems, constitute the entire disorder. Thus it is
essential that physicians pay as much systematic attention to these
problems as to disease problems.

Illness experience problems consist of the experiential, familial, economic, inter- and intrapersonal, and occupational problems engendered

Table 1. Illness Experience Problems[a]

---

1. Family problems created or worsened by sickness.
2. Financial problems created or worsened by sickness.
3. Major changes in a patient's personal identity and social role in the context of a terminal sickness or a permanent disability.
4. Lack of compliance with therapeutic regimen due to the unusual nature of a procedure or its expected outcome.
5. Maladaptive coping responses that patients and families use to manage sickness, such as denial, passive–hostile behavior, "shopping" among different doctors, and manipulative suicidal attempts.
6. Conflict in personal beliefs between patients (and family) and practitioners concerning cause or nature of sickness and expected course and objectives for treatment.
7. Inappropriate resort to sick role and illness behavior owing to psychological or social gain.
8. Conflict in cultural values concerning treatment style and interpersonal etiquette between patients and practitioners due to substantial differences in social class, lifestyle and ethnic norms.
9. Inappropriate use of alternative or indigenous health care agents and agencies.
10. Breakdown in communication between patient (and family) and practitioners.
11. Transference and countertransference problems in the doctor–patient or doctor–family relationship.
12. Life problems stemming from the particular stresses engendered by special treatment environments.

---

[a]From Katon and Kleinman (1981), p. 261.

by the disease and its treatment. For example, the onset of back pain in a laborer may necessitate a change in career and may lead to economic hardships, marital discord, a change in recreational and social pastimes, disability-related lawsuits, and significant intrapersonal distress.

In a systematic approach, these problems can be listed like disease problems to facilitate their ongoing recognition and attention by physicians or by referral to appropriate practitioners or social agencies.

Table 1 lists the major illness problems we have encountered in clinical practice. Although possible illness problems probably can be as varied as disease problems, this list touches the major areas that assess how the patient, his family, and his social network cope with illness and its treatment.

A Negotiation Model of Doctor–Patient Relationships

As can be seen from our earlier discussion, doctors and patients differ in many aspects. They differ in their area of concern, disease versus illness, and they often differ in their explanatory models. A key aspect of clinical management that is also often neglected is the development of a therapeutic alliance with the patient. Only when the doctor and the patient have reached a common agreement on the nature of the problem and therapy can meaningful medical therapy begin. Practitioners must become adept at the negotiation of discrepancies between their patients and themselves.

A clinically useful model for negotiation of doctor–patient conflicts has been described by Katon and Kleinman (1981). This model involves seven steps:

1. The physician elicits the patient's EM and assesses the problems presented by the illness.
2. The physician presents his own EM in lay terms.
3. An attempt is made to develop an EM that is mutually acceptable.
4. If an understanding cannot be reached, the physician should decide on an acceptable compromise and offer it to the patient.
5. The patient then responds to the offer and can accept or reject it or offer another plan.
6. If agreement cannot be reached, referral to another physician should be made.
7. Both the patient and the physician should monitor the agreement on an ongoing basis.

CASE 6*

Mrs. W. is a 25-year-old white female with a past history of multiple medical workups for chronic abdominal pain and back pain. She presented to the family medical center with a 6-month history of severe headaches. These headaches were most severe in the frontal region but had a bandlike distribution and seemed worsened by stress. Neurological evaluation, including a physical exam, a laboratory exam, and a skull x-ray and computer-assisted tomograph (CAT) scan were negative. Over the last 2 months she had gradually increased her use of Tylenol #3 for the headaches and often called at night to get refills. Her pain complaints all had gradually become amplified as well. She also complained of insomnia, decreased energy, decreased appetite, weight loss, and anhedonia. Mrs. W. admitted that she had been under a great deal of stress over the last 6 months. She was the mother of two young children, ages 6 months and 3 years, and her current boyfriend was an alcoholic who frequently physically abused her. They had several separations over the last few months but had recently reunited.

Mrs. W. was the oldest of five children brought up in a chaotic family. Her father was an alcoholic and was physically abusive to her mother. They divorced when she was 10 and thereafter her mother had three other marriages within 8 years. Her mother also had headaches that would cause her to go to bed for days at a time. Mrs. W. had been married twice previously,

*The authors wish to thank Dr. Wayne Katon, who provided this case illustration.

but each relationship ended in divorce owing to physical abuse by her husbands.

Past medical history revealed a history of high clinic utilization for multiple somatic complaints and two prior abdominal exploratory surgeries for abdominal pain (both with negative results). Several of her past clinic physicians expressed concern over narcotic abuse and she left the hospital against medical advice on one occasion after a confrontation about this.

Based on medical and psychiatric evaluation, it was hypothesized that Mrs. W. had the chronic maladaptive patterns of dealing with relationships and stress that are often seen in patients with chronic depression or personality disorders. Her use of somatization provided her with support from physicians as well as narcotics that eased both physical and psychological pain. Much of her pain behavior could be explained by her addiction to short-acting narcotics. Our diagnosis was the following: (1) chronic personality disorder (hysterical type), (2) chronic tension headaches, and (3) chronic somatization secondary to (4) intra- and interpersonal conflict.

We therefore entered into the following negotiation. Mrs. W.'s pain was redefined as chronic, necessitating different measures than acute pain. We explained that short-acting narcotics would temporarily block pain but would necessitate increasing dosages. Based on her experience, she readily agreed.

We proposed the following treatment program for Mrs. W.:

1. Change use of Tylenol #3 to pain cocktail with methadone on a scheduled basis. Her physician would control the dosage and slowly taper the methadone.
2. See only her primary physician on a once-a-week basis for 15- to 20-minute appointments, with a limit of one after-hours call and no refill of narcotic prescription by any other physician.
3. Refer to a community mental health clinic for counseling to learn to more adaptively deal with stress.
4. Increase child care for her two young children.
5. Enter an Alanon program to work on the relationship problems caused by her boyfriend's alcoholism.
6. Start a tricyclic antidepressant to relieve the dysphoric and vegetative signs of depression she was experiencing.

The patient agreed to this program and was successfully tapered off methadone over 1 month as an outpatient. Her after-hours visits and calls stopped, and on the scheduled visits more time was spent on psychosocial stress and less on headaches.

The negotiation process we have outlined here, as well as the other approaches, demands a shift from a physician-dominated doctor–patient relationship. The relationship that emerges from this approach is a patient-centered one where the physician provides information, understanding, and advice based on his training and experience, while acknowledging the obvious fact that the patient and his family are the ultimate arbiters.

Cultural Checklist for Clinical Assessment and Intervention

The final clinically applied anthropological method we will review is an outline for a systematic assessment of cultural influences on illness and care that the clinician can use in the patient interview to evaluate the influence of culture on the illness and the treatment. Recently Harwood has edited a handbook on ethnicity and care, written for clinical students and practitioners, that reviews this question in detail, especially with respect to the specific problems that may arise in the case of patients from a variety of different American ethnic groups (Harwood, 1981). Where practitioners routinely treat patients from one or several ethnic groups, it is their responsibility to familiarize themselves with the health beliefs and practices that characterize these groups and which may therefore influence the care they provide ethnic patients.

Cultural Influences on Stress

Ethnic patients not only must deal with the ubiquitous social and personal problems faced by every adult in American society, but may also have to confront special forms of stress. These include racial bias, language barriers, cultural obstacles found in educational institutions and in the job market, the stress of migration and acculturation, value conflicts, shifting religious affiliation, urban–rural differences, dietary problems, and particular epidemiological patterns of risk and prevalence of disease. The clinician needs to assess both universal and culture-specific stresses in each case. He may discover that inappropriate use of medical facilities and maladaptive coping (passive aggressive or open hostility, giving up, noncompliance, doctor shopping) as well as particular disease may result from or be exacerbated by culturally influenced stressors and the particular patterns of stress response they engender. The same major life event changes may be differentially perceived as more or less stressful in different groups, and this in turn will shape the response to and consequences of stressful life experiences.

Cultural Influences on Coping and Social Support

Clinicians should keep an open mind about whether ethnic coping styles are adaptive or maladaptive in particular cases. Though somatization is a favored idiom of distress and coping style for handling stress in many traditional ethnic groups, it is not necessarily maladaptive, though it may be so in particular cases. Similarly, dietary customs, rituals for treating sickness or marking life transitions, and use of traditional healers should be assessed case by case. Where they lead to maladaptive consequences, the negotiation approach can be used to try to change them (a difficult but often useful process); where adaptive, they should be supported. The clinician needs to realize that the very judgment of whether a given coping practice is adaptive or not is culturally influenced; therefore he needs to compare his evaluation with that of the patient and the family.

Our tendency is to view the extended family in which ethnic patients are often living as an important source of social support, and this is in fact frequently so. But the extended family can also be a source of considerable stress. Again, individual assessment of each case is the way to determine which social function predominates. In recent Asian-American refugees, the family, not the adult individual, may be regarded as the ultimate source of health care decisions, and this is true in other ethnic groups.

Cultural Influences on Thinking, Feeling, and Behavior

These may be profound and can range from altered psychophysiological responses and differential pharmacokinetic and pharmacodynamic reactions to cognitive orientations that make routine psychotherapy inappropriate and require culture-specific forms of counseling and support. Included in this category are cultural influences on how the emotions and bodily complaints are expressed. The former are often suppressed or displaced (externalized) and the latter amplified in members of traditional ethnic groups. Some culturally based behavior may be considered deviant in American society but appropriate in an ethnic subculture under particular circumstances. Dissociative states, trance and possession states, and hysterical outbursts are examples. Conversion symptoms, other manifestations of "classical hysteria," and catatonia are culturally constituted illness behavior responses to universally occurring psychiatric diseases that are much more common among ethnic patients in primary care than among mainstream American patients in psychiatric practice. Hence the primary care physician, not the psychiatrist or psychologist, is more likely to be the first to encounter and treat these behaviors.

Cultural Influences on the Doctor–Patient Relationship and Biomedical Treatment

Cultural norms may produce conflicts between lay expectations of interpersonal etiquette and physician expectations of patient behavior. In Mexican-American culture, for example, a strong code of modesty between the patient and the practitioner of opposite sex, especially when the physician is white, may make untenable certain parts of the physical examination. Gypsy views that the top part of the body is clean while the part below the waist is polluted translate into expectations that the physical exam not be conducted in such a manner as to cross back and forth between these symbolic domains (Shields, 1980). Elderly ethnic patients may not wish to be treated by casually attired white professionals who address them by their given names. Although it is not the responsibility of the health professional to memorize these distinctive norms, he should inquire about them and conduct the interview and examination in a way that does not contravene them.

The possibility of miscommunication is obviously more of a problem owing to the fact that English is not the native language of some patients. These clinical communication problems might involve differences in verbal fluency and comprehension, in the meaning of similar terms (Hispanic patients may interpret *hot* in symbolic rather than temperature terms), and in the use of special terms (jargon), or they might involve the ineffective use of translators. Most translators, untrained in biomedicine, may not know how to translate technical terms or may be embarrassed and fail to communicate accurately patient beliefs. Family physicians should be aware that working through translators can be a potential cause of miscommunication and should anticipate this problem, since it is so common.

Chinese and other recent Asian refugees, who regard injections as the most efficacious form of biomedical treatment, may expect the visit to the doctor to involve "shots" and may be unwilling to accept care without them. Traditionally oriented Southeast Asian and Hispanic patients may not find an egalitarian relationship with their physician acceptable. Black patients, anticipating racism, may misinterpret or overinterpret the responses of white practitioners.

In dealing with ethnic patients, practitioners must be careful so that culturally oriented interventions do not have unintended negative consequences. For example, the practitioner may stereotype the patient and treat him as an "ethnic" rather than as a "person." This danger of stereotyping can be avoided by determining whether the patient is behaviorally ethnic (i.e., maintains and acts on ethnic beliefs) or not.

The EM approach and the expectation of cultural difference can be used with all patients, not just members of exotic minority groups. Cultural conceptions are brought to the doctor–patient relationship by each patient, family, and practitioner. In this very pluralistic society there are many worlds within which individuals dwell and become sick. Patient EMs, then, are a way for the physician to enter these worlds and determine how their beliefs and values influence the illness and its treatment. There are, for example, based on fundamental differences in values, diverse orientations that characterize views of abortion, weight gain, smoking, natural foods, alcohol, drug use and abuse, pain, jogging, psychiatric problems, as well as almost all other controversial aspects of illness and care. The EM framework provides a clinical method to get at and respond to these value orientations.

Differences of class, education, religion, rural/urban background, traditional/modern orientation, political ideology, personality, and so forth, between patient and practitioner may result in tacit (and sometimes not so tacit) conflicts that may yield poor care. It is just as essential for the family physician to be familiar with these aspects of his patients' lives as it is for him to be aware of family problems. Indeed, physicians would make few mistakes by systematically eliciting family as well as patient EMs, keeping in mind that these may differ considerably and require negotiations if the treatment plan is to be accepted. Physicians should not, however, be blinded by the fact that a patient has the same background as themselves, but should instead look for other kinds of potential discrepancies in beliefs and values that may be significant clinically. It is possible, even where family supports are reasonably good, that conflicts may arise from differences among family members on how they regard a particular illness episode and its treatment. Where tensions exist in families, this approach may prove effective in the assessment of these tensions.

Finally, biomedical treatment will be affected by resort to indigenous lay and folk-expert treatment systems, as we mentioned above. Since most illness episodes are treated in the family context (Kleinman, 1980), ethnic patients may make use of special diets, food, herbs, massage, exercises, and religious treatments. Popular approaches to care, which patients from the mainstream culture also routinely use, may at times conflict with the medical treatment, resulting in noncompliance and unanticipated drug–drug interactions or side effects. Monitoring of patient and family self-treatment will clarify these alternative treatment approaches, which can then be the focus of clinical negotiation.

Additionally, folk-experts may play a major role in the treatment of ethnic patients. *Curanderas* among Hispanic Americans; root workers and spiritualist ministers among blacks; herb doctors and acupuncturists among Chinese, Japanese, and Koreans; voodoo specialists among Haitians; and medicine men among native American populations are potential allies or sources of trouble for the family physician in caring for members of these ethnic groups. Traditional healers frequently support and complement the advice of physicians; not uncommonly, however, they may also countermand or undermine this advice. While some folk healing practices have documented efficacy—for example, ephedrine in traditional Chinese medicine pharmacopeia and rauwolfia in traditional South Asian (Ayurvedic) medicine—and many others probably exert important placebo effects, there are infrequent untoward effects as well. Acupuncture, for example, has on occasion been associated with local infection and hepatitis, ginseng with gastrointestinal complaints, and faith healing rituals with the rare case of psychiatric decompensation. It is quite obviously in the interest of the physician to become aware of his patients' use of alternative healers.

Conclusion

In this chapter we have attempted to demonstrate the severe limitations of the narrowly defined biomedical model in the provision of quality health care. Only by expanding our focus to include both disease and illness can we begin to meet the needs and expectations of our patients. To achieve this end, the practitioner must broaden his own conceptual framework and move beyond a mere diagnosis and treatment of disease to a systematic inquiry and interpretation of the broader meanings of symptoms and illness for the patient. Inherent in this approach is the necessity of viewing the patient not as an isolated biological entity, but as a member of a family, cultural group, social network, and broader society. In the same way that patients with a given disease vary widely in presentation, course, and response to treatment, so do the personal and social significances vary widely (Rosen et al., 1982; Mechanic, 1975; Fabrega, 1974; Engel, 1980).

The clinical social science approaches we have outlined and illustrated offer the physician a coherent and logical approach to the study of illness. With accurate illness diagnosis, the physician is able to prescribe meaningful and efficacious treatments. Moreover, the approach trains the clinician to move between multiple and divergent perspectives on sickness episodes, to work out some useful integration that draws on the plural social constructions any sickness engenders. This we take to be the essence of a humanistic approach to medicine that is clinically practical.

We feel the benefits of this approach are multiple. For the physician, the frustration of dealing with "difficult" patients can be decreased and the potential for clinical success is increased. For the patient this approach offers a greater chance of efficacious care and for the health care system it brings out of the shadows and into the spotlight those ubiquitous psychosocial issues that are so often "hidden" and untreated at such high cost to all concerned, including the health care system itself.

References

Berkman, L.F. 1981. Physical health and the social environment: A social epidemiological perspective. In L. Eisenberg and A. Kleinman, eds.: The Relevance of Social Science for Medicine. Dordrecht, Holland: D. Reidel; pp. 51–76.

Eisenberg, L. 1977. Disease and illness. Distinctions between professional and popular ideas of sickness. Culture, Medicine and Psychiatry 1(1):9–24.

Engel, G. L. 1977. The need for a new medical model: A challenge for biomedicine. Science 196:129–136.

Engel, G. L. 1980. The clinical application of the biopsychosocial model. American Journal of Psychiatry 137:535.

Fabrega, H. 1974. Disease and Social Behavior. Cambridge, Massachusetts: MIT Press.

Good, B. J., and M. J. D. Good. 1981. The meaning of symptoms: A cultural hermeneutic model for clinical practice. In L. Eisenberg and A. Kleinman, eds.: The Relevance of Social Science for Medicine. Dordrecht, Holland: D. Reidel; pp. 165–196.

Harwood, A., ed. 1981. Ethnicity and Medical Care. Cambridge, Massachusetts: Harvard University Press.

Katon, W., and A. Kleinman. 1981. Doctor–patient negotiation and other social science strategies in primary care. In L. Eiseberg and A. Kleinman, eds.: The Relevance of Social Science for Medicine. Dordrecht, Holland: D. Reidel; pp. 253–279.

Katon, W., A. Kleinman, and G. Rosen. 1982. Depression and somatization. American Journal of Medicine, 72(1):127–135; 72(2).

Kleinman, A. 1980. Patients and Healers in the Context of Culture. Berkeley, California: University of California Press.

Kleinman, A., and R. Hahn The sociocultural model of medicine. Rockefeller Foundation Working Papers, in press.

Kleinman, A., and T. Y. Lin, eds. 1981. Normal and Abnormal Behavior in Chinese Culture. Dordrecht, Holland: D. Reidel.

Kleinman, A., L. Eisenberg, and B. Good. 1978. Culture, illness and care. Annals of Internal Medicine 88:251–258.

Leigh, H., and M. F. Reiser. 1980. The Patient: Biological, Psychological, and Social Dimensions of Medical Practice. New York. Plenum Press.

Lin, K. M., T. Inu, A. Kleinman, and W. Womack. 1982. Sociocultural determinants of help seeking. Journal of Nervous and Mental Disease 176:78–85.

Lindenbaum, S. 1979. Kuru Sorcery: Disease and Danger in the New Guinea Highlands. Palo Alto, California: Mayfield.

McKinlay, J. B. 1981. Social network influences on morbid episodes and the career of help seeking. In L. Eisenberg and A. Kleinman, eds.: The Relevance of Social Science for Medicine. Dordrecht, Holland: D. Reidel; pp. 77–110.

Mechanic, D. 1972. Social psychological factors affecting the presentation of bodily complaints. New England Journal of Medicine 286:1132.

Mishler, E., L. Amansingham, S. Hauser, R. Heim, S. Osherson, and N. Waxler, Eds. 1981. Social Contexts of Health, Illness and Patient Care. Cambridge, Massachusetts: Cambridge University Press.

Rosen, G., A. Kleinman, and W. Katon. 1982. Somatization in family practice: A biopsychosocial approach. The Journal of Family Practice 14:493–502.

Shields, M. 1980. Ethnicity and clinical care: The Gypsy patient. Physician Assistant and Health Practitioner, March, pp. 62–65.

Waitzkin, H. 1981. A Marxist analysis of the health care systems of advanced capitalist societies. In L. Eisenberg and A. Kleinman, eds.: The Relevance of Social Science for Medicine. Dordrecht, Holland: D. Reidel; pp. 333–370.

Zborowski, M. 1952. Cultural components in response to pain. Journal of Social Issues 8:16–30.

Zola, I. K. 1966. Culture and symptoms. American Sociological Review 3:615–630.

6

Somatization
in Primary Health Care

Wayne Katon, M.D.* and Harold A. Dengerink, Ph.D.†

Somatization refers to the phenomenon of patients presenting physical complaints in the absence of biological abnormalities or with discernable pathology that does not warrant either the degree of patient complaints or utilization of the health care system. In most circumstances such complaints are not totally fictitious and do not represent malingering; rather, the discomfort experienced by these patients may be very real and will require intervention, although of a different kind than that dictated by organic pathology. The discomfort or pain that leads these persons to seek medical care may stem from psychological or social distress rather than from physical diseases. This distress is interpreted as being physical or is attributed to physical causes, and thus justifies seeking medical intervention.

Somatization is one of the most common and troublesome problems physicians face. Studies have repeatedly demonstrated that as many as 50% of patients utilizing primary care clinics actually have psychological precipitants, as opposed to biomedical ones, as the main cause of their clinic visits (Stoeckle et al., 1964; Roberts and Norton, 1952; Mannucci et al., 1961). Furthermore, Regier et al. (1978) have demonstrated that most people with emotional disorders are seen and treated in primary care settings rather than by psychiatrists or psychologists. Goldberg and Blackwell (1970) have pointed out that in addition to the substantial numbers of patients whose emotional problems are recognized by their physicians, there are many whose emotional disorders go unrecognized.

*Assistant Professor, Department of Psychiatry and Behavioral Science, University of Washington School of Medicine, Seattle, Washington.
† Professor and Director of Clinical Training, Department of Psychology, Washington State University, Pullman, Washington.

These are predominantly patients who presented with somatic symptoms and who are treated symptomatically. Not only does mental disorder commonly present as a physical disorder, but early detection is especially beneficial for the severe disorders (Johnstone and Goldberg, 1976). The early detection and treatment of the somatizing patient not only shortens the course of illness, but also spares the patient unnecessary physical investigations that tend to reinforce hypochondriacal symptom patterns and thus short-circuit the significant risk of iatrogenesis.

The phenomenon of somatization occurs in several different ways, ranging from the obvious to the remarkably subtle and occurring both in acute and chronic forms. It is a phenomenon that occurs as a result of normal stress-related processes, cognitive information processing, and learning and which is facilitated by social processes and the medical professions. Clearly it is a phenomenon that requires careful diagnosis and appropriate treatment.

Types of Somatization

Classic Conversion

Historically, somatization was described as a coping or defense mechanism that protected the patient from anxiety or dysphoric emotion. By focusing on a headache or back pain, the patient was unaware of an underlying depression or psychological conflict. The prototype is the patient with a conversion reaction in which an acute neurological deficit in sensory or motor functioning develops—for example, paralysis, numbness, blindness or aphonia—that cannot be explained by known physical disorders or pathophysiological mechanisms (Lazare, 1981). Many of these patients are faced with overwhelming external stresses or internal conflicting emotions just prior to the development of the "neurological" problems—hence the term *conversion*. The implication is that a psychological problem has been converted into a physical one. Unfortunately, although this definition is accurate in many cases of conversion reactions, it tends to maintain the reductionistic Cartesian model of patient symptomatology as being all "in the head," and therefore a psychiatric problem, or all "in the body," and therefore a medical problem. Furthermore, only a minority of somatization problems fit in this classic category, although it may be more common in non-Western cultures.

Somatization Related to Psychiatric Disorders

Somatization may occur in a wide variety of psychiatric disorders: depression, anxiety, Briquet's syndrome (formerly called hysteria), obsessive-compulsive disorders, grief reactions, and hysterical personality disorders. Depression and anxiety are clearly the most prevalent. There are several studies that indicate the incidence and prevalence of affective disorders in primary care patients. Although most of these studies suffer from a lack of diagnostic clarity, there appears to be a correlation between the prevalence of depression and anxiety despite the utilization of differing diagnostic techniques. In a large study in Virginia based upon 526,196 patient visits to 118 family practitioners, depression and anxiety constituted 86.8% of the psychiatric problems seen by these physicians (Marsland et al., 1976). In two studies of over 2000 primary care patients in Philadelphia (Hesbacher et al., 1975) and London (Goldberg, 1979), a family physician in the first study and a psychiatrist in the latter each found that 87% of the combined 492 patients with a psychiatric diagnosis had an affective disorder, that is, depression, mixed anxiety and depression, an anxiety state, or an affective psychosis. While these studies indicate that depression and anxiety constitute the two major syndromes seen by physicians in primary care, they do not indicate the prevalence or incidence of depression. The study of Hoeper et al. (1979) did reveal the prevalence of mental disorder in a primary care clinic population. That group found the prevalence of mental disorder to be 26.7%, with depressive disorders (major, intermittent, and minor) and anxiety (phobic and generalized) representing over 80% of the cases. Major depressive disorder alone made up 21.7% of the psychiatric diagnoses. Raft et al. (1975) studied 300 medical patients and outpatients in a general hospital and estimated the rate of depression to be 35%. In two longitudinal studies the incidence of affective disorder (depression, anxiety–depression) in a large family practice was found to be 5–6 per 100 patients a year (Schuman et al., 1978; Ramesar et al. 1980). Major depressive disorder is present in 6% of primary care patients and thus is the most prevalent medical or psychiatric disorder, with hypertension second at 5.7%. If major and minor depressions are taken together, the rate is as high as 25% of the primary care clinic population (Marsland et al. 1976).

   Patients with depression and anxiety in the above studies experienced substantial physical symptomatology and thus often found their way to medical practitioners for consultation and treatment, yet two studies revealed that primary care physicians only diagnose depression in 0.5–4.5% of their cases (Rawnsky, 1968; Reifler et al., 1979). A substantial portion of the cases go undiagnosed. In Nielson and Williams' 1980 study the primary care physician failed to diagnose depression in 50% of the cases. The main problem appeared to be the inability of the physician to conceptualize depression as existing without the patient being able to perceive an affective state and report it voluntarily to the physician. Thus a patient who has not developed the language to label and relate his emotional states, who utilized defenses or coping styles that minimize affects, or who believes his problem to be a physical one will not be diagnosed as depressed by many physicians.

It should be noted that somatization resulting from psychiatric disorder can occur both when the disorder is acute and when it is chronic. Thus grief reactions, a reactive form of depression, can result in somatic complaints in the same fashion as chronic depression. A review of two cases will illustrate this point.

CASE 1
Mrs. S. was a 28-year-old physical therapist who presented several times over a 1-month period to her family physician, complaining of chest pain and tightness, palpitations, tremulousness, and a feeling of faintness. These symptoms came on episodically, lasting from minutes to as long as an hour, and were associated with a feeling of impending doom. The patient was convinced she was going to have either a heart attack or a stroke. Review of systems and other medical history were otherwise negative. Family history revealed that her father had died suddenly from a stroke when she was 16 and her mother had a subsequent severe depression, with the patient taking charge of the household, including care of her two younger siblings. Physical exam, blood tests, and electrocardiogram proved negative, with the exception of mild tachycardia and tremulousness. The patient was questioned about stress and revealed that she had gotten married 5 months prior to the onset of these episodes and that she and her husband had been having marital problems. Her attacks of symptoms seemed often to be correlated with arguments, especially when her husband left the house angrily. The patient admitted to worrying constantly over a possible marital separation and felt tense much of the time. She also had problems with insomnia, decreased energy, and concentration, but denied suicidal thoughts. A diagnosis of anxiety attacks with a secondary depression was made and the patient began Imipramine (an antidepressant) therapy as well as individual and marital therapy with the family physician and a consultation-liaison psychiatrist. Her symptoms rapidly abated and many of the marital problems improved with psychotherapy. On a 6-month follow-up she was off all medication and functioning well in her marriage and job.

CASE 2
Mrs. H. was a 40-year-old white female with a past history of drug abuse; 10 prior surgeries, including three negative exploratory laporatomies for abdominal pain; and 15 listed problems on her family medical center problem list. She has been coming in two to three times a week over the last month for abdominal pain and escalating her use of Tylenol #3, taking nine to ten a day. Her physical exam, laboratory tests, and a complete gastrointestinal series were unremarkable. Her review of systems showed 30 positive symptoms in nine separate organ systems.

Mrs. H. had been brought up in a chaotic family with her father a heavy drinker, who both physically and sexually abused Mrs. H. and her two younger sisters. Mother seemed ineffectual and had chronic back pain for which she visited physicians frequently. Mrs. H. was often left with her relatives for months at a time owing to her mother's "illness."

When asked about stressful life events, Mrs. H. initially became angry, stating that the pain was physical and doctors were always trying to tell her it was all in her head. When her family physician gently persisted, inquiring about stress, however, Mrs. H. admitted that her boyfriend had left her 2 months ago and she had been feeling quite anxious and depressed. In fact she had been drinking heavily and was in danger of losing her job. Mrs. H. felt that her depression was secondary to her abdominal pain and that she needed to come into the hospital.

Based on medical and psychological evaluations, it was determined that Mrs. H. had chronic maladaptive patterns of dealing with stress that are often seen in patients with chronic depression and/or personality disorders. Her use of somatization was chronic and provided her with support from physicians, as well as narcotics that eased both her physical and psychological pain.

The family physician embarked on a negotiation with the patient in which he defined her abdominal pain as a chronic problem and not an acute one. He recommended scheduling the patient for regular visits twice a week, starting a pain cocktail three times a day with a long-acting narcotic that would be slowly tapered to avoid addiction to codeine, starting an antidepressant medication, and going to Alcoholics Anonymous (AA) to deal with the alcohol problem. The physician's plan was based on the fact that the patient's problems were long term and permeated many aspects of her life and thus no single modality such as medications or AA was likely to be efficacious.

The patient agreed to the program. She did on two occasions try unsuccessfully to get more pain cocktail by "losing her prescription," but with firm limits by her family physician her abdominal pain gradually decreased. The physician gradually tapered the narcotic in her pain cocktail, as well as the frequency of visits. The patient is attending AA on a regular basis and has made several friends whom she sees regularly. She does continue to come in with frequent somatic complaints when under stress and it has been necessary to again schedule regular visits after the death of a close friend.

Somatization of Stress Without Major Psychiatric Disorder

Many patient symptoms are expressions of social and/or psychological distress. The brain is the organ that monitors external and internal threats and stresses and through the autonomic and neuroendocrine systems alerts the body's homeostatic mechanisms to danger. The prototype is the "fight or flight" response, in which the brain perceives an external threat and through neuroendocrinological mechanisms directs the release of catecholamines, causing tachycardia, hyperventilation, increased muscular blood flow, and decreased flow to the skin and splanchnic organ systems; that is, stressful conditions generate physical symptoms. Some persons selectively focus on these changes rather than upon the emotional or cognitive effects of the stress and a stressful event becomes labeled as a physical disorder.

Some conditions may be particularly likely to result in somatization. These include conditions in which the stress is not well defined or vague. It may be difficult for persons to attribute physical symptoms to stressful events when they are unable to define or describe the stressful events. Another condition that may aid in somatization is that of anticipatory stress; that is, many physiological reactions occur in anticipation of harmful or stressful events that have not yet occurred. When the stressful event has not yet occurred, persons may be less able to attribute their symptoms to those stressors. A third condition that may predispose a person to somatize is a stress that bears some negative social connotations. In addition, persons who have developed coping mechanisms that involve avoidant thinking and denial may be particularly likely to somatize these kinds of physiological stress reactions. This pattern of coping is discussed in detail in Chapter 11.

CASE 3

Mr. A. was a 45-year-old business executive who presented with a 2-week history of dizziness and headaches. Review of systems and medical history was otherwise negative. Physical exam was entirely normal and the patient was questioned about recent stressful life events. He denied any problems at work or in his family but did reveal that he had started to have nightmares. He returned for a follow-up appointment 1 week later and reported that he began to have the headaches, dizzy spells, and nightmares after accepting an invitation to speak about his Vietnam War experiences. The patient's nightmares in fact were of actual traumatic experiences in the war, where he witnessed several of his friends being killed. He had canceled the speech that he was asked to give and reported decreased dizziness and headaches over the last 4 days. The patient declined an offer of supportive counseling about his war experiences, stating he would handle the memories the way he always had, by suppressing them, and accept no further offers to speak on the war. A 6-month follow-up revealed an asymptomatic patient functioning well at work and with his family.

Somatization as a Life-style

A recent study (see Chapter 22) revealed that most persons, particularly elderly ones, have numerous physical symptoms for which they do not seek medical attention. Another reported that primary care patients experience one physical symptom every 6–7 days yet rarely present these complaints to physicians. This suggests that any person may have adequate reason to seek medical care. Most persons, however, will respond to symptoms only if these are sufficiently severe or of sufficient duration to indicate some abnormal condition. Even then the person takes such action only after consulting other persons, typically family members (McKinley, in press).

Some persons will respond to a wide variety of ailments by seeking medical attention even when these are sufficiently minor that they would be ignored by others. Such somatization can occur in the absence of any identifiable stress and without clear psychopathology; it may occur when the person lacks a social support system within which to validate his or her symptoms as medically insignificant. As a result, the medical profession becomes the first line of defense rather than the final one. In addition, some persons with an intact social network may somatize as a means to receive attention or support from that network. Physical complaints can be seen as a legitimate mechanism by which to control or manipulate one's spouse, elicit care and nurturance, avoid responsibilities or sex, and assume a dependent role. The physician may be seen by such patients as providing some validity to their complaints and may be used to facilitate interpersonal manipulation. This kind of somatization is discussed thoroughly by Loeser and Fordyce in Chapter 16.

The last three kinds of somatization listed above do not conform to the Cartesian dualism that is supported by the notion of classical conversion symptoms; rather, they suggest that somatization is a complex process resulting from several interrelated mechanisms. These processes include the biological consequences of stress reactions, the cognitive decision-making strategies of patients and physicians, the reinforcing effects of familial and medical interventions, and the social roles adopted by patients, physicians, and family members.

The Processes Underlying Somatization

The Physiological Concomitants of Stress

The most basic underlying cause of somatization relates to the natural physiological processes that are part of reactions to stress. Stress causes psychophysiological reactions with changes in the neuroendocrine, limbic, and autonomic nervous systems (Ward et al., 1979). Somatizing patients often appear more anxious or depressed than normal or can be suffering from an acute fear or grief reaction but without more thorough psychiatric syndromes. Symptoms like tachycardia, anxiety, muscle tension, diaphoresis, fatigue, insomnia, and decreased libido are common. If stress is severe enough, many patients experience distress in vulnerable organ systems. Symptoms such as headaches, backaches, epigastric abdominal pain, diarrhea and cramping, nausea and vomiting, and so on, are common, depending upon the patient's unique physiological vulnerability. On a psychobiological level there is an initial acute increase in catabolic hormones like cortisol, epinephrine, glucagon, growth hormone, antidiuretic hormone, renin, angiotensin, aldosterone, erythropoietin, thyroxin, and parathormone. Table 1 describes the bodily changes that occur with the perception of stress. Tables 2 and 3 list the reactions that occur in

Table 1. Hormonal Pattern During Arousal

Increasing catabolic hormones	Decreasing anabolic hormones
Cortisol	Insulin
Epinephrine	Calcitonin
Glucagon	Testosterone
Growth hormone	Estrogen
Renin	Prolactin
Angiotensin	Luteinizing hormone
Aldosterone	Follicle-stimulating hormone
Erythropoietin	Gonadotropin-releasing hormone
Thyroxin	Prolactin-releasing hormone
Parathormone	
Melatonin	

depression and anxiety, respectively. It should be noted that many of the reactions that occur in these affective states are symptoms of stress.

For a person to remain healthy, periods of arousal must be balanced by periods of relaxation; otherwise there would be no replenishing of resources used during catabolism. There would be no repair of damage, no vigilence against pathogens. In fact, Holme's studies of life changes have elucidated a strong relation between life stresses and reported physical illness (Holmes and Rahe, 1967). Indeed, one major role of the physician in the case of somatizing patients is to ensure that symptoms do not become more overwhelming, leading to acute medical problems such as peptic ulcer disease, asthma attacks, and hypertension or an acute psychiatric syndrome.

The relation between stress and physical processes and the use of biofeedback to treat psychophysiological disorder are described more thoroughly in other chapters in this volume.

Attribution and Somatization

Carr and Maxim in Chapter 7 imply that human beings are not passive observers of the phenomena that they experience; instead of being passive, they actively engage in labeling the various events that occur. Other peoples' behavior may be labeled as helpful, obnoxious, boring, charitable, stingy, and so on. Physical stimuli may be described as bright, painful, chilly, comfortable, and so forth. This is a very basic process and a major benefit of the language abilities that are unique to human beings, because it permits us to categorize events and store them in memory in a

Table 2. Major Depressive Disorder Reactions

Cognitive	Affective	Somatic
Thoughts of worthlessness, self-reproach or excessive or inappropriate guilt. Recurrent thoughts of death, suicidal ideation, wishes to be dead, hopelessness and helplessness.	Dysphoric mood or loss of interest and pleasure in all activities. Dysphoric mood is characterized by symptoms like: depression, sadness, hopelessness, being low or blue, and irritability.	Poor appetite or increased appetite. Weight loss or weight gain. Insomnia or hypersomnia. Psychomotor agitation or retardation Loss of energy, fatigue. Decreased ability to think or concentrate or indecisiveness. Loss of interest and pleasure in usual activities or decrease in sex drive.

Table 3. Anxiety Reactions

Cognitive	Affective	Somatic
Worry	Anxiety or nervousness	Tachycardia
Sense of foreboding		Hyperventilation (patient complains of shortness of breath)
Sense impending doom		
Exaggerating innocuous situations as dangerous		Tingling in hands and feet
		Diaphoresis
Exaggerating probability of harm in specific situations		Dizziness or syncope
		Flushing
		Muscle tension
		Tremulousness
		Restlessness
		Chest tightness, pressure on chest (pseudoangina).
		Headaches, backaches, muscle spasms

far more efficient fashion that would be possible otherwise. Furthermore, insofar as we apply the same label to similar events we are then able to respond consistently to events that have only minor differences among them.

In contrast to the kind of labeling and categorization that is now possible with computerized machinery, human labeling is not simply descriptive; that is, the labels we apply to events do not necessarily represent the events we experience in a direct fashion. Instead, for many of the events we experience we assign labels that provide some meaning or interpretation to these events (Kanouse, 1971). This process of a assigning meaning with the labels we apply is perhaps most apparent in social situations. For example, we may witness some person giving money to another person. Depending upon a number of factors, we may label that behavior as charitable or as stingy and insulting. These two labels could be applied to the same objectively perceived behavior but have very different meanings. The different meanings will then determine our emotional reactions to the event and determine the ways in which we later interact with the person who executed that behavior. A 4-year-old child who gives a nickel tip to a cab driver after a 5-mile ride will likely be regarded warmly and seen as lovable. The child's father who offers the same tip, while apparently able to offer more, will likely be considered far less favorably.

The same phenomena of providing labels for our experiences are hardly limited to social situations. We label the temperature in our rooms as chilly, warm, comfortable, and so on, rather than with more accurately descriptive terms such as 62°F, and the implications or connotations of describing a room as chilly are very different from those resulting when we describe it as being 62°F. The term *chilly* implies that it is uncomfortable and that there is some need for action, such as raising the thermostat or donning a sweater. We also apply these labels to physical symptoms that we experience—tolerable, painful, uncomfortable, pleasant, excruciating, and so forth—and we label the illness behavior of other persons in similar ways—stoic, hypersensitive, tolerant, etc. Again, these labels have different connotations than would be implied by more accurately descriptive labels.

These connotations will even influence the subjective and physiological reactions to the events that are labeled. A large number of studies have demonstrated that pain tolerance is determined by the labels one provides for those painful stimuli (e.g., Sternbach, 1966); that is, painful events are tolerated for shorter periods of time or in lesser intensities if they are labeled as painful ("strong electric shock," "intense," "painful"). Furthermore, physiological reactions such as galvanic skin responses (palmar sweating) and changes in heart rate to events will depend upon the label that is provided for those events (Lazarus, 1967; Grings, 1965). Electric shock applied to one's forearm elicits greater galvanic skin responses if it is labeled a "strong shock" than if it is labeled a "mild shock." Viewing films of aboriginal subincision rites results in less autonomic arousal if the viewing is accompanied by a commentary that minimizes the amount of pain or emphasizes the important social consequences of these rites of passage.

These points suggest that the meaning applied with the labels will depend upon the language system that is available to the person. If a language does not include terms for depression, for example, then a person who uses that language will not label his own mood states as depressed; rather, some other term with different connotations will be applied. The medical professions have a language system that is far more complex, with respect to disease and illness phenomena, than does the general public. Thus medical professionals are likely to label disease and illness phenomena with terms that have connotations very different from those that are likely to be applied to the lay person.

This process of assigning meanings in the act of labeling is an elementary form of what is referred to as attribution. In the act of labeling we not only describe but also assign or attribute other characteristics to those events. It is an elementary form because it only assigns character-istics to events experienced. More complex attributions also assign characteristics to the person who executed the act, attribute cause for the events to various possible sources, assign responsibility to one or more persons involved in the situation, and ultimately determine appropriate reactions to the perpetrator or determine the nature of one's future interactions with the person seen as responsible. Labeling an act as charitable may also cause us to believe that the person responsible for the act is a charitable individual. That belief in turn may determine our subsequent interactions with that person.

Suppose, for example, that you are suddenly bumped by a grocery cart while searching for some item in your favorite supermarket. You could label that event as an accident and the cart pusher's behavior as unintentional. Having labeled that person's behavior as unintentional, you would be very unlikely to take steps to retaliate physically even if you were lying uncomfortably on the floor of the store. In fact, you may be more likely to apologize for being in the road than to take retaliatory actions. On the other hand, if you determine that the events were nonaccidental and the person's behavior intentional, then you would be unlikely to apologize and more likely to take either verbal or physical retaliatory measures. From research on aggression, it is apparent that such behavior is very much dependent upon perceived or attributed intent. The behavior of a potential aggressor is better predicted by that person's perception of the attacker's intent than by the pain experienced from the attack (Dengerink and Covey, 1982). Clearly, legal decisions such as the discrimination between murder and manslaughter rest upon similar discriminations of intent.

The same sort of phenomena can occur for medically relevant events as well. A person with some chest discomfort may attribute that experience to a wide variety of causes: his or her smoking habits, the flu, lack of exercise, excessive exertion, tension, coronary problems, and so on. The course of action taken will depend upon the particular attributions the person makes. The physician's clinical judgment is another example of the attributional process. The physician's differential perception of a patient's pain as being appropriate physiologically versus amplified due to the patient seeking secondary gain will directly influence his or her workup and treatment.

The Process of Attribution

It is important to recognize that the processes and consequences of attributions can and do occur in the absence of any evidence to determine the accuracy of such attributions, and, once made, these attributions may be difficult to modify. One may perceive that another intended to inflict harm and react accordingly even though that perception was entirely inaccurate or in the absence of any means to determine whether the original actions were intentional or not. All that is necessary is that one make the attribution and have some degree of confidence in it. Similarly, a potential patient may determine that some chest discomfort is the result of excessive exercise and act on that attribution, when in fact it is the result of some degenerative disease process. Alternatively, the "professional patient" may be convinced that certain symptoms are attributable to a disease process and search for a physician to confirm that attribution despite repeated opinions that the attribution is inaccurate.

It is also important to recognize that attribution is a normal and ubiquitous process, not a pathological one. Everyone utilizes it and does so in regard to all events they experience, internal or external, physical or social. This is the process in which jurors engage to assign responsibility for an automobile accident and in which physicians engage to reach a diagnosis (Elstein, 1976).

Two basic processes have been proposed as governing the attribution phenomenon. The first of these is the personal knowledge model (see Maselli and Altrocchi, 1969). In this model attributions of cause, intent, and so forth, are proposed to occur based upon one's reasoning that "if I had done that, it would have been because I . . . " or "other persons whom I've seen do this have done it because . . . " This is basically an inference process that operates by analogy. In part it is an illogical process, because there is no way to determine that the analogy is appropriate or that similar events have similar causes. It is a frequent process, however, and one that is most likely to occur when information and understanding are lacking. It is the process by which primitive religions have assigned certain motivations to the gods. It is the process that occurs when two patients compare symptoms and determine that both are, correctly or not, suffering from the same disease. The same process can result in the decision that a feeling of "pressure" could be relieved by blood letting or screaming or other cathartic processes.

The second process by which attributions can occur may be referred to as the logical inference model (Jones and Davis, 1965). In this process one takes into account the events that occur, the context in which they occurred, the past history of the persons involved, and so forth, and reaches some logical conclusion. The personal knowledge model asserts that "if I only gave a nickel tip to a cabbie, I would have been very angry or felt very stingy, thus this person must have felt the same." Alternatively, the logical inference model would take into account the age of the person (a 4-year-old child), his or her ability to have caused or prevented the events (whether that was the man's last nickel after spending the rest on the cab fare), related events (an argument with the cabbie over the fare), and past history (whether this person is usually a big tipper), and so on, before making a decision. The logical inference model is the kind of process that we follow in making medical diagnoses and choosing appropriate interventions.

The logical inference model has more appeal as being accurate and respectable, at least in Western society, but it has its limitations as well. It is limited first of all by the information available. People who are unaware that stress and tension can result in physical symptoms will be more likely to attribute such symptoms to disease processes. Persons who are unaware of disease processes may attribute symptoms to mystical or magical processes. Physicians who have not been trained to understand symptoms in the context of patients' lives may diagnose and make treatment decisions without relevant psychosocial data.

Alternatively, the attribution process may be short circuited when one must process a great deal of information to reach a conclusion. For example, Table 2 lists ten major symptoms that may be experienced by a depressed patient. In addition, such persons are likely to experience social or interpersonal difficulties as well as vocational ones. When all of these are experienced simultaneously, the person may be unable to determine cause and effect.

A second difficulty of the inference model is that it is sometimes distorted by other processes such as emotional ones and is not always logical or empirical. Some conclusions may seem undesirable and are thus avoided. Patients may be unwilling to accept certain diagnoses because they have social connotations that they see as undesirable. Being diagnosed as having a degenerative disease may be undesirable because it may imply some major life changes that the person is unwilling to accept. Alternatively, being diagnosed as having a psychophysiological disorder will be unacceptable to others because the social connotations are aversive. Physicians may avoid psychophysiological diagnoses because they lack the expertise to intervene for such problems and because of the expected negative response of their patient to such a diagnosis.

A third difficulty with the inference model is that certain conclusions may seem overwhelming given the information that has been gathered. As a result, additional relevant information is not sought. Valins and Nisbett (1971) described the case of a young bride who broke out in hives while on her honeymoon. Her condition did not respond to over-the-counter medications and worsened, so she sought medical advice from a physician in the resort town where she and her husband were spending their honeymoon. The physician determined that the woman had no previous problem with rashes and that she was sexually inexperienced. The circumstances and history led him to the conclusion that her hives were psychosomatic and likely the result of stress (related to having gotten married) and perhaps related to some sexual anxieties. He prescribed tranquilizers and recommended psychiatric help. That diagnosis resulted in considerable concern for the woman and considerable difficulties for the newlywed couple.

Being unwilling to accept the psychosomatic diagnosis or the recommendation for psychiatric help, the woman returned to her family physician after the honeymoon. Her family physician was aware that this woman came from a Jewish background and had married a man of Italian descent, but rather than assume that the cross-ethnic and cross-religious marriage had contributed to the stress, the family physician asked the woman about the honeymoon and their dining activities in particular. During the honeymoon the woman had consented to her husband's choice of restaurants and had taken the opportunity to sample a variety of Italian dishes under her husband's tutelage. The family physician diagnosed a tomato allergy and instructed her to refrain from pursuing her husband's culinary preferences. When she did so, the "psychosomatic" disorder disappeared. The original evidence compelled a psychosomatic diagnosis and the strength of the evidence precluded the physician from gathering further information.

Similar misattributions often occur on the part of patients themselves and another example has been described by Valins and Nesbitt (1971). They pointed out that local anesthetics such as procaine usually include some amount of epinephrine. When used in facial areas, the epinephrine promotes vasoconstriction and thus retards dissipation of the anesthetic while prolonging its effects. In contrast, when a local anesthetic is used in other areas that are not as rich in blood (such as the digits), it is used without epinephrine. As a result, dental patients routinely receive local anesthetic along with a powerful sympathomimetic included. Thus the dental patient, who is already experiencing some anxiety in anticipation of the painful procedures, will experience even greater increases in heart rate, palmar sweating, muscle tension, dry mouth, and so forth, than he would in other situations that cause pain. Without the information that this greater arousal is a result of the medication, the dental patient is likely to attribute the symptoms to his own fear of the procedures and to believe that he is more afraid of the dentist than of other pain agents. Such misattribution may lead to even greater avoidance of the dentist. Clearly, more accurate attributions would be appropriate in this situation. Unfortunately dental patients are seldom aware that the anesthetic will make them more tense. Instead, the dentist or physician is likely to reassure the patient and tell him that the anesthetic will eliminate discomfort. Doing so may increase the likelihood that the patient will attribute fear to themselves.

This is one situation in which misattribution may be advantageous in the opposite direction. If the patient could be induced to attribute all of his arousal (including that which would occur naturally without epinephrine) to the medication, then he may consider himself to be nonanxious. Consistently, researchers have demonstrated that physiological symptoms, which occur as a result of pain, will not produce pain behavior if the person can attribute those symptoms to some other source such as medication (Schachter and Singer, 1962; Nisbett and Valins, 1971).

Changing Somatic Attributions

Attributions are a basic part of illness behavior, which has been described earlier in this volume, and part of the process by which persons generate their explanatory models for their diseases. Rosen and Kleinman (Chapter 5) have discussed some steps for negotiating between different explanatory models of the physician and the patient. One key to understanding that negotiation process is recognizing the steps by which attributions occur. Misattributions often occur when information is inaccurate or incomplete. Attributions can be changed when accurate information is provided and when logical inferences are challenged by new information. For example, a person may be induced to attribute physical symptoms to emotional causes if he or she can be shown that the symptoms wax and wane with changes in life stresses or that the symptoms disappear when stress reduction measures are taken. Still useful, but less so, is information that the symptoms do not abate when biologically based interventions are attempted. This latter information is less useful because it could be explained by inadequate intervention rather than by a misattribution on the patient's part.

One of the greatest impediments to changing patient attributions is the failure of the physician to illustrate the inference process to the patient. Typically the patient is told the end result of the physician's decision making but is not privy to the steps taken to get there. The lack of time available for office visits is part of this impediment. Another part is a failure to involve the patient in the inference process. Patients who are asked to gather data, chart improvement in symptoms, and so forth, are in a far better position to change their attributions than ones who are simply given an official and professional diagnosis.

Reinforcement for Being Sick

In Chapter 9 Carr et al. discuss the role that reinforcement can play in determining patient behavior. The consequences that physicians, family members, employers, and others provide for the actions of patients may be particularly important for chronic patients, as described by Loeser and Fordyce (Chapter 16). Somatization may be particularly sensitive to the effects of reinforcements by the medical profession and the patient's social network. To the extent that a person's somatizing behaviors result in attention, medication, and relief from a physician, in empathy, nurturance, escape from arguments or responsibilities on the part of family members, and disability payments from employers, that somatizing behavior will reoccur. It is important to recognize that physicians may facilitate the process of somatizing.

Engel (1977) has pointed out that most physicians armed with extensive training in the biomedical model often do not evaluate the psychosocial causes of physical complaints. Instead, the physician in the case of depression often works up and "treats" the "physical problem" only. To be fair, many patients will also push vigorously for a somatically oriented workup and treatment and at times react angrily to any hint by the physician that he or she thinks the sickness is due to an emotional problem. However, the major point here is that physicians, by virtue of their training, which is highly technological, are somatizers; that is, physicians preferentially look for and treat somatic complaints and often do not monitor the psychosocial aspects of their patient's lives. A significant factor is the physician's anxiety that he or she will miss an occult physical problem (a fear reinforced by the increase in malpractice suits). Marks et al. (1979) have shown that general practitioners often miss the diagnosis of depression by simply not asking the patient during the interview in an empathic manner about the psychosocial aspects of their lives.

The effect on the patient's perception of his illness of the physician's narrow somatic model is that hypochondriacal patterns are reinforced by medical concern and substantial workups. The physician's somatic focus helps "externalize" the patient's subjective dysphoria or anxiety as an "objective" bodily complaint that is often more palatable to the patient than a diagnosis of depression, anxiety, or psychophysiological syndrome, which often has moral connotations. Thus the patient's cognitive model is influenced by the physician's somatic focus and he learns that the ticket of admission is a physical symptom. The longer the patient perceives himself or herself to be somatically ill and the longer the physician focuses on the somatic aspects of the patient's illness, the more likely the patient is to develop significant secondary gain for being ill and to accept the sick role as a way of life. Certainly patients who have few coping skills and who have long been troubled by poor adaptation to work, interpersonal relationships, and troublesome family relationships are most susceptible to these secondary gains, but many people who seem to cope with life fairly well prior to beginning the somatization are also susceptible.

In considering the social context of anxiety neurosis, depression, hypochondriacal symptoms, hysteria, and parasuicide, Henderson (1974, 1980) postulated that there are substantial deficiencies in the care giving afforded such patients by others, giving rise to care-eliciting behavior to correct the deficiency in social support. Thus the patient's symptoms or illness behavior functions to increase the amount of interest, affection, or care shown to him or her by the primary social group. Learning would account for a large part of the choice of symptoms. Henderson has found a strong inverse relation between social bonds and the presence of neurotic symptoms; specifically, patients with neurotic symptoms have the fewest affectional ties. Many studies have further revealed the preventive significance of psychosocial support systems in such diverse illnesses as angina pectoris (Medalie and Goldbourt, 1976), complications of labor, (Nuckolls et al., 1972), and depression (Brown and Harris, 1978).

In Western society especially, where the extended family system is being rapidly replaced by a more mobile, isolated, and increasingly unmarried population, the physician often provides a supportive relationship that patients lack in much of the rest of their lives. In one study, over a third of the widows studied found a physician helpful during bereavement; specifically, the physician listened to and reassured them (Clayton et al., 1971). Balint (1957) has pointed out that a significant number of patients in general practice come to clinics because they are searching for someone who will show genuine interest and empathy, not because of physical symptoms. Thus the patient with depression often presents to the physician with a somatic complaint and if the affective illness is unrecognized and the patient has few social supports, he or she may value the physician as the primary support system. Indeed, this is seen recurrently with much of the urban geriatric population in primary care, where the physician may be the only empathic, caring person in their lives. The likelihood is that this supportive function of the physician will change the needy patient's cognitive system such that physical symptoms are more readily perceived and reported.

These points indicate that medical care is an interpersonal process. The interactions that occur between patient and physician or between the patient and significant others will influence the likelihood of seeking medical care, the kind of medical care provided, and ultimately the treatment outcome. The social influences in somatization, however, go far beyond interpersonal interactions, as illustrated in the next section concerning the sociocultural factors in the somatization of depression.

Sociocultural Factors

Historically in Western society somatization of depression or anxiety was the norm. Patients did not go to indigenous healers and physicians with existential depressions. They did not complain of mood or affective changes but presented with somatic and vegetative complaints. The development of "psychological mindedness" is largely a twentieth-century phenomenon in Western culture. A majority of cultures in the world even today do not value and often stigmatize the expression and perception of emotions. In many cultures stoicism is considered a virtue. Thus the ability to perceive an affective state and report it to a physician seems to be a very recent development. Cross-cultural evidence points to the fact that depression occurs in all cultures, but the form it takes varies. The core vegetative symptoms of depression are similar, but the cognitive changes, like intense guilt and self-depreciation seen in Western culture, are absent or diminished, as is the expression of depressed affect (Marsella, 1979, 1980). Racy (1970) studied depression in the Middle East and discovered that traditional Arabs presented with somatic complaints such as gastro-intestinal symptoms, loss of appetite, and decreased weight. Guilt and self-depreciation were rare. However, as Arabs became Westernized, the forms of depression became closer to that seen in the West. Pfeiffer (1968) reviewed 40 reports of depression in 22 non-European countries and found that the vegetative symptoms were always found, including insomnia, decreased libido, decreased appetite, and weight loss, but self-depreciation, hopelessness, and guilt were rare. Mezzich and Rabb (1980) compared depressive symptomatology and its sociocultural context across Peruvian and American samples of 93 and 64 adult depressive patients, respectively. A basic common core of depressive signs and symptoms was found across samples (including vegetative, cognitive, and affective symptoms), but more complaints and higher scores on somatic symptoms were found in the Peruvian group, and higher scores on suicidal manifestations in the American group. Somatization is also correlated in the United States with lower socioeconomic class, traditionally oriented ethnic groups that discourage and disparage the undisguised expression of emotions, blue collar workers, rural living, and lower educational levels (Pilowski, 1970; Bart, 1969; Hollingshead and Redlich, 1958; Lerner and Noy, 1968; Srole et al., 1962; Barsky, 1979).

It appears then that most non-Western cultures still present with physical complaints as the primary symptom of depression and that even in Western culture it is probably only a recent trend whereby patients present with self-depreciating thoughts, hopelessness, and helplessness and are able to perceive and articulate depression as a discrete affect. At present primary care physicians, not psychiatrists, still see most of the patients with mental illness (Regier et al., 1978), and the Goldberg (1979) and Widmer and Cadoret (1978, 1979) studies of primary care clinic populations suggest that most depressed patients somatize. Therefore, in Western society as well as most other cultures, somatization represents a powerful method of coping with psychosocial distress. Symptoms are communications of distress and in many cultures depression connotes weakness, moral culpability, and loss of face; besides, there are no psychiatrists and mental illness is highly stigmatized. Moreover, physical complaints are legitimate cues for obtaining care, love, sympathy, time off, and time out; that is, they possess social efficacy. Therefore it is not surprising that the affective component of depression is minimized or overtly suppressed, denied, or perhaps not experienced and the vegetative or somatic experiences highlighted.

Culture influences depression in three major ways. In many cultures there are essentially no words to describe internal emotional states. For example, when Leighton et al. (1963) studied the Yoruba of Nigeria, they found that the Yoruba had no words for depression as an emotional state or a single concept of depression as a syndrome or disorder. Tseng and Hsu (1969) reported a similar observation among the Chinese. Benoist et al. (1965) studied French-Canadians and found that only 5% labeled a case involving sadness, insomnia, fatigue, and loss of interest as depression. They defined depression as a "nervous condition," like a nervous breakdown, with the emphasis on "nerves" as a physical problem. Kleinman (1982) found that of 100 patients suffering "neurasthenia" in the outpatient psychiatric clinic at the Hunan Medical College in China, 87 had major depressive disorders, but all presented with physical symptoms as their chief problem; most regarded their disorder as neurological and due to nervous exhaustion.

Secondly, in many cultures there are strong sanctions against talking about and perceiving emotional states like depression and specific cognitive coping styles are utilized that deflect affective complaints along the channels of physical symptoms. These coping devices block intro- spection as well as direct expression feelings. They place dysphoric affects in a nonpsychological idiom. Unlike the "internal" idiom used by

Westerners, it is an "external" idiom that communicates affect indirectly as somatic, situational, or dissociated behavioral metaphors.

Chinese patients often present with the symptom *hsing-ching pu hao*, a term that refers to general emotional upset (Kleinman, 1980). This vague term functions to reduce the intensity of anxiety and depression by keeping the emotions undifferentiated. Leff (1973) studied Chinese and Nigerian subjects and found that they did not distinguish between anxiety and depression. Thus in some cultures patients use undifferentiated terms to cope with depressive states. Further evidence was provided by Tanaka-Matsumi and Marsella (1976), who compared word associations to the equivalent words *depression* and *yuutsu* ('depression' in Japanese) in three groups of patients: (1) Japanese nationals, (2) Japanese Americans, and (3) white Americans. The Japanese nationals associated more external referent terms such as *rain* and *cloud* and somatic references such as *headache* to the word *yuutsu*. Japanese Americans and white Americans associated predominantly mood state terms such as *sad* and *lonely* to the word *depression*. These findings suggest that there is cross-cultural variation in the subjective meaning and expression of depression. The association to external referents by Japanese nationals suggests that they experience depressive feelings "externally," in an indirect fashion, as related to impersonal Nature and its culturally established emotional referents.

Other related mechanisms that cope with emotions like depression include minimization to overt denial, dissociation (affects are separated from consciousness by mechanisms like trance states and hysterical behavior), and somatization. Minimization refers to the process where the intensity of emotion is suppressed by minimizing its significance. Somatizers with depression often use this coping device with statements like, "Yes, I'm depressed, but anyone with this pain would be." This process extends to frank denial whereby emotions are simply not acknowledged. When examining patients with somatized depression, many appear visibly depressed and all have the vegetative symptoms of depression and have family members who describe a change in affect, yet they vehemently deny perception of depressive mood. It is important here to point out that a subgroup of these patients seem not just to be using denial or conscious suppression but appear not to perceive and label internal emotional states; some may even lack a language to express such states. Dissociation points to a whole range of coping mechanisms where affect is separated from consciousness, cognition, or behavior or the specific stimuli provoking it. This dissociated affect is expressed in isolation most usually in a culturally sanctioned way. Kleinman (1980) has found that in Taiwan one sees angry, sad, and anxious feelings expressed via trance states or hysterical behavior or displaced to other subjects, that is, socially legitimated anger at strangers and deviants.

The third effect culture may have on the perception and expression of depression is where there are culturally idiosyncratic explanations for certain affective states. For instance, in Central and South America in people of Latin American ancestry there exists a disease called *susto* in which symptoms include weakness, decreased appetite, anxiety, insomnia, motor retardation, and decreased libido (Marsella, 1980; Kiev, 1968; Rubel, 1964). In our culture this constellation of symptoms might be labeled as agitated depression, but in Latin American culture it is labeled *susto*. *Susto* means "soul loss" and the connotation of having this disease in terms of treatment is that it has a supernatural or religious cause, for example, breaking taboos, curses, or witchcraft. Just as American cultural beliefs about depression may lead individuals not only to perceive vague symptoms as a sign of depression but to amplify or "imagine" appropriate complaints, so too perhaps in *susto* and other culture-bound disorders symptoms are construed and constructed in keeping with local beliefs about how the disease should "be felt." Thus culture provides the sick person with illness beliefs, views about how the body works, and dominant metaphors and idioms that organize his interpretation of bodily change (White, 1980).

Treatment

The importance of accurate diagnosis and treatment of somatization cannot be overstated. The cost to the medical care system and to the emotional status of the patient of misdiagnosing somatization is profound; such patients are often high utilizers of multiple medical clinics (Lipsitt, 1970; Jacobs et al., 1968). Collyer (1979) has pointed out that 3.6% of his families present with recurrent somatic complaints that take up 48% of his time and that usually one of the parents is depressed. In addition, the experience with patients with chronic pain has demonstrated the iatrogenic harm, that is, the unnecessary surgery and narcotic and hypnotic–sedative abuse that can result (Rawnsky, 1968; Chapman, 1977). Studies have also revealed the secondary gain that often occurs once the depression and somatic complaints become chronic owing to misdiagnosis by patient, family, physician, disability boards, and sociopolitical institutions (Henderson, 1974, 1980; Hudgens, 1979; Parson, 1979; Miller, 1976; Hirschfeld and Behan, 1963). The cost to society in terms of work absences, injuries, disability payments, and family discord is high, but recent data suggest that once recognized and appropriately treated, these personal and social costs can be significantly reduced (Goldberg et al., 1970; Follet and Cummings, 1967).

The key to diagnosis is taking a complete biopsychosocial history and a careful history of vegetative symptoms. In anxiety states, patients also often selectively focus on somatic manifestations of anxiety like tachycardia, subjective shortness of breath (many patients actually are hyperventilating), tingling in the hands and feet, diaphoresis, lightheadedness, muscle tension, and so forth. Again, the key to diagnosis is in questioning the patient about types and significances of life changes and the somatic as well as the cognitive and affective manifestations of anxiety, while also exploring the personal and social meanings and functions of the symptoms.

The first stage in treatment requires negotiating the clinician's bio-psychosocial view of the patient's symptoms (i.e., your headaches are due to muscle tension that has been caused by the stress of your divorce and an ensuing depression) with the patient's somatic view. It is important here not to give the message "it's all in your head" and to invalidate the patient's symptoms, but to point out the underlying psychophysiological connections between mind and body. Often it is not worth quibbling over whether the anxiety or depression is primary or secondary to the somatic symptom, but emphasizing that treatment of the psychological symptom may help alleviate the distress is essential. With acute anxiety attacks or major depression tricyclic antidepressants are extremely efficacious. Many patients can also be treated with psychotherapy and a recent review of treatment of depression found the combination of antidepressants and psychotherapy to be the most helpful (Marsella, 1979). Again, the physician must assess what is acceptable for the patient. Many patients who refuse psychotherapy are willing to try medication and vice versa. In Chapter 5 Rosen and Kleinman discussed in greater detail the strategies for negotiating differences in the explanatory models of the physician and patient.

Conclusion

Patients differ markedly in their language for describing emotions and their styles of coping with pain. Many patients minimize or deny both psychological and physical pain, while others amplify it and are apt to use the health care system frequently. Symptoms are expressions of patient distress but often do not describe whether the distress is in the social, psychological, or physical realms of the patient's life. These symptoms are often ways of enlisting and mobilizing social support from both the health care system and the family. Physical symptoms are considered out of the realm of personal causality and are sanctioned ways of receiving support, caring, and time out from life's responsibilities. There is little problem when illness is used in this way temporarily, but many patients, owing to the lack of more effective ways of enlisting care giving and owing to chronic anxieties and insecurities with life's stresses, begin to utilize somatization as a chronic strategy. The secondary gains like disability payments, opiate and Valium prescriptions, and increased caring by family members and the medical care system are often so powerful that the patient unconsciously continues to focus on somatic symptoms. This is especially true when stress is chronic, when there is underlying depression or anxiety attacks, or when the patient has maladaptive coping mechanisms to deal with chronic intense feelings of lack of self-esteem and insecurities. The clinician must learn to understand patients' symptoms in context with their life experiences. This is especially important with patient symptoms that do not fit known physiological pathways or when the patient seems to be amplifying known physiological illness.

Factors in somatization include the patient's culture, religion, family system and larger social network, work disability system, developmental history, age, history of use of the medical system (number of doctor visits and operations, history of doctor shopping), drug and alcohol use, and parental history of chronic illness or somatization. The primary care physician is perhaps in the best place to attend to these various parameters in that he or she often has treated other family members, can make home visits, and especially in a small town practice may know the patient and his or her family in other social contexts. In order to diagnose somatization in the early stages of the disorder it is essential to screen for stress and the vegetative signs of anxiety and depression. The primary care physician must weigh the physical, psychosocial, and social parameters of illness and develop a comprehensive treatment program based on this complete picture. The physician's job is to recognize that a patient's distress or dysphoria can be due to psychosocial, biological, or both types of problems, but that the patient, owing to a lack of emotional language, psychological defenses, or cultural beliefs and norms, most often presents complaints in a somatic language.

References

Balint, M. 1957. The Doctor, His Patient and the Illness. New York: International Universities Press.

Barsky, A.J. 1979. Patients who amplify bodily sensations. Annals of Internal Medicine 91:63–70.

Bart, P.B. 1969. Social structure and vocabularies of discomfort: What happened to femal hysteria. Journal of Health and Social Behavior 9:188–193.

Benoist, A., M. Roussin, M. Fredette, and S. Rousseau. 1965. Depression among French Canadians in Montreal. Transcultural Psychiatry Review 2:52–54.

Brown, G.W., and T. Harris. 1978. Social Origins of Depression: A Study of Psychiatric Disorder in Women. London, England: Tavistock.

Chapman, C.R. 1977. Psychological aspects of pain patient management. Archives of Surgery 112:767–772.

Clayton, P.J., J.A. Halikes, and W.L. Maurice. The bereavement of the widowed. Diseases of the Nervous System 32:597–604.

Collyer, J.A. 1979. Psychosomatic illness in a solo family practice. Psychosomatics 20:762–767.

Dengerink, H.A., and M.K. Covey. 1983. Implications of an escape/avoidance theory of aggressive responses to attack. In: R. Geen and E. Donnerstein, eds.: Human Aggression: Theoretical and Empirical Reviews. New York: Academic Press.

Elstein, A.S. 1976. Clinical judgement: Psychological research and clinical practice. Science 194:696–700.

Engel, G.L. 1977. The need for a new medical model: A challenge for biomedicine. Science 196:129–136.

Follet, W., and W.A. Cummings. 1967. Psychiatric service and medical utilization in a prepaid health setting. Medical Care 5:25–35.

Goldberg, D. 1979. Detection and assessment of emotional disorders in a primary care setting. International Journal of Mental Health 8:30–48.

Goldberg, D., and B. Blackwell. 1970. Psychiatric illness in general medical practice. British Medical Journal 2:439–443.

Goldberg, I.D., G. Krantz, and B.Z. Locke. 1970. Effect of short-term outpatient psychiatric therapy benefit on the utilization of medical services in prepaid group practice medical program. Medical Care 8:419–428.

Grings, W. 1965. Verbal–perceptual factors in the conditioning of autonomic responses. In W.F. Prokasy, ed.: Classical Conditioning. New York: Appleton-Century-Crofts; pp. 71–89.

Henderson, S. 1974. Care-eliciting behavior in man. Journal of Nervous and Mental Disease 159:172–181.

Henderson, S. 1980. A development in social psychiatry. The systematic study of social bonds. Journal of Nervous and Mental Disease 168:63–69.

Hesbacher, P.T., K. Rickels, and D. Goldberg. 1975. Social factors and neurotic symptoms in family practice. American Journal of Public Health 65(2):148–155.

Hirschfeld, A.H., and R.C. Behan. 1963. The accident process: I. Etiological considerations of industrial injuries. Journal of the American Medical Association 186:193–199.

Hoeper, E.W., G.R. Nyczi, P.D. Cleary, D.A. Regier, and I.D. Goldberg. 1979. Estimated prevalence of RDC mental disorder in primary care. International Journal of Mental Health 8:6–15.

Hollingshead, A.B., and F.C. Redlich. 1958. Social Class and Mental Illness: A Community Study. New York: Wiley.

Holmes, T., and R. Rahe. 1967. The social readjustment rating scale. Psychosomatic Research 11:213–218.

Hudgens, A.J. 1979. Family-oriented treatment of chronic pain. Journal of Marital and Family Therapy 5:67–78.

Jacobs, T.J., S. Gogelson, and E. Charles. 1968. Depression ratings in hypochondria. New York State Journal of Medicine 68:3119–3122.

Johnstone, A., and D. Goldberg. 1976. Psychiatric screening in general practice. Lancet 1:605–608.

Jones, E.E. and K.E. Davis. 1965. From acts to dispositions. In L. Berkowitz, ed.: Advances in Experimental Social Psychology, Vol. 2. New York: Academic Press.

Kanouse, D.E. 1971. Language Labeling and Attribution. Chicago, Illinois: General Learning Press.

Kiev, A. 1968. Curandismo: Mexican-American Folk Psychiatry New York: The Free Press.

Kleinman, A. 1980. Patients and Healers in the Context of Culture: An Exploration of the Borderland Between Anthropology, Medicine and Psychiatry. Berkeley, California: University of California Press.

Kleinman, A. 1982. Neurasthenia and depression: A study of somatization and culture in China. Cultural, Medicine, and Psychiatry 6:117–190.

Lazare, A. 1981. Current concepts in psychiatry: Conversion symptoms. New England Journal of Medicine 305:745–748.

Lazarus, R.S. 1967. Cognitive and personality factors underlying threat and coping. In M.H. Appley and R. Trumbull, eds.: Psychological Stress: Issues in Research. New York: Appleton-Century-Crofts.

Leff, J. 1973. Culture and the differentiation of emotional states. British Journal of Psychiatry 123:299–306.

Leighton, A., T. Lambo, C. Hughes, D. Leighton, J. Murphy, and D. Macklin. 1963. Psychiatric Disorder Among the Yoruba. Ithaca, New York: Cornell University Press.

Lerner, J., and P. Noy. 1968. Somatic complaints in psychiatric disorders: Social and cultural factors. International Journal of Social Psychiatry 14:145–150.

Lipsitt, D.R. 1970. Medical and psychologic characteristics of "crocks." Psychiatry in Medicine 1:15–25.

McKinley, J.B. 1983. Social network influences on morbid episodes and the career of help seeking. In A. Kleinman, and L. Eisengerg, eds.: The Relevance of Social Science for Medicine. Dordrecht, Holland: D. Reidel. In press.

Mannucci, M., S.M. Friedman, and M.R. Kaufman. 1961. Survey of patients who have been attending non-psychiatric outpatient department services for ten years or longer. Journal of the Mount Sinai Hospital 28:32.

Marks, J., D. Goldberg, and V.F. Hiller. 1979. Determinants of the ability of general practitioners to detect psychiatric illness. Psychological Medicine 9:337.

Marsella, A.J. 1979. Cross-cultural studies of mental disorders. In A.J. Marsella, R. Tharp, and T. Ciborowski, eds.: Perspectives on Cross-Cultural Psychology. New York: Academic Press.

Marsella, A.J. 1980. Depressive affect and disorder across cultures. In H. Triandis, and J. Draguns, eds.: Handbook of Cross-Cultural Psychology, Vol. 6: Psychopathology. Boston, Massachusetts: Allyn and Bacon, pp. 237–291.

Marsland, D. W., M. Wood, and F. Mayo. 1976. Content of family practice: A data bank for patient care, curriculum and research in family practice—526,196 patient problems. Journal of Family Practice 3:25–68.

Maselli, M. D., and J. Altrocchi. 1969. Attribution of intent. Psychological Bulletin 71:445–454.

Medalie, J. H., and U. Goldbourt. 1976. Angina pectoris among 10,000 men. II. Psychosocial and other risk factors as evidenced by a multivariate analysis of a 5-year incidence study. American Journal of Medicine 60:910–921.

Mezzich, J. E., and E. S. Rabb. 1980. Depressive symptomatology across the Americas. Archives of General Psychiatry 37:818–823.

Miller, J. 1976. Preliminary report on disability insurance. Public Hearings before the Subcommittee on Social Security of the Committee of Ways and Means, House of Representatives, 94th Congress, 2nd Session, May–June 1976. U.S. Government Printing Office, Washington, D.C.

Nielson, A. C., and T. A. Williams. 1980. Depression in ambulatory medical patients. Archives of General Psychiatry 37:999–1004.

Nisbett, R. E., and S. Valins. 1971. Perceiving the Cause of One's Own Behavior. Chicago, Illinois: General Learning Press.

Nuckolls, K. B., Cassel, J., and B. H. Kaplan. 1972. Psychosocial assets, life crisis and the prognosis of pregnancy. American Journal of Epidemiology 95:431–440.

Parson, T. 1979. Definitions of health and illness in the light of American values and social structure. In G. Jaco, ed.: Patients, Physicians and Illness, 3rd ed. New York: The Free Press; pp. 120–144.

Pfeiffer, W. 1968. The symptomatology of depression viewed transculturally. Transcultural Psychiatry Research Review 5:121–123.

Pilowski, I. 1970. Primary and secondary hypochondriasis. Acta Psychiatrica Scandinavica 46:273–285.

Racy, J. 1970. Psychiatry in the Arab east. Acta Psychiatrica Scandinavica Supplementum 21:1–171.

Raft, D., J. Davidson, T. C. Toomey, R. D. Spencer, and B. F. Lewis. 1975. Inpatient and outpatient patterns of psychotropic drug prescribing by non-psychiatrist physicians. American Journal of Psychiatry 132:1309–1312.

Ramesar, S., S. H. Schuman, M. J. Groh, and J. H. Poston. 1980. Detection of affective disorders in family practice: 126 assessments. Journal Family Practices 10:819–828.

Rawnsky, K. 1968. Epidemiology of affective disorders. British Journal of Psychiatry Special Supplement 2:27–36.

Regier, D. A., I. D. Goldberg, and C. A. Taube. 1978. The de facto U.S. mental health services system: A public health perspective. Archives of General Psychiatry 35(6):685–693.

Reifler, B., J. Okomoto, F. Heidrich, and T. S. Inui. 1979. Recognition of depression in a family medicine training program. Journal of Family Practice 9:623–628.

Roberts, B. H., and N. M. Norton. 1952. Prevalence of psychiatric illness in a medical out-patient clinic. New England Journal of Medicine 245:82.

Rubel, A. J. 1964. The epidemiology of a folk illness. Susto in Hispanic America. Ethnology 3:268–284.

Schachter, S., and J. E. Singer. 1962. Cognitive, social and physiological determinants of emotional state. Psychological Review 69:379–399.

Schuman, S. H., S. B. Kurtzman, J. V. Fisher, M. J. Groh, and J. H. Poston. 1978. Three approaches to the recognition of affective disorders in family practice: Clinical, pharmacological and self-rating scales. Journal of Family Practice 7:705–711.

Srole, L., T. S. Langer, S. T. Michael, M. K. Opler, and T. A. C. Rennie. 1962. Mental Health in the Metropolis: The Midtown Manhattan Study. New York: McGraw-Hill.

Sternbach, R. A. 1966. Principles of Psychophysiology. New York: Academic Press.

Stoeckle, J. D., I. K. Zola, and G. E. Davidson. 1964. The quantity and significance of psychological distress in medical patients. Journal of Chronic Diseases 17:959–970.

Tanaka-Matsumi, J., and A. J. Marsella. 1976. Cross-cultural variations in the phenomenological experience of depression: I. Word association studies. Journal of Cross-Cultural Psychology 7:379–396.

Tseng, W., and J. Hsu. 1969. Chinese culture, personality formation and mental illness. International Journal of Social Psychiatry 16:5–14.

Valins, S., and R. E. Nisbett. 1971. Attribution Processes in the Development and Treatment of Emotional Disorders. Chicago, Illinois: General Learning Press.

Ward, N. G., V. L. Bloom, and R. O. Friedel. 1979. The effectiveness of tricyclic antidepressants in the treatment of coexisting pain and depression. Pain 7:331–341.

White, G. M. 1980. Cultural Explanations of Illness and Adjustment: A Comparative Study of American and Hong Kong Chinese Students. Paper presented at the Ethnography of Health Care Decisions, 79th Annual Meeting of the American Anthropological Association, Washington, D.C.

Widmer, R. B., and R. J. Cadoret. 1978. Depression in primary care: Changes in pattern of patient visits and complaints during a developing depression. Journal of Family Practice 7:293–302.

Widmer, R. B., and R. J. Cadoret. 1979. Depression in family practice: Changes in pattern of patient visits and complaints during subsequent developing depressions. Journal of Family Practice 9:1017–1021.

7

Communication Research and the Doctor–Patient Relationship

John E. Carr, Ph.D.* and Peter E. Maxim, M. D., Ph.D. †

Communication and Conceptual Structure

It has long been recognized that the doctor–patient relationship plays a crucial role in contributing to the ultimate success of the medical intervention process. Research findings from the behavioral sciences over the last several decades have now confirmed scientifically what has been little more than a belief since the dawn of healing, that is, that the efficacy of a therapeutic procedure is a function of two primary variables: (1) the ability of the therapist to establish a condition of trust and influence over the patient and (2) the skill of the therapist to utilize within that context an array of appropriate therapeutic techniques (Strupp and Bergin, 1969). Medical education has traditionally focused upon the latter, providing the physician/surgeon-to-be with a broad armamentarium of treatment techniques, procedures, and operations, leaving the former to somehow be acquired through the more informal teaching procedures of the clinical training situation. In recent years, medical educators have come to recognize the importance of providing for the education of prospective physicians in the establishment and facilitation of the doctor–patient relationship, and have turned to their colleagues in the social and behavioral sciences to contribute to this important aspect of medical education.

Our immediate task becomes one of identifying the critical factors that define the so-called doctor–patient relationship. Attempts at definition based upon the itemization of the traits and characteristics of ideal doctors

*Professor and Acting Chairman, Department of Psychiatry and Behavioral Sciences, University of Washington School of Medicine, Seattle, Washington.

† Associate Professor, Department of Psychiatry and Behavioral Sciences, University of Washington School of Medicine, Seattle, Washington.

and ideal patients has generally proven to be noncontributory. The doctor–patient relationship, as the term implies, is not a static or even an additive phenomenon. While it is tempting to think of it in these terms, one cannot identify the ideal physician any more than one can identify the ideal patient. What must quickly be appreciated is that we must look at variables that are interactional in nature.

To establish influence and credibility with the patient, the therapist is dependent upon operationally definable conditions such as interpersonal warmth, positive regard, and accurate empathy (Truax and Mitchell, 1971). While the conditions of interpersonal warmth and positive regard are attitudinal conditions, the definition of accurate empathy is clearly unique in that it involves a communicative process, that is, (1) the ability of the therapist to understand *in the patient's own concepts* the patient's understanding of his or her conditions (2) the ability of the therapist to communicate back to the patient *in the patient's own concepts* the fact that he or she understands the patient's condition, and (3) that the patient recognizes and acknowledges that the therapist understands. What is involved here, therefore, is the capacity of the therapist to view the patient's condition from the patient's conceptual framework, to put him- or herself in the patient's shoes and to look at the world through the patient's eyes. Equally important is the ability of the therapist to communicate to the patient that in fact he or she, the therapist, is able to accomplish this.

As can be seen, this is not simply communication in the sense of a mechanical exchange of information, but a focusing upon the cognitive and conceptual bases of the communication process. Indeed, even a modest understanding of the nature of communication as it occurs between the patient and the physician requires familiarity with a complex array of variables considered by the physician in training.

In this chapter, we shall review these factors and the role they play and attempt to show how each relates to the other in the communication process. In the course of our discussion, we shall first consider the topic of verbal communication, its physiological basis and development, and the contribution of linguistic scholars to our understanding of the communication process. It is important to note that the development of language itself involves an interdependent relationship between philosophical, psychological, and sociocultural determinants. Next we shall consider nonverbal communication or paralanguage, the definitional and methodological problems inherent in studying this phenomenon, and the substantive findings of scholars in the field. We shall then consider the complex interrelation between roles and the communication process, with special attention to the impact of role expectations on the communications between doctor and patient. Following this, we shall consider a special problem of the doctor–patient relationship, treatment compliance, and will show how the very nature of the problem can be traced to factors within the communication process between doctor and patient. Throughout our discussion we will encounter a recurring theme, namely, that successful communication is largely dependent upon the degree to which the communicants share a common conceptualization of the world about them. In the final section we shall return to this important point and explore its implications in greater detail. Our review will begin with a consideration of the physiological bases for language, which distinguishes humans from other species.

Verbal Communication

Among humans, language is the primary form of communication and as such plays an essential role in the establishment and maintenance of social institutions. The capacity of symbolic representation and the sophistication of grammar allows the human to transmit an almost infinite variety of communications. Language becomes the basis not only for the conceptualization of human experience, but also the sharing of it in the form of knowledge with one another. Thus language becomes a vehicle of exchange among humans, with a high degree of potential for impacting on behavior, not only at the societal and institutional levels, but also at the individual level. It is important to distinguish language, which is the behavioral component of vocal communication. In this respect, language is a manifestation of the social norm, a representative part of the culture, whereas speaking is an individual act that takes on significance only insofar as it conforms or does not conform to the social practices of the language community (Wilson, 1975).

Linguists distinguish between "surface" structure, which refers to the phonological representation of the word units, and "base" or "deep" structure, the more complex semantic interpretation that derives from the words combined. Another way of describing this distinction is "how it reads" (surface structure) versus "what it means" (deep structure). There appears to exist within most language systems a limited number of formal principles by which words are combined to create various meanings. Children learn very quickly the "deep structure" of a language within their own culture, although the process by which these principles are acquired is not yet fully understood. The distinction between surface and deep structure, however, underlies the importance of semantics and language analysis. Here we see the linguistic basis for the common observation that what words say or to what they refer individually is not necessarily the same as what they mean combined with other words. For example, the metaphorical use of the word *pain* suggests the type of problem this poses for the physician. The complaint "a pain in the heart" may suggest an attack of angina when in actuality the patient is describing grief.

Despite their differences, languages possess certain universal properties that leave some theorists to hypothesize a biological capacity for language. The evidence for this hypothesis is limited, but quite persuasive. Lenneberg (1967) cited five reasons why biological propensities in the human for language could be reasonably assumed:

1. There is evidence of anatomical and physiological specialization in the speech mechanism and brain center that controls speech.
2. There is evidence of a regular schedule of development in all children, regardless of cultural variations.
3. There is evidence that language development generally continues despite handicaps resulting from disabilities or neglect.
4. By contrast, there appears to be a failure of nonhuman forms to develop even the most primitive forms of language.
5. There exist language universals in phonology, syntax, and semantics.

Given this innate biological capacity, what, then, motivates the child to learn increasingly complex forms of language? It has been suggested that the child's need for differentiating between and expressing a growing variety of conceptual representations of life events provides the primary motivation. Reinforcement provided by increased capacity for successful interpersonal communication seems to play a major supportive role in this language acquisition schema.

It has been shown that, developmentally, the speech of children exposed to different conditions of learning in different language systems (e.g., Russian, Japanese, and English) display identical grammatical features. According to Bellugi (1965), this course of language development appears to follow a general schema with four identifiable stages:

1. An initial stage comprised almost exclusively of deep structure sentences such as "see truck," "daddy gone." Subsequent language development involves the addition of transformations, for example, changing an affirmative sentence into a negative sentence, which, at this early stage, is accomplished by adding *no* or *not* to the affirmative statement.
2. A second stage in which there is an increase in the number of negative morphemes.
3. A third stage, essentially the same as stage 2, but with greater diversity of negative morphemes plus a number of special cases. This stage seems to represent the upper limit to which nontransformational grammar can be extended. There are few of the deep structure sentences seen in stage 1 and more advanced forms of transformational statements (e.g., "I did not hear the noise" versus "no hear noise"). The language begins to assume characteristics that are

peculiarly or distinctively English, Japanese, and so on, in grammar.

4. Stage four is characterized by the clear emergence of complex transformations.

Language and Conceptual Structure

It has been hypothesized (Whorf, 1941; Sapir, 1929) that how an individual experiences the world is shaped in part by the structure of the language one speaks:

> Are our own concepts of time, space, and matter given in substantially the same form by experience to all men, or are they in part conditioned by the structure of particular languages? (Whorf, 1956, p. 138)

While it is generally agreed that language and perception are interrelated, there has been considerable controversy as to the precise nature of this relationship. As a result, there are essentially three versions of the Whorfian hypothesis: (1) that the structure of language directly influences thought, (2) that the structure of language does not necessarily influence thought but does influence perception, and (3) that the structure of language does not necessarily influence thought or perception but does influence memory. At present, the evidence appears to best support the third version, that is, that the structure of language has less to do with the conceptual representation of experiential events per se but more, rather, with the information storage and retrieval process in cognition. Although surprising, the implications of these research findings are no less significant. The impact of culture, via language, does not so much influence how an individual perceives or thinks about what is happening to him but, rather, how he later recalls it. This gives us some indication of the reasons for the cultural richness of myths and legends as contrasted with official reports and eyewitness observations of events. Now, consider the implications: Culture and language structure will impact more significantly on what a patient remembers of past medical history than it will on immediate observations of symptomatology.

So far, we have seen that the unique communicative capacity of the human involves (1) anatomical and physiological specialization of the speech mechanism, permitting broadcast of a wide range of communicative sounds, and (2) the capacity, in part biologically based, of organizing this finite range of sounds into a system of almost infinite meaning potential on the basis of a few universal encoding rules. What remains to be described is the third component in this system, (3) the cognitive capacity for conceptualizing and organizing the referential basis for these life experiences.

Concept Formation

In this context we shall define *concept* as the cognitive basis for assigning a category label, which in turn refers to a number of specific instances or examples. The process of learning refers to any activity in which the learner must classify two or more different events or objects into a single category with some identifying characteristic in common. The development and refinement of concepts takes place over an extended period of time and is generally believed to progress from a few global, relatively undifferentiated concepts to a more highly articulated and hierarchically organized system.

Concepts in certain domains may develop more rapidly and may be more highly differentiated than concepts in other domains. For example, an engineer will have a highly differentiated set of concepts with regard to engineering principles such as stress and mechanics, but may have less differentiated concepts in such domains as medicine or marine sciences. Similarly, some patients may have highly differentiated concepts concerning the function of an organ's system, say the gastrointestinal system, while other patients may have more highly articulated notions about the functions of the respiratory system. Obviously, this articulation of concepts is tied closely to experiential events. Whereas a polar Eskimo may have a highly differentiated system of constructs with regard to experiential factors related to survival in the arctic, concepts associated with principles or events not in that realm of the Eskimo's experience are either underdeveloped or nonexistent (Berry, 1975).

Conceptual Structure and Ecology

This suggests that concepts and how they are organized are in part determined by the ecological setting in which the individual finds himself and that concepts evolve, in part, in response to the organism's attempts to adapt to environmental demands. Thus conceptual systems have survival value in that they enable the individual to predict and control life experiences (Kelly, 1955). For example, Berry (1975), Dawson (1977), and others have reported distinct differences between hunter–gatherer and agricultural societies, not only in the content of their conceptual systems, but also in the structure or manner in which information is organized.

These findings have led Berry and Dawson to hypothesize that distinct conceptual systems as well as social systems evolve in response to the specific ecological demands upon a group. In turn, these unique conceptual social systems give rise to specific social practices and values that over time become identified as cultural attributes, although the origins of these customs may never have been fully realized, or may have become obscured over the course of time. Whichever the case, latter-day explana-tions may invoke myths, religious beliefs, or simply cultural precedent—"because it has always been done that way."

It is not difficult to see that cultures may similarly produce idiosyncratic conceptual systems having to do with explanations of illness, healing, and preventive practices.

In any given individual, the acquisition of a conceptual system is a function of that individual's life experiences. Thus the nature and structure of that system are functions of the accumulation of ecological demand, cultural, and societal influences, and idiosyncratic experience. To the degree the individual is successful in acquiring useful "ecological" concepts, then to that degree will he survive in the ecological setting; to the degree that useful social and cultural concepts are attained, successful sociocultural adaptation will follow; to the degree that useful but socially acceptable idiosyncratic concepts are acquired, then to that degree will the individual survive as a psychologically as well as physically independent organism. It is perhaps this latter category of determinants that accounts for the unique individual differences we all enjoy: individual differences not just in values, beliefs, attitudes, and behaviors but, more importantly, distinct and unique differences in the ways we organize, categorize, and process information. It is this very important individual difference in conceptual structure that is the key to understanding the human commu-nication process so essential to efficacious health care.

Nonverbal Communication

At the outset one must distinguish between meaning and message in discussing nonverbal behavior. A message is the information transmitted through the production of a behavioral code from a "sending" or "encoding" person to a "receiving" or "decoding" person. The messages in behaviors that constitute such a communication system are presumably known by all people who participate as senders and receivers. Meanings in a communication system are more than the messages sent. The meaning that the encoder attaches in his or her mind to the behavior being produced consists of the encoders' feelings, ideas, memories, and views of the world at the moment that the behavior is codified and transmitted. The message carried in the behavior is only a small part of the meanings the encoder intended,however. Similarly, the meaning that the decoder attaches to the received behavioral message is different from the message itself, owing to the decoders' memories of past relationships, current goals, moods, and views of the world. It should be also noted that the decoder can attach an ascribed meaning to behaviors when those behaviors, in fact, have no codified message.

This disparity between message and meaning is greater in nonverbal than in verbal communication systems. Nonverbal communication systems are formal systems. The number of possible messages is finite; messages are fixed to particular gestures, facial expressions, and body positions. The message of each nonverbal behavior remains fixed and passive, so that stringing behaviors together does not appear to create new messages, and other past or future nonverbal behaviors do not define a context determining the meaning of an individual's behavior. In contrast, verbal communication can be viewed as an informal system. It is open ended in the number of possible messages that can be constructed. The message carried by each word is active, so that stringing words together creates new messages not found in the constituents alone, and the string of words is itself a context that further refines the message of the constituents. Thus the verbal systems' messages can more closely match the complex meanings attached to them by encoder and decoder through the flexibility of serial message ordering.

An early issue in discussing nonverbal behavior, then, is to determine which behaviors constitute a communication system bearing messages. The universe of nonverbal behaviors can be usefully divided into those that are idiosyncratic, and possibly meaningful, but have no message, and those which are communicative and carry commonly understood messages. Idiosyncratic behaviors might convey a particular meaning to a single receiver, but not to others. A physician, for example, will ascribe significance to an idiosyncratic behavior, based on his experience, although the behavior may have no meaning at all to the casual observer.

It is generally agreed that the sum total of distinguishable nonverbal signals that can be used in nonverbal communication is in excess of 100 (Brannigan and Humphries, 1974; Birdwhistle, 1970; Grant, 1969). This repertoire is larger than that of most animals by a factor of 2–3, although it exceeds only slightly the repertoire of the rhesus monkey and chimpanzee (Wilson, 1975). Included in such a repertoire are three coding principles as defined by Ekman and Friesen (1968b): arbitrary codes, iconic codes, and intrinsic codes.

Someone who closes his fist and hits someone is delivering an intrinsically coded message: It is not a message similar to aggression, it *is* aggression. Intrinsically coded behaviors are those in which the behavior and its message are the same. A person who raises a clenched fist in a salute or who runs a finger under his throat to signify "an unfortunate outcome" is performing iconically coded behavior. Iconically coded behaviors carry the clue to their message in their behavior. The message is clear and understood by everyone in the culture. These two classes of nonverbal behaviors are so obvious in their messages as to be easily decodable by the physician and not particularly useful. The third class of behaviors, those with arbitrary coding, are of special interest because they are commonly observable in doctor–patient relationships. Their messages bear no visual resemblance to what they signify and they consist of gestures, gaze directions, facial expressions, body positions, and body postures. Research in nonverbal communication in recent years has focused on these behaviors and attempted to define their messages. Early attempts at definition were very simplistic and ranged from the highly specific to the highly general; for example, "the particular movements are found to be correlated with particular indices for a particular person in a particular context" (Dittman, 1962); "movements in general express affect in general" (Sainsbury, 1955).

Though research in the last ten years has developed more sophistication in methodology then is implied by the above statements, reviews by Wiener et al. (1972) and Harper et al. (1978) underscore the conceptual and methodological problems inherent in this research. Wiener et al. concluded, "There is little consensus about any set of behaviors which can be considered to serve communication functions, and the literature consists, for the most part, of a fragmented and unsystematic array of reports, with almost any conceivable behavior considered by one or another investigator to have some communicative significance" (p. 186). This difficulty of reaching a consensus on the catalog definitions of nonverbal behaviors is matched by the difficulty in logically defining the messages contained in such behaviors.

Three research strategies have had prominence in this area. Birdwhistle (1970) has attempted to analyze the meaning of nonverbal behaviors, especially movement, in a fashion analogous to the treatment of language by linguistic scholars (e.g., what are the minimum basic units required to communicate a message?). His approach makes no distinction between message and meaning or between idiosyncratic and communicative behaviors as defined above. This approach attempts to tie meaning to every movement and to discover a system of meaning peculiar to the particular people involved and their relationship. Birdwhistle has been relatively unsuccessful in his attempts to specify a catalog of behaviors that have generality to many people, and to specify messages contained in such behaviors apart from the meanings embedded in the social context, the personality variables of the participants, and their verbal exchanges.

A second research strategy is exemplified by the work of Ekman and Friesen (1968a,b). This group has focused primarily on the study of facial expressions. The facial expression message is assumed to be a particular affect such as anger, fear, sadness, surprise, happiness, or disgust. The research tasks then focus on the degree to which static poses of facial expressions can be decoded correctly by people from diverse cultures or the degree to which different facial features affect the decoding of the previously defined affect message. This research has gone far to validate the premise that facial expressions carry arbitrarily coded messages of affect. It has additionally distinguished part–whole distinctions in non-verbal behavioral that are confused in the work of Birdwhistle; that is, this work points out the degree to which particular facial features contribute to the whole facial gestalt, while noting that it is the whole gestalt alone that carries the message, not partial features. This work, however, has been restricted to looking only at facial expressions, only in static, not interactive situations, and only with previously defined messages.

A third and more promising line of research, developed by writers such as Scheflen (1964, 1966), Watzlawick et al. (1967), Eibl-Eibesfeldt (1970), and Smith et al. (1974), emphasizes behavior in an interpersonal setting as the communication model. This research assumes that arbitrarily coded nonverbal behavior represents an older, evolutionarily earlier mode of expression than verbal language. It further assumes the existence of behavioral message continuities in human and mammalian nonverbal communication. Much previous work on primate social communication has led to a methodology for defining behavioral catalogs, which is adaptable to human nonverbal catalogs. For example, work with rhesus and pigtail monkeys has produced a method for defining messages contained in nonverbal behavior. The researcher collects examples of particular behaviors seen in different monkeys and relates them to co-occurring subsets of social contexts in which they invariably occur. Message statements for human gaze, gestures, and facial expressions have similarly been derived by collecting examples of the co-occurrence of nonverbal behaviors with verbal statements (Maxim, 1982b). Verbal content analysis schemes developed by Gottschalk et al. (1969), Viney and Westbrook (1976), and others allow one to then categorize the verbal discourse. In a recent study, Maxim examined over 3000 co-occurrences of 51 common gaze–gesture combinations and 500 verbal content categories taken from videotaped discussions between 30 pairs of human subjects. Each gaze–gesture combination was found to co-occur with a subset of verbal content categories. Thus Maxim developed a "message statement" for a particular gaze–gesture combination by assuming that there was a close similarity between the message contained in the nonverbal behavior and the message contained in the verbal content catalog. Table 1 gives a tentative list of some of these gaze–gesture combinations and their derived message statement. As can be seen, the messages appear to address relationship issues on three dimensions: affiliation–disaffiliation, assertive-ness–submissiveness, and certainty–uncertainty.

While the above lines of research hold promise, considerable work remains to be done in this area before the physician can be assured he or she knows what messages accompany particular nonverbal behaviors observed during interactions with patients.

Table 1. A Partial List of Gaze–Gesture Combinations and Their Messages[a]

Gaze–gesture combination	Message
Look at, shake head at	I want you and the others to listen and change my views.
Look at, eyebrow flash	Look at all the trouble these others have caused and how they are being blamed for it.
Look at, extend palms	Let's agree on this.
Look at, nod no	I think your views are wrong on this.
Look at, shoulder shrug	I feel anxious because I don't know enough; I feel you put me on the spot, but I'm not angry; I like you.
Look at, eyebrow raise	They and I agree; you and the others should view it this way too.
Look at, finger flag	This is why I think this way and your way is wrong.
Look away, smile	I partly agree with you and perhaps should do this differently, but their way is ridiculous.
Look away, nod no	I can't decide what to think of all these conflicting views.
Look away, settle	I'm anxious about our disagreeing.
Look away, groom	I think I disagree with you about this, but I don't have enough information to decide.
Look away, rub nose	I think we would get along if you weren't so inept.
Look away, mouth cover	I am embarrassed at not knowing enough about this and that you know it.
Look away, no gesture	I am unsure of myself and of our relationship.
Look at, slow blink	Why don't you appreciate me and give my ideas a chance?
Look at, smile	I think we agree this is the way to proceed, even if others don't.
Look at, self-gesture	Despite all that has been said, this is why my view will prove correct.
Look at, no gesture	I am being open and want a relationship.
Look at, steeple	I think you are generally right in your views and I side with you but feel defensive.
Look away, nod yes	I guess I agree with some of what you say, but I'm not sure I side with you.
Look at, lick lips	I feel ashamed and sorry about the way I've been thinking and acting.
Look at, head tilt	Maybe we could be on the same side on part of this.
Look at, swing leg	Don't blame me or the others, we already feel badly about this.
Look at, bite lip	You are right and I have been wrong about this.
Look at, nod yes	I side with you.

[a]Modified from Maxim (1982b).

Paralinguistic Communication

This label is generally assigned to aspects of verbal behavior not explicitly a part of language itself but that serve to contribute to or amplify the message in the communication, as well as provide information about the sender. Paralinguistic characteristics such as pitch, tone, volume, articulation, resonance, tempo, modulations, and so forth, provide information that may be essential to correctly understanding the intent of a message. A number of studies have also shown that the vocal characteristics of an individual relate to personality type, as measured by a personality test or inferred by an observer (Harper et al., 1978). However, it would be naive to conclude that such relations are sufficiently robust to permit indiscriminant prediction. For one thing, paralinguistic characteristics and their meaning may vary between ethnic, socioeconomic, or geographic groups, and without awareness of these differences can lead to confusion and misinterpretation in communications.

Of greater interest to researchers has been the hypothesized role of paralinguistic characteristics in communicating the emotional state of an individual. In general, the reported relation between vocal cues and affect appears to be far more substantial than the relationship to personality. Davitz (1964) has shown that sensitivity to emotional paralinguistic cues is related to perceptual and cognitive factors (auditory discrimination of tone and rhythm, verbal intelligence, spatial analytic ability, and knowledge of focal characteristics) but is unrelated to 33 personality variables measured on four different psychological tests. This is not surprising, since affective states (e.g., love, hate, joy, and fear) have more immediate social and survival value and therefore are more likely to have social referent cues with high consensual validation. Personality characteristics, by contrast, have less social communicative value and are more idiosyncratic in their development and nature.

Dittman and Wynne (1966) conducted an extensive study of the role of paralinguistic cues in interviews; they coded linguistic junctures (dividing points in the flow of speech), stress (the increase and decrease in loudness with clauses), and pitch (the rise and fall of fundamental frequencies of the speaker's voice) and attempted to correlate these variables with different emotional states. While trained judges could reliably agree on changes in these variables and the emotion they thought was being conveyed, the change in these variables showed no consistent pattern with any particular emotion. These investigators also coded paralinguistic vocalizations of three types: vocal characterizers (laughing, crying, voice breaking, etc.), vocal segregates (*uh, hum, uh huh,* etc.), and vocal qualifiers (extra increase in loudness, pitch, and duration placed on some words), but reported that vocal characterizers and vocal segregates occurred too infrequently to be useful in correlating them with a particular speaker's emotion. They also tried to code voice quality (tempo, rhythm, precision of articulation, breathing, etc.) and voice set (fatigue, age, and other physiological pecularities of the speaker's voice), but were unable to demonstrate any consistent relation between coded paralinguistic cues and any particular emotional states. One of the difficulties encountered was an inability to obtain reliability in judges' ratings of certain cues.

Among the range of emotional states, anger, anxiety, sadness, and happiness have been more reliably judged than fear, love, and surprise, which are the more difficult emotions to identify. Those individuals who are more sensitive to decoding emotional paralinguistic cues tend to be more adept at expressing affect via such cues. Zuckerman et al. (1975) had 64 college men and 37 women encode six emotions by trying to imitate emotions of anger, happiness, sadness, fear, surprise, and disgust in their videotaped facial expressions and audiotaped statement of, "I have to leave now." Each person was then asked to classify the emotion portrayed visually and verbally by the others. The results indicated that those with the best ability to encode emotions were the best at decoding it, although no one had outstanding ability. In making auditory judgments, men and women did better rating the emotions of those of the same sex. However, in making visual judgments, men and women did better rating emotions of those of the opposite sex. Women were found to be slightly better overall in both encoding and decoding emotions than men. A similar study by Buck et al. (1974) also found that women were better encoders than men, as evidenced by the greater accuracy with which both male and female judges could decode female emotions. Rosenthal and DePaulo (1979), however, found that women lost their encoding–decoding advantage when their facial or verbal cues were presented for briefer periods of time, more closely approximating the way cues are seen in everyday life.

From the physician's perspective, anxiety and depression rank among the most significant of affective states, not only because they represent important clinical conditions per se, but also because they are often critical indicators of the patient's emotional and cognitive response to disease and treatment. For a variety of reasons, ranging from individual personality to cultural role, patients are not always candid about their worries, fears, and depression relative to medical care. A subtle behavioral cue may be the physician's first and only indication that the patient is anxious and subsequent inquiry may reveal a distorted impression of the nature of his or her disease, misunderstanding as to the purpose of the surgical procedure and its outcome, or misinformation about his or her chances for survival.

There is no simple relation between anxiety and behavioral cues that can be applied indiscriminantly to all people. Sociocultural prescriptions for the meaning of cues may vary and individual responses to both the intensity and quality of the affective state can cover a wide range. On the basis of such findings, we may conclude, as did Davitz (1964), that the communication of affective meaning via paralinguistic cues is a function of the observer's cognitive and perceptual abilities rather than his other personality traits or the personality traits of the observed. Such perceptual–cognitive abilities are not necessarily related to verbal meaning or the linguistic aspects of the communication. The ability to accurately perceive the emotional implications of an individual's paralinguistic cues, within the context of various social interactions, is a perceptual or cognitive capability of the observer that has little to do with personality and which is quite distinct from the language facility of the observed. It is an interpersonal perceptual–cognitive skill and, like any skill, improves with practice and training (Carr, 1982). Thus, contrary to the popular notion among physicians that emphathic ability is a fixed quantum that must be conserved by rationing it to one's patients, relevant research indicates that empathic ability, like any skill, can only be maintained and increased through exercise. Indeed, failure to do so can only lead to its decrease and eventual disuse.

Factors in Interrupted or Blocked Communication

Perhaps it is a commentary on the state of the art that more can be said about what can go wrong with communication than about what will guarantee that it will go right. In general, however, researchers on communication agree as to some basic categories of barriers to effective communication (e.g., Parry, 1967; Miller, 1967; Watzlawick et al., 1967).

1. *Lack of a communication medium.* From a pragmatic standpoint, the most basic kind of problem is a lack of communication facilities. In a physician's practice, it may be simply a lack of commonality in language, for example, an English-speaking physician with a Spanish-speaking patient. Or the problem may be more subtle; for example, in his or her hurry to complete the physical examination, a physician provides no opportunity for communication between him- or herself and the patient.

2. *Information overload.* If we assume that a medium for communication exists, problems may occur if the receiver lacks the capacity to receive and process the information. This may be the result of limitations on the receivers of an intellectual, linguistic, social, or experiential nature. Or it may be the result of too much information or information that is too complex; for example, the receiver may be faced with a problem of having to deal with competing stimuli incoming at the same time.

3. *Distraction.* In communication theory terms, this is often referred to as "noise" and includes the various kinds of phenomena that are not relevant to the message being communicated but which may interfere with its transmission or receipt. These include affective

states such as anxiety, depression, conflict, preoccupation with distracting ideas or messages, and other forms of internal stress, as well as external or environmental stressors.

4. *Confused presentation.* While at first glance this would appear to be a problem that is self-evident, all too often it is a problem that is ignored by the physician. The physician may have well in mind the specific points he or she wishes to make to the patient regarding the treatment regimen or information about the disorder in question; however, a confused or disjointed presentation, lacking in logical sequence, fully illustrated with the use of highly technical jargon, lengthy sentences, and unfamiliar idiomatic phrases may completely obscure the meaning of the message the physician wishes to impart.

5. *Intrusion of personal motives and idiosyncratic habits.* The physician has only to experience the seemingly cooperative and compliant patient who somehow inevitably manages to sabotage the treatment regimen to realize that things are not always as they seem. Intrusion of unconscious thoughts, affect, and motivation into the doctor–patient relationship is a problem of which the physician must be constantly aware.

6. *Unstated assumptions.* Inevitably in any communicative interaction, the sender may be especially liable to make certain assumptions about the receiver and therefore to cast the message in these terms. If these assumptions are unwarranted, then the receiver may be operating under a distinct handicap in being able to receive and process the information. For example, the physician may assume that the patient is familiar with certain technical or medical terms that he or she is using to describe the patient's current disorder. If that assumption is unwarranted, then the physician's highly technical explanation will be totally misunderstood by the patient. Similarly, the patient can entertain unstated assumptions about the physician; for example, that on the basis of a minimal description of symptoms the physician is totally familiar with the patient's condition or that in referring the patient to a specialist, the patient's family physician has fully informed the specialist as to the patient's condition, family background, and so on.

7. *Incompatibility of conceptual systems.* Related to the previous item, this is probably the most important yet least attended to of the potential barriers to meaningful communication. Both doctor and patient bring to the doctor–patient relationship a highly idiosyncratic conceptual or belief system reflective of highly individualized life-learning experiences. In large part, the ability of two people to communicate successfully depends on the degree to which there is similarity in the conceptual systems they each bring to the communication situation. The degree to which one person, the physician, may influence the life

of the other person, the patient, is similarly dependent upon the degree to which the conceptual systems are compatible, permitting facilitative communication (Kelly, 1955).

Social Roles and Communication

In our discussion of the communication process between doctor and patient, we will now consider the impact on that process of the social roles played by both the physician and the patient. Much has been written about the doctor and patient roles and the pressures on the individual that are inherent in each. One is tempted to assume that the differences in these roles are largely a function of difference in education and expertise with regard to the practice of medicine. If this assumption were correct, we might conclude that since doctors know about good health practices, they know how to be good patients. In fact, whether or not the physician successfully fulfills his professional role in no way implies that he is capable of successfully assuming the patient role, and numerous studies have shown that physicians are as a rule abysmally poor patients. For example, while almost all physicians recommend annual physician exams for their patients, between one-third and two-thirds of them fail to practice what they preach. It would be naive to assume that this reflects either the physicians' lack of need for medical attention or their ability to self-diagnose. Logic dictates that the physician is as subject to having significant asymptomatic problems as anyone in the population at large and some studies even suggest that the level of undetected significant asymptomatic problems may run significantly higher among physicians than among comparable groups of business executives. Since such problems are generally picked up through routine physical examinations, the physician's ignoring of his or her own advice can hardly be justified on the assumption of lack of need. What is perhaps more significant, however, is the fact that physicians with diagnosed disorders tend to ignore these symptoms or wait twice as long from their outset to seek medical help as do lay persons.

Numerous statistics are often cited to illustrate the impact of physician role demands upon the individual. Drug abuse is much more common among physicians than among the general public, one-third of all physician hospitalizations are generally caused by alcohol and drug use, the suicide rate for physicians is double that of the general adult population, physician pilots are involved in fatal light plane crashes at a rate four times that of civilian noncommercial pilots, and so on. While these statistics suggest that the concept of role is indeed a significant factor in the physician's existence, they provide us with little insight into the nature of the role itself or the mechanics by which it evokes such dramatic consequences.

While we have come to associate the concept of roles with research in the social sciences, historically the term is borrowed directly from the theater and was used there as a metaphor intended to denote that conduct which adheres to certain parts in a drama rather than to the players per se who read or recite the parts. Thus, in contrast to the main body of psychological inquiry, the study of the isolated individual is not the focus of our concern here; instead, as Sarbin and Allen (1968) have suggested, the questions that should guide our observations of social behavior and its consequences are of this type: (1) Is the conduct appropriate to the role? (2) Is the enactment proper? That is, does the overt behavior meet the normative standards that would serve as evaluational criteria for the observer? Is the performance to be evaluated as good or bad? (3) Is the enactment convincing? That is, does the enactment lead the observer to declare unequivocally that the incumbent is legitimately occupying the position?

It is apparent from the nature of these questions that our concern here is with constellations of behavior that are consensually agreed upon by members of a social or cultural group and that behaviors are sufficiently discrete and therefore identifiable as to be capable of being communicated from one person to another, and from one generation to another, within that cultural group. We know that any member of any organized society or culture group must develop more than a single role. If he or she is to successfully function within that group, then what is required is a repertoire of well-practiced, realistic, and socially accepted roles. A person with such a repertoire is thus much better equipped to meet the societal demands placed upon him than is a person whose repertoire of roles is quite meager. Thus the roles define the social structure by which interpersonal interactions are carried out within the societal group and involve a complex constellation of behaviors, affects, cognitions, postures, statuses, and even distinct language forms. The very nature of the concept of role implies that not only are there prescriptions for what behavior is to occur in an interpersonal interaction, but also prescriptions for the communication. The best example of this, of course, is that in many cultures various roles will have distinct linguistic forms associated with them so that the individual, in assuming a role, also assumes a readily identifiable language form.

Since the notion of interpersonal interaction is inherent in the concept of role, it is necessary to look at the way in which role expectations impact upon the behavior of the participants in this interaction. By role expectations we refer to that conceptual bridge that connects social structure on the one hand with the role behavior of the participants on the other hand. Role expectation refers to those rights and privileges, duties, and obligations of the person who occupies a role as perceived by other persons in complementary roles. Once an individual has been identified as occupying the physician role, the person in the complementary role, the patient, immediately invokes certain expectations (beliefs, constructs, or concepts about the nature of the physician role) about the physician's anticipated behavior that then influence the way the patient shall behave. As can be seen, these role expectations may or may not have anything to do with the individual who is occupying the physician role. As a result, there is potential for a breakdown in communication if the physician is either unaware of the expectations or is unable to fulfill them.

Role expectations vary along several dimensions, the most important of which include (1) the degree of generality or specificity, (2) their scope or extensiveness, (3) their degree of clarity or uncertainty, (4) their degree of agreement or disagreement among those persons in the complementary roles, and (5) the degree to which they relate to formal or informal positions within the social structure.

If we look at each one of these dimensions with regard to the physician role, we observe that the role is fairly specific; that is, we are able to specify precisely required behavior, how and where the behavior should be executed, and the exact penalty for nonadherence to the role expectation. Also, the role is fairly restricted in scope, having relevance to a narrowly circumscribed area of a person's life. Next, the role certainly possesses a high degree of clarity, and there is a great deal of consensus among other persons concerning the role expectations with regard to physicians' behavior. Finally, the role expectations clearly relate to a highly formal, social position within the social structure. The physician's role is one about which almost every member of our society has a great deal of knowledge and for which there is a high degree of consensus about the role and expectations associated with it.

What specifically are the mechanisms by which the role expectations of the patient affect the role enactment of the physician? We have already implied that the role expectations are, in fact, specifications for adherence to group norms. In some respects they are culturally defined job descriptions. Therefore, assuming that there is social consensus as to the nature of this job description, the patient will be judgmentally concerned with the appropriateness and propriety with which the physician fulfills the role obligation. There is no question that patients expect physicians to behave in particular ways. Social interaction, therefore, should be effective and satisfying so long as both participants behave in accordance with those rules and expectations. According to Sarbin and Allen (1968), "clarity of role expectation can be defined as the differences between the optimal amount of information needed about role expectations and the amount actually available to a person." Certainly the amount of information impinging on the lay public via the various media sources concerning the physician's role is sufficient to provide clarity with regard to role expectations for the physician.

This is not to say that roles and role expectations do not change. Under certain circumstances, roles go through a natural evolutionary course, as can be seen from the variety of role changes associated with the developmental process throughout adolescence and early adulthood. Certainly this must represent problems in interpersonal communication, for role change must by necessity be accompanied by changes in role expectations, role demands, and the form of communication between the participants. Much has been written about the impact and consequence of change in life-styles upon an individual and specifically of the impact of these changes upon interpersonal relationships and the ability to communicate (Sheehy, 1976). The most frequently mentioned by-products of such role changes are dissolutions of relationships and social realliance.

Attention has recently been focused upon the complex interaction between sex and role expectation, especially in light of the dramatic alteration in traditional feminine roles now occurring within our own culture. The transition from the student to the doctor role is sufficiently traumatic, but add to that the complicating situation of transition from female coed to doctor and one can begin to appreciate the complexity and sometimes apparent incongruity in role expectations in our culture required by individuals in complementary roles.

In large part, the precipitation of role expectations and the appropriateness of those expectations are dependent upon the successful completion of an earlier process of role identification or role perception. By these terms, we refer to the accuracy with which the individual is able to perceive interactional behavioral cues and draw from them conclusions about the role of the other person. The cues to which we refer are quite variable and may include such things as gross skeletal movements or verbal acts, physique, posture, clothing, and perhaps even facial expressions. They may also refer to adornments or visible emblems and badges of office, uniforms, and so on. Thus we concern ourselves here not only with accuracy of perception, but a more important cognitive variable, that is, the ability to correctly deduce from the cue the appropriate information relevant to the carrying on of the interpersonal interaction. It is an established principle in social–psychological research that the accuracy with which an individual is able to perceive such interactional cues in others is directly related to the accuracy with which that same individual is able to perceive his or her own role. This empirical relationship between the perception of self and that of others once again demonstrates the important role played by cognitive process in interpersonal relationships and communication.

As we have already said, the concept of role is a metaphor for denoting socially appropriate behavior or modes of interpersonal interaction in social situations. Thus whether or not an individual is able to successfully carry out the practice of a role is not only dependent upon his or her ability to learn the appropriate aptitudes and behavioral skills involved in the carrying out of that role, but also on the ability to perceive accurately, for example, to infer validly from available cues the social positions of others as well as of the self and to infer appropriate role expectations for the positions involved.

Communication and the Problem of Noncompliance

The problem of patient noncompliance with the therapeutic regimen is one of the most critical issues faced by the practicing physician attempting to deliver efficacious health care. While there is a tendency to define noncompliance as a "management problem," a review of the available literature quickly reveals that a major contributing factor in compliance is the ability of the physician to communicate effectively with the patient.

To date, the most comprehensive treatment of the subject has been provided by Sackett et al. (1976), who reviewed 185 original studies of noncompliance. The literature shows that patients who enter the health care system with symptomatic complaints tend to keep approximately 90% of their initial appointments, whereas patients who are nonsymptomatic (i.e., patients who are referred into the health care system for routine screenings, physical exams, etc.) keep only about 50% of their appointments. Compliance with short-term medication regimens declines rapidly over time, almost on a day-to-day basis, until that rate stabilizes at about 50% for patients who are on long-term medication. Of course, these generalizations are subject to variable interpretations, depending on a variety of conditions in the doctor–patient relationship. For example, compliance rates deteriorate rapidly, especially in instances of acute illness where the patient's condition has been suddenly responsive to the medical regimen. What is remarkable is that eventually the reported rates appear to converge at about the 50% level.

Evaluations of the literature are especially difficult because of the enormous methodological problems in an area that has only recently begun to receive attention from researchers. To begin with, definitions of compliance vary significantly. For some physicians, noncompliance may be defined in terms of any patient who deviates from a prescribed regimen of treatment. For other physicians compliance with 75–80% of the treatment program may be deemed an unqualified success. Methodological problems, however, go beyond simple definition of the nature of the beast. For example, it may be that to insist upon a single universal definition of the noncompliant patient, applicable to the full range of potential treatment regimens, is overly simplistic and unrealistic. The required level of compliance by a patient for efficacious treatment of a condition such as a cold may be quite different from the level of compliance for efficacious treatment of a condition such as emphysema. Therefore one needs to look at the range of parameters involved in compliance to better appreciate its nature.

It is tempting to assume that noncompliance is a problem belonging entirely to the patient and that a review of the available research literature would reveal to us the demographic characteristics of a noncompliant patient, allowing us to make predictions about which patients are likely to be most problematic. In his review of the determinants of patient compliance, Haynes (1976) found that demographic features (e.g., age and sex) of patients are not directly related to compliance. However, he did find evidence that they affect the patient's accessibility to the health care system, thereby indirectly relating to ultimate compliance rates.

Are compliance rates a function of diagnosis or disease? There does not appear to be any consistent evidence to support the notion that compliance rates are related to the nature of the illness or diagnosis. It is often assumed that psychiatric patients in general tend to be less compliant, especially those with diagnoses of schizophrenia or personality disorder. However, Berg et al. (1982) have recently reported that diagnoses of schizophrenia and personality disorder had no relation to medication compliance in a clinic population where 30% of patients suffered schizophrenia, 24% neurotic depression, 22% personality disorder, 12% major affective disorder, and 12% schizoaffective disorder. The overall clinic compliance rate was 59%.

Is compliance a function of the nature of the therapy program? The literature consistently supports the hypothesis that compliance is a direct function of certain features of the therapy program. For example, treatment regimens that require more extensive behavioral changes on the part of the patient (especially where such behavioral changes involve long-standing life-style or habit patterns) are more likely to be associated with significantly reduced compliance rates. Similarly, treatment programs that involve highly complex features are more likely to result in reduced compliance. The same thing can be said of treatment programs that tend to be long term. There does not appear to be any clear relation between compliance and side effects, although the problem has not been extensively studied.

Is compliance a function of the patient–therapist interaction? Again, the literature provides some fairly consistent findings in this area. In general, the closer the degree of medical supervision over the treatment regimen, the more likely the patient is to comply. This finding is based upon research comparing compliance rates for outpatient, day-care, and hospitalized patients, and also on a number of outpatient studies in which the degree of medical supervision was varied. A variant of this finding is that the longer a patient has to wait for any aspect of the treatment program, the less likely it is that there will be compliance.

Some of the most extensive work with regard to the relation between patient–therapist interaction and compliance rate has involved the patient's perceived level of satisfaction with the therapist. Compliance is a function of the level of satisfaction, which in turn is a function of the degree to which the patient's expectations are met by the therapist and are unrelated to the attitude the patient holds toward either the health care system or doctors in general.

In their study, Berg et al. (1982) found that 75% of patients who subsequently were noncompliant to prescribed medication dosage would indicate prospectively that they were not going to be compliant; for example, they gave negative or equivocal answers, at the time the medication was prescribed, to questions regarding their willingness or ability to take the medication. Furthermore, they gave clear reasons as to why they probably would not comply: They felt they were being coerced; they have no money; they though they were getting too little or too much medication; or they predicted that they would forget to take it. Such reasons, should the physician take the time to elicit them, are probably correctable by active intervention and negotiation, thereby leading to much better compliance.

In his review of the sociobehavioral parameters of compliance, however, Becker (1976) argued that the "health belief system" a patient maintains has a direct influence on the patient's acceptance of preventative health care recommendations, whereas the patient's knowledge of diseases and therapy does not. Becker concluded that compliance with one aspect of the treatment program favors the probability that there will be compliance with other aspects of the program, with the critical element in predicting compliance being the presence or absence of a stable and supportive family structure.

The available literature appears to support a health belief model that contains three essential elements:

1. The patient's evaluation of a health condition as determined both by his perceived likelihood of getting the disease and his perceptions of the probable severity of the disease. The result is a state of "readiness to take action."
2. The patient's evaluation of the recommended health behavior in terms of its feasibility and efficacy weighed against estimates of the physical, psychological, financial, and other costs of, or barriers to, the proposed behavior.
3. A "cue to action" must occur to trigger the recommended health behavior; this stimulus can be either internal (e.g., symptoms) or external (e.g., advice from family, friends, mass media, and other communications).

Some further insight into the possible determinants of the compliance problem may be gained by a review of types of programs that have proven to be successful when reducing noncompliance. In general, a review of the literature along these lines suggests that behavioral and multiple strategies hold a substantial edge over educational strategies in terms of both increases in compliance and improvements of therapeutic outcome. In assessing the implications of this finding, we must keep in mind that the majority of studies have found no association between patients' knowledge about their diseases and compliance. Nor is there any evidence to suggest a relation between intelligence and compliance. This suggests that the critical element is indeed communicational, but not simply in terms of the clarity of the message being communicated. Rather, consistent with the evidence cited earlier, the clarity of the message and *its consistency with the patient's existing health care belief system* are essential. Thus the literature suggests that probability of compliance should be increased in those cases where the physician is able to accurately perceive the health care belief system of the patient and formulate treatment recommendations and a description of the treatment regimen in terms that are consistent with that system.

Ley (1977) has reviewed psychological studies of doctor–patient communication and similarly concluded that improved communication appears to depend upon the ability of the physician to (1) accurately determine the patient's fears and worries, (2) assess the patient's expectations and communicate to the patient whether or not these expectations can be met and why, (3) provide information about the diagnosis, its meaning, and its implications with regard to the cause of illness, (4) adopt a friendly rather than a businesslike attitude, (5) avoid medical jargon, and (6) spend time in conversation regarding nonmedical topics. The emphasis in these six points is less upon the communication of factual medical information than it is upon the establishment of a condition of trust and influence with regard to the patient. Ley pointed out that in order to increase the understanding of the patient with regard to his or her condition, materials concerning the condition and the treatment regimen should be presented to the patient in a straightforward and concrete fashion. Patients often lack the elementary, technical, and medical knowledge required to understand many treatment regimens; furthermore, they often have misconceptions that militate against proper understanding (e.g., the patient's belief system about health care practices). Ley contended that the chief problem in patient compliance is the tendency of the patient to forget up to 40–50% of the intended message anywhere from 5 to 80 minutes following the consultation, but other research suggests that the problem is less one of forgetting and more one of inadequately understanding the initial message. To ensure maximal understanding and recall of treatment instructions, Ley emphasized the following points:

1. Whenever possible, provide the patient with instructions and advice at the start of the information session; that is, make the critical points initially.

2. When providing instructions and advice, stress the importance of the instructions.
3. Use short words and sentences.
4. Use explicit categorizations wherever possible.
5. Repeat things wherever possible.
6. When giving advice, make it specific, detailed, and concrete.

In studies where these recommendations were tested, recall and understanding on the part of the patients increased by 10–20%.

The issue often arises as to whether or not the patient should be told all of the details of his or her disorder. Surveys indicate that the majority of physicians believe that patients should not be told (69–90%), but in fact, when questioned, the majority of patients indicate that they do want to know as much as possible about their illness, even if it is fatal (77–89%). Furthermore, outcome studies indicated that life adjustment following illness was far better among informed patients than among those who had been uninformed or misinformed.

The work of Janis (1958, 1971) has underscored the significance of the relation that exists between the degree to which the patient is informed and the patient's adjustment to illness and/or health care procedures. In his studies of factors affecting patients' recovery from surgery, Janis found that patients with prior information about the specific unpleasant outcomes they might expect showed better pre- and postoperative adjustment than those patients who received no information. Informed patients showed less fear prior to the procedures, less anger, greater confidence in the outcome and in the skill of the doctor, and less emotional disturbance overall. Janis hypothesized that by having such information available prior to the surgical procedure, the patient was able to anticipate the fear he would experience and to rehearse adapting and coping responses in the face of perceived danger. By being uninformed, the patient was deprived of the opportunity to anticipate this fear and adequately prepare for it. As a result, he was left to feel helpless when the danger actually appeared. This, in turn, led to the expectation of vulnerability, disappointment and distrust in the physician, and, consequently, feelings of fear and anger.

Clearly, by providing the patient with full and complete information about the sensations, pain, uncomfortable exercises, or unpleasantness of various treatment regimens, the physician may evoke some degree of fear and anticipatory anxiety in the patient. However, as Janis pointed out, this may in fact prove to be adaptive for the patient in that when these events do occur there will be no surprises, no feelings of loss of control or that events are proceeding outside of the realm of expectation, and therefore no basis for anger or fear in response. The patient does not feel that he or she has been deceived, misled, or worse, perhaps, that something is going wrong, since the outcome is proving to be not what the physician had led the patient to expect.

Conclusions

Social and behavioral scientists have long acknowledged that an individual's success in coping with the social environment is largely determined by the degree to which that person is able to develop a sufficiently differentiated cognitive representation of the environment (Zajonk, 1968). The principle has far-reaching implications for medical practice and indicates that research focusing upon the cognitive processes in social interactions should prove valuable in advancing our understanding of what contributes to successful therapeutic intervention. Furthermore, the success of a social interaction is also a function of the degree to which there is compatability among the participants in the level of differentiation of their cognitive structures.

This "cognitive compatability" has been defined as one person's (e.g., the doctor's) ability to accurately perceive and communicate within the system of cognitive dimensions used by another (e.g., the patient) to conceptualize his or her experience (Landfield and Nawas, 1964) and is the fundamental psychological process underlying the concept of *empathy*. Cognitive compatability is defined not only in terms of similarity in the concepts used in conceptualization but, more importantly, similarity in the degree to which their conceptual dimensions are differentiated (Triandis, 1960). The physician and patient may share a common dimension such as painful–nonpainful, but for one individual (the patient) the dimension may be poorly differentiated, allowing him to make few discriminations among a given group of stimulus conditions ("everything causes pain, doctor"), whereas for another it may be highly differentiated, permitting him to perceive a greater number of differences among the same group stimulus condition. Whether doctor and patient agreed that a given condition was painful would not necessarily depend upon whether or not they used the same semantic label, but whether they shared a relatively common degree of differentiation of that conceptual dimension. Therefore the more meaningful "functional" similarity of their conceptual structure could be distinguished from merely the "semantic" similarity and operationally defined in terms of the degree to which the level of differentiation of one approached the level of differentiation of the other (Carr, 1982).

The principle of cognitive compatability offers a possible explanation for several of the dilemmas of health care research. We have suggested that cognitive incompatibility could account for problems of noncompliance and the failure of doctor and patient to agree about the outcome of the treatment (Rogers, 1967; Carr and Whittenbaugh, 1969). Nawas and Landfield (1963) hypothesized that most improved patients should show a significant increase from pre- to posttherapy in the number of concepts borrowed from the doctor, whereas least improved patients should show a decrease. Instead they found that improved patients showed a *decrease* in the number of constructs borrowed from the doctor. In a subsequent study, Landfield and Nawas (1964) found that a minimal degree of communication between the patient and the therapist *within the patient's language dimensions* was essential to treatment success, but that communication within the therapist's language dimensions was not.

If patients are concerned with whether they are understood by the doctor and base their judgment of the treatment outcome on this perception, then their ability to assume the doctor's frame of reference is less relevant to the treatment process than the doctor's ability to assume theirs. Furthermore, while a meaningful understanding of the patient's life situation, problems, and modes of adjustment may require the doctor's appreciating the patient's cognitive dimensions and their level of differentiation, this does not necessarily imply that the doctor uses the patient's vantage point when it comes to the task of evaluating outcome. Indeed, in response to the demands for "professional" evaluation, the doctor is more likely to shift back to the more familiar personal conceptual structure or a "professional" vantage point comprised of the theoretical or conceptual dimensions acquired through professional training.

The research on doctor–patient cognitive compatibility has shown that not only is it a critical factor in predicting the success of treatment outcome, but that it plays an important role in the teacher–student relationship in medical school training. The relationship is far more complex, the teacher's cognitive structure appearing to be a primary variable, yet compatability is still an important determinant. In other research with community action groups, cognitive compatability has been shown to determine the nature and type of decision or behaviors carried out by these groups.

Results of these studies have more far-reaching implications with regard to health care delivery in general, but especially in multiethnic societies. While we have often observed that a physician of white American background may have considerable difficulty in comprehending a Mexican-American or black patient's conceptualization of illness, we have been able to say little about the nature of the relationships involved other than that differences in the ethnic or socioeconomic background appear to affect one's perceptions. Indeed, the literature and our current findings suggest that cognitive process is the intervening variable required to account for the interaction between ethnic and culture variables and behavior. Furthermore, an understanding of the nature of that relation requires not simply an appreciation of the ethnic/cultural factors involved but, more importantly, an appreciation of the indigenous conceptual framework and the cognitive processes by which those factors are assigned meaning.

References

Becker, M. 1976. Sociobehavioral determinants of compliance. *In* D. Sackett and R. Haynes, eds.: Compliance with Therapeutic Regimens. Baltimore, Maryland: Johns Hopkins Press.

Bellugi, U. 1965. The development of interrogative structures in children's speech. *In* K. Riegel, ed.: The Development of Language Functions. University of Michigan Language Development Program. Report No. 8, pp. 103–137.

Berg, J., P. Maxim, and J. Brinkley. 1982. Unpublished manuscript, Dept. of Psychiatry, University of Washington, Seattle, Washington.

Berry, J. 1975. Ecology, cultural adaptation and psychological differentiation: Traditional patterning and acculturative stress. *In* R. Brislin, S. Bochner, and W. Lonner, eds.: Cross-Cultural Perspectives on Learning. New York: Wiley, pp. 207–230.

Birdwhistle, R. 1970. Kinesics and Context: Essays on Body Motion and Communication. Philadelphia, Pennsylvania: University of Pennsylvania Press.

Brannigan, C., and D. Humphries. 1974. Human nonverbal behavior, a means of communication. *In* N. G. Burton-Jones, ed.: Ethological Studies of Child Behavior. Cambridge, England: Cambridge University Press, pp. 37–64.

Buck, R., R. E. Miller, and W. F. Carl. 1974. Sex, personality, and physiological variables in the communication of affect via facial expression. Journal of Personality and Social Psychology 30:587–596.

Carr, J. 1982. Personal construct theory and psychotherapy research. *In* A. Landfield and L. Leitner, eds.: Personal Construct Approaches to Cognitive Therapy. New York: Wiley, pp. 233–270.

Carr, J., and J. Whittenbaugh. 1969. Sources of disagreement in the perception of psychotherapy outcome. Journal of Clinical Psychology 25:16–21.

Davitz, J. 1964. The Communication of Emotional Meaning. New York: McGraw-Hill.

Dawson, J. 1977. Theory and method in biosocial psychology: A new approach to cross-cultural psychology. *In* L. Adler, ed.: Issues in Cross-Cultural Research. New York: New York Academy of Science, pp. 46–65.

Dittman, A. 1962. The relationship between body movements and moods in interviews. Journal of Consulting Psychology 26:480.

Dittman, A., and L. C. Wynne. 1966. Linguistic techniques and the analysis of emotionality in interviews. *In* L. A. Gottschalk and G. Auerbach, eds.: Methods of Research in Psychotherapy. New York: Appleton-Century-Crofts, pp. 146–152.

Eibl-Eibesfeldt, I. 1970. Ethology: The Biology of Behavior. San Francisco, California: Holt, Rinehart, and Winston.

Ekman, P., and W. Friesen. 1968a. Nonverbal behavior in psychotherapy research. *In* J. Shlien, W. Hunt, J. Matarazzo, and C. Savage, eds.: Research in Psychotherapy, Vol. 3. Washington, DC: American Psychological Association, pp. 179–216.

Ekman, P., and W. Friesen. 1968b. The repetoire of nonverbal behavior: Categories, origins, usage, and coding. Semiotica 1:49–98.

Gottschalk, L. A., C. N. Winget, and G. C. Gleser, 1969. Manual of Instructions for Using the Gottschalk–Gleser Content Analysis Scales: Anxiety, Hostility and Social Alienation–Personal Disorganization. Berkeley, California: University of California Press.

Grant, E. Human facial expression. Man 4:525–536.

Harper, R., A. Weins, and J. Matarazzo. 1978. Nonverbal Communication. New York: Wiley.

Haynes, R. 1976. A critical review of the "determinants" of patient compliance with therapeutic regimens. In D. Sackett and R. Haynes, eds.: Compliance with Therapeutic Regimens. Baltimore, Maryland: Johns Hopkins Press, pp. 26–39.

Janis, I. 1958. Psychological Stress: Psychoanalytic and Behavioral Studies of Surgical Patients. New York: Wiley.

Janis I. 1971. Stress and Frustration. New York: Harcourt, Brace, and Jovanovich.

Kelly, G. 1955. The Psychology of Personal Constructs. New York: W. W. Norton.

Landfield, A., and M. Nawas. 1964. Psychotherapeutic improvement as a function of communication and adoption of therapist's values. Journal of Counseling Psychology 11:336–341.

Lenneberg, E. 1967. Biological Foundations of Language. New York: Wiley.

Ley, P. 1977. Psychological studies of doctor–patient communication. In S. Rachman, ed.: Contributions to Medical Psychology, Vol. 1. Oxford, England: Pergamon, pp. 9–42.

Maxim, P. E. 1982a. Contexts and messages in macaque social communication. American Journal of Primatology 2:63–85.

Maxim, P. E. 1982b. Messages in Human Nonverbal Communication. Journal of Personality and Social Psychology, in press.

Miller, G. 1967. The Psychology of Communication. New York: Basic Books.

Nawas, M., and A. Landfield. 1963. Improvement in psychotherapy and adoption of the therapist meaning systems. Psychological Reports 13:97–98.

Parry, J. 1967. The Psychology of Human Communication. London, England: University of London Press.

Rogers, C. 1967. The Therapeutic Relationship and Its Impact. Madison, Wisconsin: University of Wisconsin Press.

Rosenthal, R., and B. M. DePaulo. 1979. Sex differences in eavesdropping on nonverbal cues. Journal of Personality and Social Psychology 37:273–285.

Sackett, D. 1976. The magnitude of compliance and noncompliance. In D. Sackett and R. Haynes, eds.: Compliance with Therapeutic Regimens. Baltimore, Maryland: Johns Hopkins Press, pp. 9–25.

Sainsbury, P. 1955. Gestural movement during psychiatric interview. Psychosomatic Medicine 17:458.

Sapir, E. 1929. The status of linguistics as a science. Language 5:207–214.

Sarbin, T., and V. Allen. 1968. Role theory. In D. Lindzey and E. Aronson, eds.: Handbook of Social Psychology, Vol. 1. Reading, Massachusetts: Addison-Wesley, pp. 488–567.

Scheflen, A. 1964. The significance of posture in communication systems. Psychiatry 27: 316–331.

Scheflen, A. 1966. Natural history method in psychotherapy: Communicational research. In L. A. Gottschalk and H. A. Auerbach, eds.: Methods of Research in Psychotherapy. New York: Appleton-Century-Crofts, pp. 263–289.

Sheehy, G. 1976. Passages. New York: Dutton.

Smith, J., J. Chase, and A. Lieblich. 1974. Tongue showing. Semiotica 11:201–246.

Strupp, H., and A. Bergin. 1969. Some empirical and conceptual bases for coordinated research in psychotherapy: A critical review of issues, trends and evidence. International Journal of Psychiatry 7:18–90.

Triandis, H. 1960. Cognitive similarity and communication in a dyad. Human Relations 13:175–183.

Truax, C., and K. Mitchell. 1971. Research on certain therapist interpersonal skills in relation to process and outcome. In A. Bergin and S. Garfield, eds.: Handbook of Psychotherapy and Behavioral Change. New York: Wiley, pp. 299–344.

Viney, L. E., and M. T. Westbrook. 1976. Cognitive anxiety: A method of content analysis for verbal samples. Journal of Personality Assessment 40:140–150.

Watzlawick, P., J. Deavin, and D. Jackson. 1967. Pragmatics of Human Communication. New York: W. W. Norton.

Whorf, B. 1941. The relation of habitual thought and behavior to language. In L. Spier, ed.: Language, Culture and Personality, Manasha, Wisconsin: Sapir Memorial Publication Fund.

Whorf, B. 1956. In J. B. Carrol, ed.: Language, Thought and Reality, Cambridge, Massachusetts: MIT Press.

Wiener, M., S. Devoe, S. Rubinow, and J. Geller. 1972. Nonverbal behavior and nonverbal communication. Psychological Review 79:185–214.

Wilson, E. 1975. Sociobiology. Cambridge, Massachusetts: Harvard Press.

Zajonk, R. 1968. Cognitive theories in social psychology. In G. Lindzey and E. Aronson, eds.: Handbook of Social Psychology (rev. ed.), Reading, Massachusetts: Addison-Wesley, Vol. I, pp. 320–411.

Zuckerman, M., M. S. Lipets, J. H. Koivumaki, and R. Rosenthal. 1975. Encoding and decoding nonverbal cues of emotion. Journal of Personality and Social Psychology 32:1068–1076.

8

The Unity of Biomedical
and Psychosocial Issues in Individual
and Family Health Care

Gabriel Smilkstein, M. D.*

Introduction

The biopsychosocial concept of health care, which unifies the physical, psychological, and sociocultural assessment of a patient's health problems, represents the ideal in patient care (Engel, 1977, 1980). The purpose of this chapter will be to review systems for evaluating and analyzing data that permit the physician to aim for this ideal. The challenge for physicians who accept the rationale of these evaluation systems will be to make them functional by incorporating them into patient assessment and care. In order to meet this challenge, physicians must visualize the patient as functioning within the context of family and community (Richardson, 1945; Litman, 1974; Smilkstein, 1977).

Comprehensive Health Care

In 1966 the American Medical Association's Ad Hoc Committee on Education for Family Practice suggested that "comprehensive health care services include preventive, diagnostic, therapeutic, rehabilitative, and health maintenance services" (Lee, 1974). This definition deals primarily with the range of services offered to the patient. Comprehensive health care, however, is more than the totality of desirable health services; it is also an attitude of total care with which the individual doctor, specialist, or generalist approaches the patient (Somers and Somers, 1961).

In his assessment of a community's health orientation, Murphy (1975) defined comprehensive health care as that which encompasses "physical

*Professor, Department of Family Medicine, University of Washington School of Medicine, Seattle, Washington.

and sociopsychological health needs, and . . . environmental health activities." This definition further broadens the scope of comprehensive health care, for in addition to focusing on physical and emotional health problems, it also suggests that deliverers of comprehensive health care must be concerned with home and community environmental problems.

Physicians who wish to be advocates for a comprehensive health care program are challenged by the limitations of time and resources that restrict the extent to which they may develop plans for the comprehensive management of patients' problems. Furthermore, some patients may not wish to extend their contract with the physician beyond their presenting problems, since they may not be emotionally, physically, or financially prepared to participate in a prolonged encounter. These limitations suggest that frequently the realities of medical practice prevent the physician from developing a total care program for every patient; however, they do not preclude physicians from offering the fullest measure of care possible within the contraints of the practice situation.

How does a clinician avoid the frustrations of the added burdens of a comprehensive health care program? The first step is to utilize a schema that gives an overview of the components of comprehensive care. Such a schema should identify the components and indicate how they may interact to yield improved health care. Utilizing guidelines drawn from such a schema, clinicians will be more utilitarian in their approach to comprehensive health care, gathering appropriate data and setting pragmatic priorities for planning total patient care.

Figure 1 demonstrates a comprehensive health care schema that is based on three categories of the problem-oriented medical record (POMR) (Weed, 1968). This is a medical system with which most physicians are familiar. The POMR consists of three components into which comprehensive care concepts are woven: (1) data base on patient, family, and community; (2) assessment of physical, psychological, and sociological problems; and (3) plans for curative (plus rehabilitative), preventive, and (health) promotive activities.

Data Base

While a data base on the individual patient is the usual focus of the medical workup, to consider the data base comprehensive, an evaluation of the patient's family and community milieu is essential. The value of the study of the patient within the context of family has been well documented (Richardson, 1945; Litman, 1974; Geyman, 1977; Schmidt, 1978; Haggerty and Alpert, 1963).

One of the elements desirable in establishing a family data base is the family folder with records of medical histories and reports of physical examinations of members of the family (Grace et al., 1977; Froom et al.,

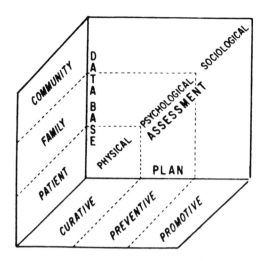

Figure 1. A model for teaching comprehensive health care based on the problem-oriented medical record (POMR). A complete data base includes information about the patient within the contexts of family and community. Assessment includes an integrated view of physical, psychological, and sociological problems, while the plan utilizes the patient's personal, family, and community resources to cure and prevent disease, as well as promote health. From Smilkstein (1977).

1977). Such family folders may be strengthened with a record of the family tree and a family problems list, both physical and psychosocial. Most medical charts contain only the structural information that details a patient's family members' sex, age, and biomedical data on illnesses, surgeries, accidents, and deliveries. Few offer a comprehensive approach to medical record keeping that includes functional information on family member interaction.

The clinician who wishes to obtain family information must develop strategies to gain such data. The functional status of the family may be revealed to the physician overtly through the interview process if a patient elects to describe a stressful family conflict. However, patients seldom volunteer information about family interaction. For example, they may covertly represent their family or interpersonal conflicts through the process of somatization—the use of physical symptoms as a maladaptive technique of achieving aid for unresolved anxiety related to stressful psychosocial life events. Some of the clues that may suggest the possibility of somatization are to be found in the patient who presents "a laundry list" of symptoms and who has a history of doctor shopping and, in general, a history of high utilization of health care facilities. This issue of somatization is discussed more thoroughly in Chapter 6.

166

Family APGAR questionnaire
Part I

The following questions have been designed to help us better understand you and your family. You should feel free to ask questions about any item in the questionnaire.

The space for comments should be used when you wish to give additional information or if you wish to discuss the way the question is applied to your family. Please try to answer all questions.

Family is defined as the individual(s) with whom you usually live. If you live alone, your "family" consists of persons with whom you now have the strongest emotional ties.

For each question, check only one box.

	Almost always	Some of the time	Hardly ever
I am satisfied that I can turn to my family for help when something is troubling me.	☐	☐	☐

Comments: _____

I am satisfied with the way my family talks over things with me and shares problems with me.	☐	☐	☐

Comments: _____

I am satisfied that my family accepts and supports my wishes to take on new activities or directions.	☐	☐	☐

Comments: _____

I am satisfied with the way my family expresses affection and responds to my emotions, such as anger, sorrow, and love.	☐	☐	☐

Comments: _____

I am satisfied with the way my family and I share time together.	☐	☐	☐

Comments: _____

Figure 2. Family APGAR questionnaire, Part I. Adapted from Smilkstein (1978a).

Family APGAR questionnaire

Part II

Who lives in your home*? List the persons according to their relationship to you (for example, spouse, significant other,† child, or friend).

Check the column that best describes how you now get along with each member of the family listed.

RELATIONSHIP	AGE	SEX

WELL	FAIRLY	POORLY

If you don't live with your own family, list the persons to whom you turn for help most frequently. List according to relationship (for example, family member, friend, associate at work, or neighbor).

Check the column that best describes how you now get along with each person listed.

RELATIONSHIP	AGE	SEX

WELL	FAIRLY	POORLY

*If you have established your own family, consider your "home" as the place where you live with your spouse, children, or "significant other" (see next footnote for definition); otherwise, consider home as your place of origin, for example, the place where your parents or those who raised you live.

†Significant other is the partner you live with in a physically and emotionally nurturing relationship but to whom you are not married.

Figure 3. Family APGAR questionnaire, Part II. Adapted from Smilkstein (1978a).

For the busy practitioner, assistance in gaining information on the status of family interaction may be obtained through the use of a utilitarian screening test for family function, the Family APGAR (Smilkstein, 1978a, 1980a; Good et al., 1979). This five-item questionnaire will give the physician an instrument that examines the patient's perception of five components of family function (see Figs. 2 and 3). As with any laboratory test, the Family APGAR results must be put into context with the information the physician obtains from the history and physical examination.

Each item in the Family APGAR is scored 2 (almost always), 1 (some of the time), or 0 (hardly ever). The total score of the responses of the five items will range from 0 to 10. Validation studies on various clinical and nonclinical populations have shown that most individuals score in the 8–10 range. Thus moderately to severely dysfunctional families with scores of 0–7 are highlighted. These norms permit the clinician to identify those family members who may be at high risk for problems associated with family or support system dysfunction. A growing body of literature suggests that these individuals with dysfunctional support systems will demonstrate increased utilization of health care facilities, morbidity, and mortality (Cobb, 1976; Gore, 1978; Berkman and Syme, 1979).

If the physician determines that family dysfunction is a major component of the patient's disability, appropriate measures may be taken to assist the patient. The decision for therapy will vary according to the nature of the family's problem as well as the physician's expertise with psychosocial issues. The physician's intervention may range from facilitating patient ventilation of family conflicts to involvement in family therapy, to referral to appropriate agencies.

Assessment

Assessment should include problems and diagnoses drawn from the physical, emotional, and sociological components of the patient's data base. The patient's physical and emotional problems tend to be standard items in a POMR report; however, physicians should also search for those sociocultural factors that contribute to an understanding of ill health (Kleinman et al., 1978). Some of these are family dysfunction, absence of a social support group, unusual health-seeking behavior, nontraditional health belief concepts, and adverse environmental conditions (Smilkstein, 1980b; Mauksch, 1974; Kleinman and Smilkstein, 1980). Knowledge of the patient's cultural, educational, economic, and environmental resources will significantly improve the effectiveness of the physician's plan for the management of the patient's problem.

Plan

The plan for patient care should include curative, preventive, and promotive components. Curative medicine, the major business of the health care industry, is based on what Breslow (1972) called a "complaint-response system." But comprehensive medicine requires an expanded plan that goes beyond a curative response to the patient's chief complaint. The plan should include, as needed, recommendations for the rehabilitation of the postacute and chronically ill, continuity of care, patient education for disease and accident prevention, the promotion of health through physical fitness and improved nutrition, and attention to family and community environmental factors that may have adverse effects on patients' health. That is, effective planning will take into account the effect of psychosocial systems and biomedical phenomena as well as that of the biomedical processes and the medical intervention on the patient's psychosocial system.

A model of comprehensive health care would not be complete without taking into account the influence of cross-cultural factors (that is, the interaction of the sociocultural milieus of the health care recipient and deliverer). Physicians need to understand their patients' perception of health care and disease, as well as offer the patient an explanation of the medical assessment and plan. Mutual understanding between the recipient and the deliverer allows for negotiations of priorities between patient and doctor. When this attitudinal ideal in health care is achieved, optimum patient compliance may be anticipated.

Family: The Principal Support System

The biomedical literature tends to treat patients in isolation from their environment. In general, the process of reductionism is in effect, with only a portion of the patient, the pathological and biological part, being examined. Comprehensive medicine requires an expanded view of the patient. This necessitates an understanding of the family or support system in which the patient functions.

Assessment and management of family dysfunction is an area of study that has been ascendent during the past decade (Crawford, 1971; Bauman and Grace, 1977; Minuchin, 1974; Pratt, 1976). In family medicine the aim has been to use these studies to develop a body of knowledge that will allow physicians to approach the patient's family problems with the same competency they apply to biomedical problems (Cowan and Sbarbaro, 1972; McWhinney, 1972; Curry, 1977; Ransom and Vandervoort, 1973). To facilitate the utilization of knowledge from family studies, a model is needed that demonstrates the interrelation of components that are critical to an understanding of the family in trouble.

The cycle of family function (Smilkstein, 1980b) is a conceptual framework that presents an empirical view of the responses that may result when a family experiences a stressful life event. It offers the student, resident physician, and family physician a common language with which to discuss family function, as well as a format that addresses the data base needed to assess and care for the family in trouble. Terms used in the cycle of family function are defined in Table 1. These definitions represent an empirical synthesis of concepts from the writings of medical and social scientists who have contributed to the study of the family.

Table 1. Definition of Terms Used in the Cycle of Family Function[a]

Equilibrium	A state of family homeostasis in which member interaction results in emotional and physical nurturement, thus promoting growth of family members and the family unit
Stressful life events	A life experience that requires the family's use of resources for coping or adapting not usually required by the family members for the management of daily activities
Crisis	A state of family disequilibrium that results from failure to identify resources adequate to allow family members to cope with a stressful life event
Disequilibrium	A state of impaired functioning, nurturing, or role complementarity in which a family, for the time being, can neither escape nor solve problems with their customary problem-solving resources
Resources	Those assets that serve the process of family nurturing and fall in the general categories of familial and extrafamilial social, cultural, religious, economic, educational, environmental, and medical support systems
Adaptation	The process by which family members utilize their resources to effect a resolution of a stressful life event and return to nurturing family function or equilibrium
Maladaptation	The process by which a family in crisis or disequilibrium chooses abnormal defense mechanisms to achieve some measure of equilibrium in family function
Pathological equilibrium	A state of impaired interaction or nurturing within a family that follows the utilization of abnormal defense mechanisms to escape from anxiety of unresolved family crisis (Families in pathological equilibrium may have members who are so isolated from their fellow members that they cannot receive help, or individuals who are so adhesive to their family members that independent function is paralyzed.)

[a]From Smilkstein (1980b). Reprinted with permission of Appleton-Century-Crofts.

Definition of Family

An agreement on the meaning of family is essential for any discussion about this biopsychosocial unit. The physician requires a definition of family that is discipline specific (i.e., a definition that clarifies the structure and function of the patient's family as it relates to the health problems of the patient under study). Biomedical problems such as genetic abnormalities are best understood by establishing a structural definition of the family (Table 2). In order to study psychosocial issues, however, the physician requires a definition of family that permits an understanding of family function as perceived by the patient. The study of the biomedical and psychosocial problems of the patient within the context of the family requires, therefore, that both structural and functional components be included in the definition of family.

The definition of family that applies to the conceptual model described in this paper is as follows: *The family is a sociocultural system in which members have a commitment to nurture each other emotionally and physically. The commitment is usually one to share resources such as time, space, and finances and is made between two or more adults with or without children or between single adults with children.*

Once the unit under study (the family) is established, the physician requires a standard for the family in health. In this chapter, *a family in health is one whose members perceive it as cohesive and offering the nurturement and resources that are necessary for personal growth and sustenance. A family in health offers its members reasonable limits and guidelines and supports its members as they challenge life.* The critical words in this definition are *cohesive* and *nurturement. Cohesive* suggests that the family is a unit that cooperates to supply resources for its members; *nurturement* is included to indicate that family members require physical and emotional support for continuing growth.

Table 2. Structural Definitions of Family[a]

Family of orientation	The nuclear family in which a person has had the status of child
Family of procreation	The nuclear family in which a person has or had the status of parent
Extended family	Any grouping whose members are related by descent, marriage, or adoption; broader than the nuclear family
Joint family	Various groups of nuclear families, usually related biologically, who share property rights
Polygamous family	Two or more nuclear families affiliated by plural marriage (e.g., one man and two women and progeny)

[a]From Smilkstein (1980b). Reprinted with permission of Appleton-Century-Crofts.

Family Resources

The cycle of family function is a model that reflects the manner in which family member interaction ebbs and flows in response to the impact of life events. The impact of a stressful life event on a family in health will serve as a starting point in the study of the conceptual model of the cycle of family function.

A nurturing family maintains equilibrium by utilizing its intrinsic resources on a day-to-day basis to meet the needs of its members (see Table 3). Stressful life events, however, induce a measure of disequilibrium that requires a special coping response on the part of family members. Success in coping depends primarily on the integrity of the principal family resources—social, cultural, religious, economic, educational, environmental, and medical (or technological). These resources, to which the acronym SCREEEM may be applied, are considered effective in a family when the following conditions are met:

Social interaction and communication are evident among family members. Family members also have well-balanced lines of communication to extrafamilial groups such as friends, sport groups, clubs, and other community organizations.

Cultural pride or satisfaction can be identified, especially in distinct ethnic groups.

Religion offers satisfying spiritual experiences as well as contacts with a like-minded extrafamilial support group.

Economic stability is sufficient to provide both reasonable satisfaction with financial status and an ability to meet the economic demands of usual life events.

Education of family members is adequate to allow members to solve problems that arise within the format of their life-style.

Table 3. Adaptive or Coping Behavior in Functional/Nurturing Families with Adequate Resources

Resources pooled

Points of view shared—listening skills employed

Individual growth and change accepted

Affection shared

Time, space, and money shared

Role changes accepted (orchestrated)

Nurturing family rituals utilized

Appropriate humor part of the family's life-style

Environmental conditions are such that the family is favored by clean air and water and space to satisfy its needs for work, play, and home life.

Medical or technical resources, are, in general, available through channels that are easily established and which have previously been experienced satisfactorily.

Variation in Response to Stressful Life Events

There is substantial evidence that stressful life events requiring social readjustments may lead to illness (Wolff, 1953; Dohrenwend and Dohrenwend, 1974; Gunderson and Rahe, 1974). Masuda and Holmes (1978), chief architects of the theory, cautioned that when relating life changes to illness in individuals, significant variability may be expected. They stated that, in general, there is concordance in cross-national and cross-cultural rank orderings of life events; however, "the individual's perceptions of the significance and impact of life events are clearly tempered by the uniqueness of his nature and environmental experiences." Factors identified by Masuda and Holmes as influencing the social readjustment rating scale are age, marital status, sex, ethnicity, education, and frequency of experience.

The value of relating both psychosocial stresses and resources to outcome in health care was noted by Nuckolls et al. (1972) in a study of complications of pregnancy. The study revealed that, taken alone, neither life stresses as measured by the life change units score (Masuda and Holmes, 1978; Holmes and Rahe, 1967) nor resources (Table 4) were significantly related to complications of pregnancy. However, when these

Table 4. Resources Examined in Assessing Patient's Assets[a]

Self	Ego strength, loneliness, adaptability, trust, hostility, self-esteem, crying, perception of health
Marriage	Duration of marriage, marital happiness, concordance of age and religion
Extended family	Relationship of subject with own parents, siblings, and in-laws; confidence in emotional or economic support if needed
Social resources	Adjustment to community, friendship patterns, and support
Definition of pregnancy	Extent to which pregnancy was desired or planned, feelings about pregnancy and childbirth, confidence in physician, fear of labor, anticipation of baby, confidence in outcome

[a]Adapted from Nuckolls et al. (1972).

variables were considered conjointly, women who had experienced major life stresses but who had high resource scores had only a third the complication rate of women with equal values for life stresses but low resource scores.

Transition into Crisis

Hill (1949, 1965) and colleagues (Hill and Hansen, 1960), who have made seminal contributions to the study of family function, formulated a conceptual framework for the factors that make families prone to crisis. Hill stated that, "A, the event, interacting with B, the family's crisis-meeting resources, interacting with C, the definition the family makes of the event, produces X, the crisis."

It is important to recognize that the physician who wishes to understand the family's crisis clearly must investigate factors A, B, and C. All too often stress is equated with outcome. Analysis of the stressful life events alone will not adequately facilitate understanding of the crisis. Information must also be obtained on family resources and function, as well as what Kluckholn (1958) called the family's orientation to the stressful life event that induced the crisis. Elucidation of a family's orientation to a crisis is important to the family physician, for it will help clarify the family's explanatory model or sociocultural view of an illness or psychosocial crisis (Kluckholn, 1958; Kleinman, 1975). Knowledge of the patient's explanatory model is valuable to family physicians, for it establishes the congruence of the patient's view with that of the physician. Lack of congruence may lead the family physician to attempt to resolve a family crisis with resources that the patient may consider inappropriate. The consequences are usually noncompliance and prolongation of the crisis (Lipsitt, 1970; Snow, 1974; Freud, 1946).

Families with Inadequate Resources: Pathological Defenses

When families lack adequate resources, the consequence of stressful life events may be crisis. Identification and assessment of psychosocial crises are vital functions of the family physician, for a family physician is frequently the extrafamilial resource family members call upon to assist in resolving crises.

In order to relieve the stress and pain of the chaotic feelings that result from a family crisis, family members, unable to find resources with which to appropriately cope, adopt some form of ego defense. Some of the primary defenses described by Anna Freud (1946) are listed in Table 5. Of

Table 5. Psychological Defense Mechanisms Utilized by Family Members When Resources Are Inadequate or Inappropriate for Managing a Family Crisis[a,b]

Avoidance	Postponing
Conversion	Projection
Denial	Rationalization
Displacement	Repression
Identification	Somatization
Masking	Transference

[a]These defense mechanisms may be used at times by highly functional families. In dysfunctional families the duration of use of these defense mechanisms is prolonged and the mechanisms chosen are usually more pathological (e.g., denial).
[b]From Smilkstein (1980b). Reprinted with permission of Appleton-Century-Crofts.

these, the most common defense mechanisms the physician will identify in patients are somatization and projection.

Pathological Equilibrium and Terminal Disequilibrium

Pathological equilibrium exists in those families that have accumulated a series of unresolved crises and have incorporated into their family system pathological defense mechanisms. These defenses allow some family nurturing, but the families are usually symptomatic. The physician may recognize members from families in pathological equilibrium, since they will frequently report such symptoms as depression, fighting, scapegoating, criticizing, or arguing. Although treatment of symptoms may be appropriate to ease the pain that such behavior generates, it should be recognized that the symptoms reflect the family's pathological equilibrium. Therapy, if desired by the family or family member, should be directed at the cause. The physician should identify the stressful life events and resource deficiencies that triggered the dysfunctional process. The physician who has identified the etiology of a family's problems will be in the best position to assist the family in improving its level of physical and emotional health.

It is important to recognize that diseases and medical interventions, such as hospitalizing a patient, are sources of stress for the patient and the family. These stresses may add to existing psychosocial stresses and mobilize the patient's and family's coping and defense mechanisms. If the coping abilities are marginal or pressed to the limit, then the disease and medical interventions may precipitate a crisis.

For some families, the cycle of family function is ever downward owing to failure to resolve crises, the discomfort of living with pathological defense mechanisms, and the poor nurturing environment of a family in pathological equilibrium. In this terminal state, nurturing functions are not discernible and family dissolution frequently occurs. Not all families can or should be saved, but it is hoped that a decision for termination is made after a meaningful assessment of the family's problems and their potential for improved function.

In summary, the purpose of the cycle of family function is to demonstrate how, following a stressful life event, the outcomes of family function are influenced by family resources, extrafamilial resources, and defense mechanisms.

The Biopsychosocial Formula for Health Care Outcome

Whereas the cycle of family function is designed to give emphasis to psychosocial issues related to the interaction of stressful life events and resources, the final model in this chapter is designed to give an integrated view of the biomedical and psychosocial forces at work in shaping a patient's illness behavior outcome. The components of the final formula is outlined as follows:

Biomedical risk factors	+ Psychosocial risk factors	= Predicted biomedical and illness behavior outcome
Age	Significance of stressful life event as determined by patient and members of family	
Immunological defense status, genetically and environmentally determined		
	Duration of stressful life event	
State of health prior to biomedical insult	Number of other stressful life events experienced by family, especially unresolved stressful life events	
Seriousness of insult		
Duration of biomedical insult		
	Status of family function	
	Resources of patient and family (SCREEEM items)	

Biomedical outcomes of disease processes are well described in textbooks of the various medical disciplines. Illness behavior (Kleinman et al., 1978; Kleinman and Smilkstein, 1980; Lipowski, 1976) represents an area of study that is newer to medicine and, in general, is not part of the

Table 6. Illness Behavior Problems Identified in Assessment
of Psychosocial Issues

Psychosocial issues	Examples of illness behavior problems
Stressful life events	Experience rated by family members as overwhelming, unexpected, or never before experienced
Significance of stressful life event	Viewed as threatening to ego or role function, e.g., role modification due to sickness not acceptable
Explanatory model	Stressful life event or sickness seen in narcissistic terms—only a "why me" response
Duration of stressful life event	Exhausted resources result in maladaptive behavior such as being overly dependent or demonstrating transference or somatization
	Noncompliant, passive, or hostile behavior
Resources Sociocultural/religion	Belief system of patient in conflict with that of physician, noncompliance frequently a result, e.g., religious taboo against use of blood products for therapy
Family function	Dysfunctional family with little commitment to give emotional or physical support to patient
Education	Limited education, a factor inhibiting the patient–physician negotiation of a therapuetic plan
Economical/medical	Anxiety generated by cost of medical care accentuates health problems
Environmental	Hospital environment that features restrictions, controls, and routine contrary to patient's life-style frequently results in conflict
Medical	Patient and family from medically underserved community with barriers due to poverty, language, or health belief.

routine assessment carried out by practicing physicians. Table 6 indicates some of the illness behavior problems that may be played out by patients.

The hypothesis upon which the biopsychosocial formula for health care is based is that clarification of disease and illness problems will best be found by identifying both the biomedical and the psychosocial risk factors.

The following examples highlight interaction of components of the biopsychosocial model.

1. Example of the biomedical component as the principal active variable. A 10-year-old
   child, previously in good health, reports a sore throat. The child has symptoms of fever,
   sore throat, and malaise, and medical aid is sought. A diagnosis of β-hemolytic
   streptococcus throat infection is established. There is no family history of diabetes or
   unfavorable experience with infection. The family is cohesive and functional with good
   social support.

Biomedical risk factors	+ Psychosocial risk factors	= Predicted biomedical and illness behavior outcome
Age—favorable, since child probably has already had some experience with illness and defense response established	Stressful life event and significance of stressful life event to family—little anxiety is associated with this illness, since it has been experienced before by family members with good results following therapy	Predict favorable illness behavior and medical outcome, since medical aid is sought early, patient is cooperative, and family is supportive
Genetic predisposition—favorable, since no personal family history exists to suggest hereditary problems with immunological defenses	Other stressful life events—other than for usual day-to-day encounters with stress, family is not dealing with any major unresolved conflict situations	
Biomedical insult—favorable, since child is in good state of nutrition and active in exercise.	Resources of patient and family (SCREEEM)—family is highly functional (i.e., cohesive and has economic, educational, and medical resources to manage problem)	
Seriousness of insult—epidemiological information suggests chances for complication minimum with early medical attention and treatment		

2. Example of biomedical component influenced by psychosocial variable to produce
   unexpected biomedical outcome[a]: A 10-year-old child with a history of recurrent sore
   throats (β-hemolytic streptococci cultured) reports a sore throat. Previous biomedical
   evaluations, including studies of the family, revealed no genetic or environmental
   explanation for the recurrent infections. The child was taken to the doctor early by his
   anxious parents. Later psychosocial evaluation revealed the family to be dysfunctional
   with overt evidence of parental conflict.

Biomedical risk factors	+ Psychosocial risk factors	= Predicted biomedical and illness behavior outcome
Same as for previous case, except for recurrent episodes	Stressful life event and significance of stressful life event yielded a high level of anxiety in the parents; overtly explained as consequent to the child's recurring throat infection	Biomedically unexplained recurrent β-hemolytic streptococcus throat infections may be related to
No genetic or environmental explanation for recurrent throat infections		

Other stressful life-events—family unit reflects interactional conflict between parents with a history of failure of resolution of problems	child's increased somatic vulnerability due to psychosocial family stresses and child being identified patient, a victim of the projection of parental problems
Resources (SCREEEM)—satisfactory except for poor social support group; family function perceived as poor by parents; child perceives family life as unhappy	

[a]Model based on studies of Meyer and Haggerty (1962).

The examples noted serve to illustrate how biomedical and psychosocial elements may be integrated into a formula that predicts disease and illness behavior outcome. The elements of the formula are not new to health studies. The purpose of the formula is to emphasize that just as biomedical data is gathered and weighted to allow a prognosis of outcome and to facilitate medical management, so may psychosocial data be treated; that is, a definitive psychosocial data base must be gathered and weighted and combined with biomedical data to permit optimum outcome predictions.

The rationale for this approach to health care has its historical roots in the psychosomatic writings of Dunbar (Smilkstein, 1977) and Alexander (Alexander, 1950). More recent conceptual support comes from Minuchin et al. (1975), Medalie and Goldbourt (1976), and Berkman and Syme (1979). The reason for the failure of general application of the bio-psychosocial approach to health care is complex; however, the solution may lie in the present difficulty of demonstrating how psychosocial components may be identified and weighted in a utilitarian manner.

The Future of the Biopsychosocial Model in Health Care

The future of biopsychosocial medicine may require that we learn how to apply that which we have been given. The elemental components of the psychosocial data base have been enunciated by Hill (1949) and Hill and Hansen (1960) (stressful life events, the significance of the stressful life events, and the resources available to the patient and family). Through the years, these basic components of psychosocial analysis have maintained that their worth in crisis analysis are felt to be essential to the physician's assessment of the influence of psychosocial factors on a patient's health status (Imig, 1981).

The identification and weighting of stressful life events have already been pioneered by Masuda and Holmes (1978) and Holmes and Rahe (1967). The principle of the significance of stressful life events was established by Kluckholn (1958) and Hill and Hansen (1960). Modern investigators feel the most accurate way to weight the significance of a stressful life event is to require the patient and family members to give their personal assessment of the impact of life change induced by the stressful life event (Sarason et al., 1978). The final component in the formula, resources, is being studied to ascertain its impact on biopsychosocial health status. It is likely that social support, primarily family and friends, will prove to be the resource that most significantly moderates stress (Nuckolls et al., 1972; Cobb, 1976).

Summary

The worth of a biopsychosocial approach to health care has been established by numerous investigators. The resistance in practice to the application of the unified concept to health/illness assessment is probably related to the need for a utilitarian approach. The three models offered in this chapter give an instructional basis for students and teachers interested in the biopsychosocial approach to health care. The future application of the concept depends on the development of pragmatic techniques for the gathering and weighting of a data base that integrates the biomedical and the psychosocial.

References

Alexander, F. 1950. Psychomatic Medicine: Its Principles and Applications. New York: W. W. Norton.

Bauman, M. H., and N. T. Grace. 1977. Family process and family practice. Journal of Family Practice 1:24–26.

Berkman, L. F., and S. L. Syme. 1979. Social networks, host resistance, and mortality: A nine-year follow-up study of Alameda County residents. American Journal of Epidemiology 109:196–204.

Breslow, L. 1972. The organization of personal health services. Milbank Memorial Fund Quarterly 50:365.

Cobb, S. 1976. Social support as a moderator of life stress. Psychosomatic Medicine 38:300–314.

Cowan, D. L., and J. A. Sbarbaro. 1972. Family-centered health care: A viable reality? Medical Care 10:164–172.

Crawford, C. O. 1971. The family and health: A paradigm for analysis of interface dynamics. In C. O. Crawford, ed.: Health and the Family. New York: Macmillan.

Curry, H. B. 1977. The family as our patient. Journal of Family Practice 4:757–759.

Dohrenwend, B. S., and B. P. Dohrenwend. 1974. Stressful Life Events: Their Nature and Effect. New York: Wiley.

Engel, G. L. 1977. The need for a new medical model: A challenge for biomedicine. Science 196:129–136.

Engel, G. L. 1980. The clinical application of the biopsychosocial model. American Journal of Psychiatry 137:535–544.

Freud, A. 1946. The Ego and the Mechanisms of Defense. New York: International Universities Press.

Froom, J., L. Culpepper, C. R. Kirkwood, V. Boisseau, and D. Mangone. 1977. An integrated medical record and data system for primary care, Part 4: Family information. Journal of Family Practice 5:265–270.

Geyman, J. P. 1977. The family as the object of care in family practice. Journal of Family Practice 5:571.

Good, M. J. D., G. Smilkstein, B. S. Good, T. Shaffer, and T. Arons. 1979. The family APGAR index: A study of construct validity. Journal of Family Practice 8:577–582.

Gore, S. 1978. The effect of social support in moderating health consequences of unemployment. Journal of Health and Social Behavior 19:157–165.

Grace, N. T., E. M. Neal, C. E. Wellock, and D. D. Pile. 1977. The family-oriented medical record. Journal of Family Practice 4:91.

Gunderson, E. K. E., and R. H. Rahe, (eds). 1974. Life Stress and Illness. Philadelphia, Pennsylvania: Charles C. Thomas.

Haggerty, R. J., and J. J. Alpert. 1963. The child, his family, and illness. Postgraduate Medicine 34:228.

Hill, R. 1949. Families Under Stress. New York: Harper and Brothers.

Hill, R. 1965. Generic features of families under stress. In H. J. Parad, ed.: Crisis Intervention. New York: Family Service Association of America.

Hill, R., and S. A. Hansen. 1960. The identification of conceptual frameworks utilized in family study. Marriage and Family Living 22:299–311.

Holmes, T. H., and H. Rahe. 1967. The social readjustment rating scale. Journal of Psychosomatic Research 11:213–218.

Imig, D. R. 1981. Accumulated stress of life changes and interpersonal effectiveness in the family. Family Relations 30:367–371.

Kleinman, A. M. 1975. Explanatory models in health care. In Proceedings of International Health Conference 1974: Health of the Family. Washington, D. C.: National Council for International Health.

Kleinman, A. M., and G. Smilkstein. 1980. Psychosocial issues. In G. M. Rosen, J. P. Geyman, and R. H. Layton, eds.: Behavioral Science in Family Practice. New York: Appleton-Century-Crofts.

Kleinman, A. M., L. Eisenberg, and B. Good. 1978. Culture, illness and care: Clinical lessons from anthropologic and cross-cultural research. Annals of Internal Medicine 88:251–258.

Kluckholn, F. R. 1958. Variations in the basic values of family systems. Social Casework 39:63.

Lee, P. R. 1974. What are comprehensive health services? Israeli Journal of Medical Science 10:55–66.

Lipowski, Z. J. 1976. Physical illness, the individual and the coping process. Psychiatry in Medicine 1:91–102.

Lipsitt, D. R. 1970. Medical and psychological characteristics of "crocks." Psychiatry in Medicine 1:15.

Litman, T. J. 1974. The family as a basic unit in health and medical care: A social–behavioral overview. Social Sciences and Medicine 8:495–519.

McWhinney, I. R. 1972. An approach to the integration of behavioral science and clinical medicine. New England Journal of Medicine 298:384–387.

Masuda, M., and T. H. Holmes. 1978. Life events: perceptions and frequencies. Psychosomatic Medicine 40:236–261.

Mauksch, H. O. 1974. A social science basis for conceptualizing family health. Social Sciences and Medicine 8:521–528.

Medalie, J. A., and U. Goldbourt. 1976. Angina pectoris among 10,000 men: II. Psychosocial and other risk factors as evidenced by a multivariate analysis of a five-year incidence study. American Journal of Medicine 60:910–921.

Meyer, R. J., and R. J. Haggerty. 1962. Streptococcal infections in family. Pediatrics 29:539–549.

Minuchin, S. 1974. Families and Family Therapy. Cambridge, Massachusetts: Commonwealth Fund, Harvard University Press.

Minuchin, S., L. Baker, B. L. Rosman, R. Liebman, L. Milman, and T. C. Todd. 1975. A conceptual model of psychosomatic illness in children. Archives of General Psychiatry 32:1031–1038.

Murphy, M. J. 1975. The development of a community health orientation scale. American Journal of Public Health 65:1293–1297.

Nuckolls, C. H., J. Cassel, and B. H. Kaplan. 1972. Psychosocial assets, life crises and the prognosis of pregnancy. American Journal of Epidemiology 95:431.

Pratt, L. 1976. Family Structure and Effective Health Behavior: The Energized Family. Boston, Massachusetts: Houghton Mifflin.

Ransom, D. C., and H. E. Vandervoort. 1973. The development of family medicine: Problematic trends. Journal of American Medical Association 225:1098–1102.

Richardson, H. 1945. Patients Have Families. New York: Commonwealth Fund.

Sarason, I. G., H. G. Johnson, and H. M. Siegel. 1978. Assessing the impact of life changes: Development of the life experience survey. Journal of Consulting and Clinical Psychology 46:932–946.

Schmidt, D. D. 1978. The family as the unit of medical care. Journal of Family Practice 7:303–313.

Smilkstein, G. 1977. A model for teaching comprehensive health care. Journal of Medical Education 52:773–775.

Smilkstein, G. 1978a. The Family APGAR: A proposal for a family function test and its use by physicians. Journal of Family Practice 6:1231–1239.

Smilkstein, G. 1978b. The family in crisis. In R. D. Taylor, ed.: Family Medicine: Principles and Practice. New York: Springer-Verlag.

Smilkstein, G. 1980a. Assessment of family function. In G. A. Rosen, J. P. Geyman, and R. H. Layton, eds.: Behavioral Science in Family Practice. New York: Appleton-Century-Crofts.

Smilkstein, G. 1980b. The cycle of family function: A conceptual model for family medicine. Journal of Family Practice 11:223–232.

Snow, L. 1974. Folk medical belief and their implications for care of patients: A review based on studies among black Americans. Annals of Internal Medicine 81:82–96.

Somers, H. M., and A. R. Somers. 1961. Doctors, Patients and Health Insurance: The Organization and Financing of Medical Care. Washington, DC: The Brookings Institution.

Weed, L. L. 1968. Medical records that guide and teach. New England Journal of Medicine 278:593–600.

Wolff, H. G. 1953. Stress and Disease. Springfield, Illinois: Charles C. Thomas.

9

Behavioral Medicine:
Basic Concepts and Clinical Applications

John E. Carr, Ph. D.,* Dean Funabiki, Ph. D.,† and
Harold A. Dengerink Ph. D.‡

Knowledge of behavioral medicine concepts and clinical application of
these principles are emerging as essential components of competent
medical practice. In recent years major interdisciplinary organizations for
the development of behavioral medicine have been established, (e.g., The
Academy of Behavioral Medicine, The Society of Behavioral Medicine),
specialized journals (e.g., *The Journal of Behavioral Medicine, Behavioral
Medicine Abstracts*) now publish a proliferation of research-based articles
relevant to the field, and an increasing number of books on behavioral
medicine are now being published. As in the development of any
interdisciplinary field, there is the risk of conceptual ambiguity and
confusion resulting from differences among the various disciplines in
knowledge base and definitions of basic concepts.

At present, the most precise definition for behavioral medicine has been
proposed by Pomerleau and Brady (1979, p. xii):

> (a) the clinical use of techniques derived from the experimental analysis of
> behavior—behavior therapy and behavior modification—for the evaluation,
> prevention, management, or treatment of physical disease of physiological
> dysfunction; and (b) the conduct of research contributing to the functional
> analysis and understanding of behavior associated with medical disorders and
> problems in health care.

It should be noted that this conceptualization assumes that behavioral

*Professor and Acting Chairman, Department of Psychiatry and Behavioral Sciences,
University of Washington School of Medicine, Seattle, Washington.
† Assistant Professor, Department of Psychology, Washington State University, Pullman,
Washington.
‡ Professor and Director of Clinical Training, Department of Psychology, Washington State
University, Pullman, Washington.

principles derived from the particular specialities of behavior therapy and behavior modification, rather than from the behavioral sciences in general (e.g., personality theory, medical sociology, and cultural anthropology), play a significant historical role in the development of behavioral medicine. Although the other behavioral sciences undoubtedly have an important impact on medical practice, these disciplines "have constituted a necessary but not sufficient condition for the development of behavioral medicine" (Pomerleau and Brady, 1979, p. xii). The remainder of this chapter will provide a short review of basic behavioral concepts and then describe selected behavioral medicine interventions.

Basic Concepts

Behavior

Behaviors may be defined as any activity of an individual that can be observed or measured, and may include overt, motoric, or verbal responses involving the striated musculature (e.g., engaging in physical exercises, taking medications, swallowing liquids, making grimaces or verbalizations of physical discomfort or pain), as well as internal responses involving the glandular or smooth musculature (e.g., heartbeats, bladder distension, vasoconstriction, pupillary dilation). From this perspective behavior is a very broad category of events ranging from ones that may be organ specific to others which may be actions of the whole organism.

Thus it can be seen that behavioral and biological processes may combine and interact in the medical arena. From the biological perspective, elevations in blood pressure may be seen as the result of disease processes (atherosclerosis, kidney failure) or the result of either the baroceptor reflex or of the renin–angiotensin–aldosterone system. From a behavioral perspective such blood pressure elevations may be seen as one component of emotional behaviorals, such as anxiety or fear, resulting from stressful environmental conditions. Both perspectives are correct, but each alone is insufficient. The importance of the interaction is evident when one considers that many disease processes (obesity for example) are the result of patient behaviors and that most medical interventions require some behavior change on the part of the patient.

For both practical and scientific reasons, certain limitations are frequently placed on the category of events referred to as behavior. The term behavior is limited to actions that are measurable. A principle reason for limiting the class of behaviors to observable or verifiable ones is to avoid the trap of misattribution. For example, assume that a 57-year-old man has been hospitalized following emergency surgery for kidney stones. The man has proven to be a difficult patient on the ward, frequently using the call button, demanding that his doctors be summoned immediately and threatening to check out against medical advice. In this example threats to leave the hospital and pushing the call button would be considered as behaviors that in turn may be dependent upon emotional behaviors or states. However, one could attribute these behaviors to either fear, anger, or boredom, all with equal accuracy. The man may be able to verbalize his emotions to provide some more objective measure of his underlying emotional state, but his descriptions may be inaccurate or he may not be able to provide that information (e.g. following a stroke). Acting upon the assumption that the behaviors reflect boredom will result in very different interventions than will the assumption that they reflect fear. Such misattributions can be avoided if one limits consideration to only events that are observable either directly or through the aid of instrumentation. The important issue is not the restriction of behaviors considered, but the emphasis on the verification of the behavior's occurrence and on the avoidance of assumptions concerning their causes.

KINDS OF BEHAVIOR

Two basic kinds of behavior have been identified. These are operant and respondent behaviors. Respondent behaviors are those that occur only in response to some stimulus. They are usually considered to be involuntary and behaviors classified as such are often reflexes like the leg jerk in response to a pin prick during a neurological exam. Respondent behaviors are often (though not necessarily) limited to organ systems rather than being responses of the whole organism. The consistent distinguishing feature, however, is that these are behaviors that *require* some preceding stimulus.

Operant behaviors are so classified because they have some effect upon (operate on) and may be affected by the environment. They may occur in response to a stimulus event, but the distinguishing feature is that they are controlled by events that follow the behavior rather than by events that precede it. They are typically considered to be voluntary behaviors and are sometimes referred to as being emitted rather than elicited. To some extent this distinction is arbitrary, since any given behavior sequence will likely include components of both. For example, as will be seen later, chronic pain problems may incorporate both respondent and operant pain behaviors. The behavioral reactions to nociceptive stimuli are respondent and may include alterations in posture or gait as a consequence of the pain. At the same time persons may emit postural or gait behavior in order to avoid painful experiences, the latter being operant behaviors. The distinction between operant and respondent behaviors is important to the physician because the procedures required to change these two classes of behavior are different.

ACQUISITION OF BEHAVIOR

Respondent Behavior. Although respondent behaviors may begin as reflexes, they are not static, rather, they change in magnitude or intensity, frequency, and latency as a result of changes in the stimuli that elicit them and in the conditions which surround them. The procedure for modifying such stimuli requires pairing the stimulus that initially elicited the behavior—the unconditional stimulus (US)—with another stimulus—the conditional stimulus (CS)—for a series of presentations.

For example, if a nail in your shoe causes you to limp for several days, you may find yourself limping whenever you put on that pair of shoes, even after the nail has been removed. This is most likely to occur if you are not aware that the nail has been removed. Reactions like pain behaviors may be conditioned to otherwise neutral stimuli. All that is necessary is that the CS occur along with the US for a series of trials. The conditional pain behavior is most likely to occur if the CS occurs just slightly before the US.

Another example is that of conditioned hypoglycemia. Woods (1976) has demonstrated that measured blood sugar levels decrease in the presence of an olfactory stimulus (the conditioned stimulus) when that smell was repeatedly paired with insulin injections (the unconditioned stimulus for hypoglycemia). The decreased serum glucose levels then may function as stimuli for eating and may contribute to obesity (Rodin, 1977).

Operant Behavior. The acquisition of operant behavior is, at least conceptually, more complex than that of respondent behaviors. Since operant behaviors are distinguished by and controlled by their effect on the environment, the primary mechanism for changing or acquiring these behaviors is to modify the consequences. Patients who continue to smoke do so because the act provides them with some positive social consequences or physiological effects. Pain patients may take increasing dosages of medications because doing so permits them to escape from the pain or discomfort they experienced.

There are several different categories of consequences that are important in the acquisition of operant behaviors. *Reinforcement* is any event or stimulus consequence that increases the strength or probability of the behavior that it follows. The maximum effect occurs when the reinforcement follows the behavior immediately. Positive reinforcement refers to events that, when applied, increase the likelihood of the behaviors on which they are contingent. Money, praise, favorite foods, and so on, are clear reinforcers, at least for some persons and in some circumstances. But so may be other events such as television viewing, driving a car (particularly for teenagers), or finding out that you were correct in answering quiz items. It is important to recognize that positive reinforcement is defined by the procedures and effect (increasing the likelihood of behavior).

Negative reinforcement refers to events that, when withdrawn or withheld, have the effect of increasing the likelihood of the behavior upon which it is contingent. Persons will engage in a wide variety of behaviors in order to escape from an unpleasant or aversive event, such as criticism, work, or pain. Again, the criteria for considering something as a negative reinforcer is defined by the procedure (withholding some event) and the consequence (increases likelihood of behaviors). Negative reinforcement can result in behaviors that appear to be bizarre if one is unaware of the person's history—particularly in an avoidance situation, where the reinforcer is never presented. The casual observer may thus be unaware of the consequences because the person's behavior prevents their occurrence.

Punishment is likewise defined by its effect on behavior. Punishment results in a decrease in the frequency or magnitude of behavior, in contrast to reinforcement, which results in an increase. One form of punishment that has proven to be very effective in modifying children's behavior is "time out." Time out refers to a procedure of withholding or eliminating reinforcers for behavior one wishes to reduce in frequency or eliminate, such as fighting. Frequently time out is employed by requiring that the child sit for 5 minutes in the bathroom (without destroying the fixtures) after each objectional behavior such as a temper tantrum.

Punishment and negative reinforcement are both effective procedures for changing behavior. They are particularly useful when some immediate change in behavior is desired. They have some negative attributes, however. Their effectiveness in producing immediate change can be very reinforcing to the change agent and their use by that person may increase (owing to reinforcement). The person who is repeatedly subjected to negative reinforcement or punishment may (insofar as possible) learn to avoid not just the consequences, but the change agent as well. Particularly in voluntary relationships such as that between a physician and a patient, avoidance of the change agent rather than modification of the behavior may be the most likely behavior change. Finally, the use of aversive means of changing behavior may result in imitation by the recipient of the procedures. Thus parents who rely extensively on coercive means of behavior change will find that their children use similar techniques to influence siblings, friends, and parents.

Other Basic Concepts

There are several additional concepts that are important for understanding the basic principles of behavior modification. One of these is the distinction between primary and secondary reinforcements or punishments. Primary refers to events that have their effects on behavior without any prior conditioning. These usually are related to certain biological processes and reflexes and include food, water, warmth, sexual stimulation, and pain. The term *secondary* refers to consequences that have their effect because of previous association with primary consequences. These are all "learned" consequences and include social attention, praise, money, social disapproval, and so on.

Operant conditioning results most rapidly if the reinforcement occurs every time the behavior occurs, a condition referred to as continuous reinforcement. Reinforcement that is intermittent (occurring only periodically after the behavior) results in slower learning, but the resultant behavior is more permanent, or more difficult to eliminate, than in the case with continuous reinforcement. In fixed-ratio schedules reinforcement occurs after the target behavior has been emitted a *fixed* number of times. In variable-ratio schedules the reinforcement occurs after the behavior has been emitted a *varible* number of times. Fixed-interval reinforcement provides a consequence for the first target behavior that occurs after a given time period. Variable-interval reinforcement has a time contingency, like fixed-interval reinforcement, but the interval can vary within certain defined limits.

In addition to providing more durable behaviors, schedules of partial reinforcement also help to avoid the problem of satiation. Continued use of reinforcement at a high rate will deplete the reinforcement value of that consequence. Too much food, candy, water, praise, and so forth, will obviously deplete the reinforcing value of those events.

Another important concept in reinforcement is the principle of "shaping." Frequently some desired response, particularly a set of complex responses (e.g., an exercise regimen prescribed for a pain patient), is not likely to be fully realized and therefore reinforced. Instead, approximations to the desired terminal response are successively reinforced. In this way, behaviors that gradually assume the nature or frequency of the terminal response are successfully shaped.

It was noted earlier that respondent behaviors, as opposed to operant ones, are controlled by stimuli, or preceding events. But stimuli have an important function for operant behaviors as well. Stimuli act as cues for operant behaviors. They are signs or indications that reinforcement is available in this situation. Thus one will learn that behavior of a given kind may "work" (lead to reinforcement) in one situation and not in another. People learn to respond to threats because these threats indicate that a punisher or negative reinforcement will follow. People may learn to describe their physical complaints to a physician but not to friends because the former and not the latter is able to provide some relief (negative reinforcement.)

This phenomenon of persons learning to respond in the presence of some stimuli and not in the presence of others is referred to as discrimination. A related concept is that of generalization. Generalization occurs when one learns to respond in the presence of one stimulus and then emits that behavior in the presence of similar stimuli. Thus one may acquire the habit of taking analgesics for nociceptive pains and generalize by taking similar medications for other discomforts, such as frustrations or anxiety.

A special class of stimulus events is referred to as modeling. Modeling simply refers to the behavior of a person that may then be imitated by another. This is a special class of stimuli because it can be used to prompt and markedly accelerate the acquisition of behaviors. It is especially useful in teaching novel and complex behaviors.

Some Clinical Applications
of Behavioral Principles

The remainder of this chapter will attempt to illustrate a selected sample of medical problems to which behavioral principles have been applied; each study will convey to the reader an application of the basic behavioral principles. The studies that will be considered here will not delineate the technical aspects involved in determining a treatment program and evaluating gains; more comprehensive treatment of behavior modification principles and applications are discussed elsewhere (e.g., Rimm and Masters, 1979; Bandura, 1969). The reader interested in more intensive treatment of behavioral medicine is referred to more specialized texts, such as those by Ferguson and Taylor (1980–1981), Pomerleau and Brady (1979), Katz and Zlutnick (1975), and Rachman (1977).

Broadly speaking, many medically relevant behaviors are maintained by their consequences. Although some behaviors, such as asthmatic responding, a knee buckle or limp, or a pain grimace, may have initially started as respondents to nociception, they may be readily maintained as operants as a result of consequences of their occurrence, such as attention, time out from some aversive activity, and the like. Fordyce (1976), in his comprehensive book on behavioral conceptualizations for chronic pain syndromes, identified several sources of reinforcement for pain behaviors. Some of these may be conceptualized as positive reinforcement of pain behavior (e.g., attention, a back rub, the bringing of a heating pad, or medication), compensation and litigation issues, iatrogenic reinforcement (medications or therapy on a PRN basis), negative reinforcement of pain behavior (e.g., discontinuing or avoiding exercise, household chores, or work activity that is unpleasant), and nonreinforcement of healthy behavior (e.g., excessive prescription for rest and activity restriction).

The importance of identifying and seeking to change consequences for illness behaviors is illustrated in the case study (Munford and Liberman, 1978) of a 13-year-old boy who developed a fever with coughing. Although he was not febrile a week later, the cough persisted. During waking hours the cough rate was 20–40 coughs per minute and this continued for a period of 6 months. Psychosocially, the patient was experiencing difficulties in adjusting to a new school and showing deficiencies in age-appropriate social skills. In addition, because of the coughing, he was excused from school and was permitted to receive school instruction at home. With no biomedical evidence of pathology, an inpatient operant program was instituted in which the coughing was ignored and age-appropriate behaviors other than coughing were rewarded with praise, attention, and points toward discharge. Following four treatment days, the cough rate decreased to zero, except for a slight increase to one to three coughs per minute just prior to discharge. To generalize treatment effects to the home setting, several parent training sessions were conducted to teach the parents to provide differential attention to coughing and other behaviors. That is, rather than attend to their son's coughing, the parents were trained to ignore the coughing while attending to appropriate social and other healthy behaviors. The patient remained symptom free at 3-year follow-up. In this case, there were two important indicators that the coughing was an operant behavior: (1) The patient did not cough when asleep and did not awaken from sleep and (2) the rate of monitored coughing was much higher when he knew he was being observed (an average of 2.07 coughs per 2 minutes) than when he was unaware (0.44 coughs per 2 minutes).

Operant principles of reinforcement have also been shown to be important factors in the maintenance of certain cases of asthma. Asthma has an incidence of approximately 5% in the general population and is the leading cause of restricted activity among those under 17 years of age (Hindi-Alexander, 1974). The role of parental factors in the reinforcement of asthmatic responding was demonstrated in the case study reported by Neisworth and Moore (1972). The patient, a 7-year-old boy, was diagnosed as asthmatic at age 6 months and had a history of frequent hospitalization, for periods of 1–4 weeks at a time, for asthmatic episodes. Despite seeing a medical specialist on a monthly basis from ages 2 to 7, and despite various medications and dietary restrictions, the asthmatic responding persisted. A behavioral analysis suggested that the parents provided a great deal of attention for asthmatic symptoms, and asthmatic responding increased when more attention was given.

The parents were trained to ignore asthmatic behaviors, such as coughing and wheezing, while simultaneously reinforcing behaviors incompatible with asthma attacks. This resulted in a dramatic decrement in asthma attacks, which increased when a reversal was imposed (the original contingencies for asthmatic responding were reinstated). Continuation of treatment reduced asthmatic responding considerably, with therapeutic effects maintained at an 11-month follow-up with no apparent negative side effects. The treatment of asthma using behavioral methods has been described further by Alexander and Solach (1981) and a more extensive consideration of the major applications of behavioral approaches in pediatrics has been presented by Christophersen and Rapoff (1980, 1979).

Risch and Ferguson (1981) have critically reviewed current behavioral applications in treating skin disorders, including neurodermatitis and other psychosomatic dermatoses and trichotillomania. Their major conclusion was that a wide variety of skin disorders of long-standing duration and that were recalcitrant to biomedical approaches "were significantly improved and often 'cured' by the use of behavioral treatments" (p. 269). Various behavioral techniques have been employed for treating skin disorders. Some programs were designed to treat stress-related conditions concomitant to the dermatoses and included training in progressive muscle relaxation, systematic desensitization, and assertive training. Others more directly involved operant conditioning procedures, such as positive reinforcement, negative reinforcement, and aversive conditioning (contingent presentation of an aversive stimulus). A salient feature in most dermatoses is scratching behavior, which can be a major factor in causing or aggravating the condition. As Risch and Ferguson (1981) pointed out, the pruritus, erythema, and papules characteristic of neurodermatitis are exacerbated by scratching, which produces abrasions, lichenification, and scaling. Case studies involving both adults (e.g., Walton, 1960) and children (e.g., Allen and Harris, 1966; Bar and Kuypers, 1973) have demonstrated that in some instances even simple attentional factors may maintain the scratching behaviors; differential attention (by the child's parents or the adult's spouse) for nonscratching behaviors resulted in cessation of scratching. Similarly, Dobes (1977) implemented a behavior self-modification program in which the patient, a 28-year-old female with a 15-year history of an itchy, inflamed rash on the back of her neck, solicited social reinforcement from peers for instances of decreased scratching behavior. The eczema improved, with scratching decreasing steadily across 4 weeks, from a base-line rate of 70 instances per day to 0. There was a period when the rate increased to 13 instances per day, which coincided with the patient's mother visiting. However, the rate decreased shortly thereafter, and subsequent visits apparently had no adverse effect. Extinction of the scratching behavior, along with amelioration of the eczema, was maintained at 2-year follow-up.

Another behavioral strategy that has been applied to reduce scratching behaviors is the shaping of resonses that are incompatible to scratching. For example, Watson et al. (1972) described the treatment of a patient with a 17-year history of eczema. Treatment required the patient to first develop the dominant response of stroking, instead of scratching, the affected area. Once this behavior was well established, the patient substituted touching instead of stroking. At this point, the patient was able to extinguish the touching response entirely.

Considerable progress has been made in defining effective behavioral programs for treating obesity. Weight control programs (e.g., Stuart, 1972) typically include multiple components for treatment. Self-monitoring procedures are used in which the patient learns to monitor and record caloric intake as well as body weight on a daily basis. An exercise regimen, implemented in the context of a reward system, along with behavioral skills training to change specific eating behaviors (e.g., changing the topography of eating behaviors, such as an increased number of chews, is usually included). Finally, principles of conditioning are imposed in placing eating behavior under stimulus control. For example, the patient learns to eat meals only at certain times and places, for example, mealtimes, at the kitchen table, or seated at a particular chair. Weight control is discussed more thoroughly in Chapter 10 by Brigham and Dengerink.

Numerous single-subject design programs describing successful behavioral treatment of anorexia nervosa have been reported, along with some group studies, most notably the Stanford Program (Agras and Werne, 1977). Vigersky's (1977) edited text is an excellent source of background reading on anorexia nervosa. In his recent review of behavioral treatments for anorexia nervosa, Ferguson (1981) identified several factors that appear important in treatment, such as careful patient and family preparation for a contingency contract, wherein specific goals for weight gain are specified. Desired behaviors are positively reinforced in inpatient programs, with increased access to attention and pleasurable activities, and negatively reinforced by fewer restrictions. High-rate behaviors, such as physical exercise and watching television, are identified and made contingent on low-rate behaviors, like consuming a greater variety and larger amounts of foods; high-probability behaviors can be used to accelerate low-probability behaviors, a principle of learning termed the "Premack principle" (Premack, 1959).

In one noteworthy study, Garfinkel et al. (1973) treated five hospitalized female anorexia nervosa patients, each of whom had a weight loss of greater than 25% of normal body weight, an aversion to food with "conscious dietary restriction," and amenorrhea. Individually tailored programs for each patient were developed, involving a system of positive reinforcement for attainment of daily and weekly weight gains. Rewards included physical activity, opportunities for socializing off the ward, and other privileges. Rapid weight gain was observed in each patient, with a minimization of patient discomfort and no reported side effects. However, there is a paucity of follow-up studies; the available data strongly suggest that greater attention should be given to programming maintenance of therapeutic gains once the patient leaves the hospital setting. It appears that frequent information feedback to the patient, with regard to attainment of goals (e.g., caloric intake) is also important. As Kellerman (1977) correctly noted, because of the seriousness of the problem, behavioral programs for anorexia nervosa, although the treatment of choice, need be carefully implemented. Finally, Ferguson (1981) underscored the importance of dealing with interpersonal and other psychosocial factors in working with this patient group.

Taylor (1981) identified several areas where behavioral approaches show promise in the treatment of gastrointestinal problems, including persistent vomiting and nausea, diarrhea, irritable bowel syndrome, fecal incontinence, and peptic ulcer disease. One noteworthy application is illustrated by the development of effective treatments for ruminative vomiting in infants, a life-threatening condition. The death rate has been reported to be as high as 20% owing to malnutrition and dehydration. Some reports have demonstrated success in treating this disorder with the contingent application of aversive electrical stimulation (e.g., Lang and Melamed, 1969; Cunningham et al. 1976). Behaviors related to ruminative vomiting are frequently chained, such that a stereotypic, distinct set of precursor responses reliably occur just prior to ruminations. Sajwaj and colleagues squirted lemon juice into the infant's mouth when he began tongue-thrusting movements; ruminations were reduced dramatically. It appears, given certain cautions in treatment (see Ruprecht et al., 1980; Rast et al., 1981), that this aversive conditioning procedure may be the treatment of choice for this disorder.

The interruption of chained behaviors as a form of treatment has been applied to other clinical problems as well, most notably in the treatment of functional seizure disorders. Zlutnick et al. (1975) treated patients for epileptic seizures. Each patient exhibited seizures at least once a day. Baseline data were collected to clearly identify chained behaviors that reliably preceded seizures. These preseizure behaviors were punished with an aversive stimulus. For example, for one adolescent patient this required that the classroom teacher, upon observing a stiffening of the arms and staring behavior, would immediately shake the boy and command him to stop. Marked decreases in the seizures were demonstrated for four of the five patients; effects were maintained at follow-up.

Other Applications

Noncompliance rates to prescribed medical regimens are known to vary from 20 to 80%, with an overall average of 50% noncompliance (Pomerleau, 1979). A number of factors are believed to influence patient compliance, including the patient's motivation, education, and information level; the quality of the physician–patient relationship; environmental factors; as well as the complexity of the regimen (Dunbar and Agras, 1980; Ley, 1977; Haynes et al., 1979). Recently the Surgeon General's Report (Public Health Service, 1979) identified patient compliance as a major goal of future efforts in medicine. Weinstein and Stason (1976) determined that, from a cost–benefit standpoint, funds directed toward improving compliance of hypertensive patients to their drug regimen would have greater clinical impact than the same amount directed toward identifying and treating new cases of hypertension. Dunbar and Agras (1980) described a number of strategies, many of which are based on behavioral principles, to improve patient compliance.

Prevention strategies represent another major application of behavioral medicine concepts. Primary prevention programs are designed to change the life-style behaviors that are likely to result in reduced risk for medical problems. Targets for change may include, for example, behaviors related to diet, level of physical activity, smoking, and alcohol intake (Pomerleau, 1979). The three-community study by Nash and Farquhar (1980) is a prime example of applying behavioral principles in a preventive program. In that program a comprehensive, media-based information, education, and behavioral skills acquisition program was implemented to alter behaviors that would reduce the risk for heart disease. Residents of the communities received information via a media campaign (e.g., radio and television spots, newspaper stories and columns by physicians and dieticians) and/or more intensive, face-to-face instruction and modeling of behavioral skills training for reducing risk. The general results were quite promising and demonstrated the cost effectiveness of developing methods for promoting behavior change on a large-scale basis.

Another trend in behavioral medicine is the preparation of patients for invasive or highly stressful medical interventions, such as surgery or diagnostic procedures. For example, Melamed and Siegel (1975) reported the effective use of modeling procedures to reduce pre- and postoperative fear arousal among children about to undergo surgery for hernias, tonsillectomies, and urinogenital tract problems. The children in the treatment group viewed a therapeutic modeling film that depicted a peer being hospitalized and receiving surgery. The peer modeling nonfearful behaviors that served to reduce anxiety responses.

Biofeedback involves direct feedback of physiological responses to the patient. This includes, for example, electromyography (EMG), galavanic skin response (GSR), and skin temperature ("thermal") feedback for treating a variety of problems related to the musculoskeletal system (e.g., stress-related disorders, tension headaches, temporomandibular joint syndrome), the cardiovascular system (e.g., essential hypertension, migraine headaches, cardiac arrhythmias, Raynaud's disease), the respiratory system (e.g., asthma,), and the gastrointestinal system (e.g., peptic ulcers, functional diarrhea, spastic colon). A comprehensive review of biofeedback treatments, in the context of relaxation training, has been offered by Silver and Blanchare (1978). Additionally, Steger (Chapter 14) reviews the use of biofeedback in medicine.

Conclusion

This chapter provides a review of basic behavioral principles and examples of their application to medical practice. The examples do not nearly begin to cover the variety of patient behaviors that may be modified by behavioral techniques; nor are they intended to describe rigid regimes which should be applied in similar cases. Rather, the physician, with a basic understanding of the principles, will find it necessary to design tailored programs for specific problems. Such behavioral interventions can clearly be a major adjunct to the typical physician's skills. As the examples demonstrate, significant improvement in health can be achieved by judicious use of these behavioral principles.

References

Agras, S., and J. Werner. 1977. Behavior modification in anorexia nervosa, research foundation. *In* R. A. Vigersky, ed.: Anorexia Nervosa. New York: Raven Press.

Alexander, A. B., and L. S. Solanch. Psychological aspects in the understanding and treatment of bronchial asthma. *In* J. M. Ferguson and C. B. Taylor, eds.: The Comprehensive Handbook of Behavioral Medicine, Vol. 2. New York: SP Medical and Scientific Books.

Allen, K. E., and F. R. Harris. 1966. Elimination of a child's excessive scratching by training the mother in reinforcement procedures. Behaviour Research and Therapy 4:79–84.

Bandura, A. 1969. Principles of Behavior Modification. New York: Holt, Rinehart and Winston.

Bar, H. J., and B. R. M. Kuypers. 1973. Behavior therapy in dermatological practice. British Journal of Dermatology 88:591–598.

Christophersen, E.R., and M. A. Rapoff. 1979. Behavioral pediatrics. *In* O. F. Pomerleau and J. P. Brady, eds.: Behavioral Medicine: Theory and Practice. Baltimore, Maryland: Williams and Wilkins. pp. 99–123.

Christophersen, E. R., and M. A. Rapoff. 1980. Biosocial pediatrics. *In* J. M. Ferguson and C. B. Taylor, eds.: The Comprehensive Handbook of Behavioral Medicine, Vol. 3. New York: SP Medical and Scientific Books.

Cunningham, C. and T. Linscheid. 1976. Elimination of chronic infant ruminating by electric shock. Behavior Therapy 7:231–234.

Dobes, R. W. 1977. Amelioration of psychosomatic dermatosis by reinforced inhibition of scratching. Journal of Behavior Therapy and Experimental Psychiatry 8:185–187.

Dunbar, J. M., and W. S. Agras. 1980. Compliance with medical instructions. *In* J. M. Ferguson and C. B. Taylor, eds.: The Comprehensive Handbook of Behavioral Medicine, Vol. 3. New York: SP Medical and Scientific Books.

Ferguson, J. 1981. The behavioral treatment of anorexia nervosa. *In* J. M. Ferguson and C. B. Taylor, eds.: The Comprehensive Handbook of Behavioral Medicine, Vol. 2. New York: SP Medical and Scientific Books.

Ferguson, J. M., and C. B. Taylor. (eds.). 1980–1981. The Comprehensive Handbook of Behavioral Medicine, Vols. 1–3. New York: SP Medical and Scientific Books.

Fordyce, W. E. 1976. Behavioral Methods for Chronic Pain and Illness. Saint Louis, Missouri: C. V. Mosby.

Garfinkel, P., S. Kline, and H. Stancer. 1973. Treatment of anorexia nervosa using operant conditioning techniques. Journal of Nervous and Mental Diseases 157:428–433.

Haynes, R. B., D. W. Taylor, and D. L. Sackett. 1979. Compliance in Health Care. Baltimore, Maryland. The John Hopkins University Press.

Hindi-Alexander, M. 1974. The team approach in asthma. Journal of Asthma Research 12:79–88.

Katz, R., and S. Zlutnick. (eds.). 1975. Behavior Therapy and Health Care: Principles and Applications. Elmsford, New York: Pergamon Press.

Kellerman, J. 1977. Anorexia nervosa: The efficacy of behavior therapy. Journal of Behavior Therapy and Experimental Psychiatry 8:387–390.

Lang, P., and B. Melamed. 1969. Avoidance conditioning therapy of an infant with chronic ruminative vomiting. Journal of Abnormal Psychology 74:1–8.

Ley, P. 1977. Psychological studies of doctor–patient comunication. *In* S. Rachman, ed.: Contributions to Medical Psychology, Vol. 1. Oxford, England: Pergamon Press. pp. 9–42.

Melamed, B. G., and L. J. Siegel. 1975. Reduction of anxiety in children facing hospitalization and surgery by use of filmed modeling. Journal of Consulting and Clinical Psychology 43:511–521.

Munford, P., and R. Liberman. 1978. Differenitated attention in the treatment of operant cough. Journal of Behavioral Medicine 1:289–295.

Nash, J. D., and J. W. Farquahar. 1980. Application of behavioral medicine to disease prevention in a total community setting: A review of the three community study. *In* J. M. Ferguson and C. B. Taylor, eds.: The Comprehensive Handbook of Behavioral Medicine, Vol. 3. New York: S.P. Medical and Scientific Books.

Neisworth, J. T., and F. Moore. 1972. Operant treatment of asthmatic responding with the parent as therapist. Behavior Therapy 3:95–99.

Pomerleau, O. F. 1979. Behavioral medicine: The contribution of the experimental analysis of behavior to medical care. American Psychologist 34:654–663.

Pomerleau, O. F., and J. P. Brady. (eds.). 1979. Behavioral Medicine: Theory and Practice. Baltimore, Maryland: Williams and Wilkins.

Premack, D. 1959. Toward empirical behavior laws, I. Positive reinforcement. Psychological Review 66:219–233.

Public Health Service. 1979. Healthy People: The Surgeon General's Report on Health Promotion and Disease Prevention. Department of Health, Education, and Welfare (PHS) Publication No. 79-55071.

Rachman, S. (ed.). 1977. Contributions to Medical Psychology, Vol. 1. Oxford, England: Pergamon Press.

Rast, J., J. M. Johnston, C. Drum, and J. Conrin. 1981. The relation of food quantity to rumination behavior. Journal of Applied Behavior Analysis 14:121–130.

Rimm, D. C., and J. C. Masters. 1979. Behavior Therapy: Techniques and Empirical Findings, 2nd ed. New York: Academic Press.

Risch, C., and J. Ferguson. 1981. Behavioral treatment of skin disorders. In J. M. Ferguson and C. B. Taylor, eds.: The Comprehensive Handbook of Behavior Medicine, Vol. 2. New York: SP Medical and Scientific Books.

Rodin, J. 1977. Research on eating behavior and obesity: Where does it fit in personality and social psychology? Personality and Social Psychology Bulletin 3:333–355.

Ruprecht, M. J., R. H. Hanson, M. A. Pocrnich, and R. J. Murphy. 1980. Some suggested precautions when using lemon juice (citric acid) in behavior modification programs. Behavior Therapist 3:12.

Silver, B. V., and E. B. Blanchard. 1978. Biofeedback and relaxation training in the treatment of psychophysiological disorders: Or are the machines really necessary? Journal of Behavioral Medicine 1:217–239.

Stuart, R. B. 1972. Trick or Treatment: How and When Psychotherapy Fails. Champaign, Illinois: Research Press.

Taylor, C. B. 1981. The gastrointestinal system: Practices and promises of behavioral approaches. In J. M. Ferguson and C. B. Taylor, eds.: The Comprehensive Handbook of Behavioral Medicine, Vol. 2. New York: SP Medical and Scientific Books.

Vigersky, R. A. (ed.). 1977. Anorexia Nervosa. New York: Raven Press.

Walton, D. 1960. The application of learning theory to the treatment of a case of neurodermatitis. In H. J. Eysenck, ed.: Behavioral Therapy and Neuroses. London, England: Pergamon Press.

Watson, D., R. G. Tharp, and J. Krisberg. 1972. Case study in self-modification. Suppression of inflammatory scratching while awake and asleep. Journal of Behavior Therapy and Experimental Psychiatry 3:213–215.

Weinstein, M. C., and W. B. Stason. 1976. Hypertension: A Policy perspective. Cambridge, Massachusetts: Harvard University Press.

Woods, S. C. 1976. Conditioned hypoglycemia. Journal of Comparative and Physiological Psychology 90:1164–1168.

Zlutnick, S., W. J. Mayville, and S. Moffat. 1975. Behavioral control of seizure disorders: The interruption of chained behavior. In R. Katz and S. Zlutnick, eds.: Behavior Therapy and Health Care: Principles and Applications. Elmsford, New York: Pergamon Press.

10

Self-Management
of Health-Related Behaviors

Thomas A. Brigham, Ph. D.* and
Harold A. Dengerink, Ph. D.†

The need for self-management health maintenance programs becomes readily apparent when the conditions that the physician must deal with in everyday practice are examined. Previous chapters have discussed the contribution to medical practice that can be made by a combined biopsychosocial model and have at least alluded to the need to change patient behavior. Such changes may seem relatively simple when they are conducted in hospital settings. When a person is hospitalized, the medical and paramedical personnel have considerable control over stimulus variables (reminders to take medications, to attend physical therapy, etc.) and over reinforcers (attention, television, reading material, visiting privileges, etc.) for the patient. That is, in highly structured, physician-dominated environments such as a hospital, changes in patient behavior may be effected relatively easily.

But there are some important limitations to the incorporation of behavioral techniques in general medical practice. The behavioral interventions typically described in the literature often require extensive involvement of other persons such as physicians, nurses, and physical therapists. Such involvement, of course, is terminated or severely reduced when the person leaves the hospital environment. Frequently interventions that rely heavily upon some other person are not continued once that other person is no longer involved. For example, persons who begin self-injections of insulin for diabetes in the hospital may do well as long as they remain in the hospital, but once they are on their own, they may

---

*Professor, Department of Psychology, Washington State University, Pullman, Washington.
† Professor and Director of Clinical Training, Department of Psychology, Washington State University, Pullman, Washington.

poorly control their insulin levels. Clearly some set of procedures is needed to ensure that such gains are maintained or continued after the disengagement of other persons.

Another major limitation to behavioral intervention in medical practice stems from the fact that the majority of medical interventions are conducted on an outpatient basis. Under these conditions, the person actually carrying out the intervention is the patient or possibly a close family member. This reliance on the patient to carry out the medical intervention has some important implications. First, it means that the behavioral contribution to effective health care is multiplied. It is perhaps even more important that an outpatient's behavior rather than that of a hospitalized patient be directed or modified. But reliance upon the patient to carry out the medical intervention also means that the medical professionals have less control over that behavior. Not only do patients themselves execute the medical intervention, but they do so away from the office, making it impossible to directly monitor their behavior. Furthermore, the physician's influence over patient behavior is based on an office visit that will likely last no more than 15 minutes; and these visits may have long intervals between them, ranging up to several months or even years. Consequently, the physician's ability to monitor, correct, or reinforce patient behavior is severely limited.

The importance of modifying patient behavior, relative to the execution of medical interventions, is evidenced by the many reports that patients do a poor job of executing the physicians directives. The National Heart Lung and Blood Institute (NHBLI) estimates that at least 50% of those who are aware of having hypertension are not taking prescribed medication. Frequently people are quick to dismiss this problem as being one that occurs when patients are not experiencing any immediate symptoms of their illness. Indeed, the frequency of "noncompliance" appears to be highest for conditions that are relatively symptom free, such as hypertension. The most frequent rates of noncompliance have been reported for prescriptions of iron supplements. A review of Stimson's (1974) analysis, however, indicated that frequent noncompliance also occurs in regard to prescribed antibiotics.

The importance of changing patient behavior outside of the physician's immediate control is also underscored by the increasing realization that a patient can readily create a need for medical intervention by his or her own behavior. Life-style and emotional behaviors appear to contribute to the development of coronary-related diseases and a variety of psycho-somatic disorders. Excessive alcohol consumption as well as smoking obviously contribute extensively to the need for medical interventions. A recent Surgeon General's report goes so far as to assert that over 50% of the symptoms leading to a patient seeing a physician can be related directly to that person's life-style. Therefore the role that the patient's general behavior plays in determining his or her overall health cannot be ignored in prevention or in the treatment plans for the patient's current disorder.

Some Perspectives on Self-Control

Before self-management techniques can be utilized in a knowledgeable and systematic manner as components in medical practice, some basic issues about self-control must be understood. The first and most basic issue concerns the interpretation of the term *self-control* itself. It is generally assumed that self-control is something possessed by the individual that causes the individual to act in a particular manner. In short, the possession or lack of self-control may be used to explain why a person does or does not do something. However, this commonly used notion of self-control as an internal state affecting behavior is overly simplistic and unsupported by research findings.

Because self-control connotes a seemingly commonsense but erroneous interpretation, the less value laden term *self-management* will be used instead to refer to those responses or skills that enable an individual to cope personally and effectively with life problems. The term *self-management* focuses the analysis on the responses, skills, and responsibility of the individual. A basic assumption in our research is that behaviors or skills that allow the individual to better deal with the environment can be taught. Stated in another way, people with self-management problems lack certain skills in dealing with their environment and can be taught those specific responses.

Individual or patient responsibility is another area where a misconception of self-management can interfere with effective treatment. For instance, despite the apparent importance of modifying and directing patient behavior apart from the physician's direct medical supervision, and despite the apparent poor job that patients appear to be making of it, responsibility for such direction and modification of behavior is often assigned to the patients themselves; that is, the responsibility for modifying and directing behavior is given totally to the patient. It often appears that the physician sees his or her role as merely one of giving advice and leaves the patient in a position of following or not following that advice as he or she sees fit. The position taken here is that effective health care requires a negotiated alliance between the patient and physician, with both working supportively toward the same goal.

Although it is both necessary and appropriate to hold the individual responsible for his or her behavior, the practical realities of the situation must not be ignored. The patient having difficulty controlling such behaviors as smoking, overeating or drinking, not exercising, or failing to comply with a particular medical regimen will not improve simply because he or she is enjoined to take responsibility for those behaviors. Rather, the physician must provide specific instructions or ensure that the patient receives self-management training related to the particular problem for there to be any real chance that the patient's behavior will change.

Finally, a popular view of human behavior holds that a real commitment to change will form not only a necessary but also a sufficient basis for change. If a person wants to change a behavior badly enough, he or she will be able to do so. This conception of commitment should be recognized as a variation on the willpower theme and suffers from the same failings. On the other hand, commitment can be taken simply to mean that there are good reasons in the person's life for him or her to change a particular behavior or set of behaviors. Within this context, before the individual will attempt to modify a personal behavior, he or she needs some motivation to do so. The commitment must be based on objective personal and environmental factors and not on inferred or implicit factors that may have no meaning to the patient. For example, persons who are instructed to continue taking antibiotics until after the symptoms have disappeared may have no rational explanation for this instruction. They may simply believe that the physician is being overly cautious and giving them more than they really need. Although they may appreciate the apparent excessive concern, they may stop too early because they believe there is no need to continue. In one survey the NHLBI reported that more than 60% of the hypertensive patients who had stopped taking their medications did so because they wrongly believed their physician had indicated they no longer needed to take it.

The commitment or desire to change behavior also depends upon the degree that patients experience or expect immediate benefits for doing so. A 25-year-old patient may feel little need to stop smoking when he knows that the effects of smoking will not be noticeable until many years have passed. People who are overweight find it much easier to lose weight for some specific event that is only a few weeks away than to do so for benefits which will not be realized for many years.

The degree to which an individual manages personal behavior will also depend upon the degree to which that person has competing commitments. A person may wish to modify her hostile striving to get ahead, but not do so because she has an even more intense desire to achieve the next goal. A patient who is instructed to remain in bed for several days, owing to chronic back problems, may have every intention of doing so until some emergency occurs at work or the inlaws visit.

Furthermore, commitment alone is not enough. A recent television newscast reported that the Billy Graham crusades were not very effective in prodding people to become active churchgoers. Persons who made public (in front of thousands of witnesses) professions of faith and promises to begin attending church did so infrequently; only 15%

eventually joined a church. Public commitments are often taken as a measure of intense desire to change one's errant ways. But the following article appeared in the *Denver Post* on January 1, 1976:

> The briefest New Year's resolution: White House press secretary Ron Nessen announced to the press on New Year's morning that he had given up smoking. Ordinarily a two-to-three-pack-a-day man, he had not drawn on a filter for 10½ hours. Clearly pleased with himself, Nessen then walked down the hall to his office, automatically and apparently unconsciously lighting up as he did so.

People also often lack other means of dealing with situations and will not be able to change their behavior without further assistance. Smokers often have no other means of dealing with the tension they experience. Obese people often habitually eat when bored and have no other means of entertaining themselves. Undesirable behaviors may become so automatic, as apparently in Nessen's case, that the desire to change alone cannot produce other competing behaviors. Or persons such as hypertensives who have taken little other medication may not have the habit of taking medications and may need some reminder system. Thus, even when commitment or desire is high, people have difficulty directing or modifying their behavior.

As a consequence, the patient must not only be motivated on his own and/or given sufficient reasons to change a behavior from a medical standpoint, but must also be taught the skills that will produce behavior change. For instance, a middle aged female having difficulties (lower back pain, high blood pressure, shortness of breath, etc.) related to being overweight seeks medical advice. She is an excellent cook and prides herself on the elegant meals she makes. Her husband is also overweight and they have two teenage sons who eat ravenously. After appropriate medical testing the standard treatment likely would be to prescribe medication to control the hypertension and instruct the woman to lose some weight. The physician might go further and place her on a particular diet or program. Although medically sound, studies show that this treatment seldom works. Our hypothetical patient simply cannot do it! In addition to a commitment to control her blood pressure and weight, she must be given some minimal self-management skills related to those behaviors.

Self-Management Problems

Having discussed some common misconceptions about self-management, the next step in our examination of these phenomena is an analysis of those situations that cause individuals difficulty. The majority if not all of the situations where an individual is said to have a self-management problem involve some difference between the immediate consequences of a response and its delayed consequences. Smoking is a good example of a response the immediate consequences of which are positive for most smokers, but the accumulated delayed consequences of which are clearly negative. Smoking is further complicated because the delayed negative consequences, even when they occur, are not easily discriminated by the individual. Later, when clearly discernable consequences such as coughing, sore throat, and shortness of breath do appear, smoking has been additionally strengthened by other behavioral processes to the point where the response is still difficult to eliminate when the consequences change. A process that contributes to such problems is antecedent stimulus control. In the case of smoking, the response is easy to emit concurrently or in conjunction with other responses in a wide variety of settings. Because smoking occurs consistently in many situations, these stimuli set the occasion for subsequent smoking. For example, many people smoke while drinking coffee. Because the two responses occur together, engaging in one may become a cue for the other. Later, when the smoker attempts to quit, the coffee provides a powerful antecedent stimulus for smoking.

To reiterate, in a self-management problem, some immediate consequence controls a response, while later consequences for the response or alternative incompatible responses have opposite effects from the immediate consequences. Most problems of overconsumption (i.e., eating, drinking, drug abuse, smoking) fit this set of contingencies. Both contingencies must be present to produce a self-control problem. If it were not for heart disease, lung cancer, emphysema, and the like, few people would worry about smoking. Thus smoking would no longer be a behavioral problem.

There are three other basic variations of these contingencies. A response may have immediate aversive consequences, but failure to make the response may have even greater delayed aversive consequences, as in the example of undergoing uncomfortable dental treatment. A similar set of contingencies are in effect when an individual whose initial social interactions have been punished in the past is, as a consequence, less likely to make social advances. Here the reduction of important behavior by small immediate aversive consequences may lead to the long-range loss of greater positive social interactions within an increased sphere of friends and acquaintances (i.e., if the individual had emitted the approach responses, they may have led to new friends and enjoyable activities). Finally, a response may produce a small, immediate positive consequence, but not emitting that response and emitting instead an alternative response may produce a larger, delayed positive consequence. Behavior such as saving money in small amounts may eventually result in a large reinforcer, while spending each small amount immediately might produce only small reinforcers.

Although behavioral psychologists have tried to avoid analyzing phenomena in terms of nonresponding, nonresponding appears to be an important component in analyzing self-management problems. In every such situation, the problem is a particular response that is either occurring or not occurring. Thus it is important to examine the contingencies for both the occurrence and nonoccurrence of the target response. The four sets of immediate and delayed consequences for the target response are summarized in Table 1. The first two instances are situations where the self-control problem is the occurrence of the target response, while in the second two it is the nonoccurrence of the response that constitutes the problem. The contingencies in Table 1 are identified in terms of both stimulus and operation; a response can affect either a reinforcing or an aversive stimulus.

An important feature of self-management is made explicit by these examples. The immediate contingencies involve small but relatively assured consequences, either positive or negative, while the delayed consequences are all major but potential. Cases are well documented of individuals who smoked two packs of cigarettes a day throughout their adult life and died of old age at 95 without any major health problems related to smoking. Similarly, regular visits to the dentist will not invariably avoid serious dental problems.

A less obvious aspect of self-management follows from the nature of the consequences for the responses that need to be changed. The required

Table 1. Responding (R_1) and Non-responding (R_0) Alternatives in Self-Control and Their consequences for Each Alternative. The problem response is indicated by an asterisk (*).

Response	Example	Immediate consequence	Delayed consequence
*R_1	Smoking	Minor reinforcing event	Major aversive event
R_0	Not smoking	No reinforcing event	No aversive event
*R_1	Spending money	Minor reinforcing event	No reinforcing event
R_0	Not spending (saving)	No reinforcing event	Major reinforcing event
R_1	Going to dentist	Minor aversive event	No aversive event
*R_0	Not going to dentist	No aversive event	Major aversive event
R_1	Making new friends	Minor aversive event	Major reinforcing event
*R_0	Not meeting new people	No aversive event	No reinforcing event

direction of change is a function of immediate consequences: When the consequences are positive (e.g., smoking or other substance abuse), the target response needs to be decreased in frequency, and when the consequences are negative (e.g., going to the dentist, self-injections of insulin), the target response needs to be increased. To accomplish these changes, the individual obviously must use different strategies. When decreasing the frequency of a response, a twofold approach appears to be effective. First alternative incompatible responses that will produce reinforcers need to be found, and the individual must avoid situations which in the past were discriminative for the target behavior. In the case of increasing the frequency of a response, the environment must be analyzed and restructured to make both the occurrence and the reinforcement of the response more probable. The later section on self-management programs will provide more details on dealing with specific self-management problems.

Self-Management: Component Responses

Self-management consists of skills related to self-observation, analysis of the behavioral environment, and changing the environment. This fairly simple statement obviously covers a range of very complex responses. These responses are ordinarily acquired as a function of daily living. When a person lacks self-management skills, however, the skills must be taught in a systematic manner. Such instruction requires a formal analysis and treatment of self-management.

Analysis of the Behavioral Environment

The most important component of the behavior analysis approach to changing behavior is reinforcement. Therefore a central task of self-management is learning to analyze the environment in terms of reinforcement contingencies. From this perspective the first component in self-management is the ability to recognize those contingencies in one's own life. Observation and analysis can be used to discriminate reinforcement and punishment contingencies. Observation can consist of the systematic recording of behavior and its antecedents and consequences or simply noting another person's reaction to a particular response or set of responses as a way of determining how to interact with the person.

Related to the ability to observe one's own behavior/environment interactions is the recognition of mutual influences of one's responses on the environment and of the environment on one's responses. This, of course, is the concept of reciprocity. In the case of self-management it refers, in the first person, to my recognizing that how I behave affects the way people react to me and vice versa. Although this may appear an overly simple point, people vary tremendously in how well they understand it. In general, individuals characterized as lacking self-management skills display little or no understanding of this essential interdependency.

Finally, an important product of the ability to observe objectively one's own behavior is the understanding of personal private events. The individual skillful at self-observation can discriminate relations between behavior–environment interactions and private feelings. The individual who can recognize the source of his or her feelings of anger in the behavior–environment interplay has a much greater chance of dealing with the problem than the individual who can only report feeling angry.

The person who possesses these analytical skills will then be able to recognize the various immediate and delayed contingencies involved in self-management problems discussed earlier. The student who recognizes that he is not studying enough because other incompatible responses are immediately reinforced by some friends while the consequences for studying are delayed has taken the first step in solving the problem. Similarly, the problem drinker who understands that some friends may provide the immediate consequences for abusive drinking by encouraging and reinforcing it may then be able to take steps to change the problem behavior.

Self-Monitoring

Self-monitoring refers to recording the occurrence of behaviors one is attempting to change and the conditions surrounding the occurrence of that response. Self-monitoring has two basic functions. Self-monitoring increases the individual's awareness of the specific response and provides some consequences (reinforcement or punishment) for that behavior. Persons are often unaware of how often they engage in a behavior that is causing them problems. Asking people to monitor their own behavior forces them to become aware of the frequency or intensity of that behavior. Frequently problem behaviors that need to be decreased have become sufficiently habitual that people are unaware of engaging in them. For example it has been found that obese people underestimate the amount of food they eat. Even when they are not attempting to cover up, they underestimate. In a very creative study obese people reported how much they remembered eating for a particular period of time. They were then placed in the hospital and fed that amount. Under those conditions, they all lost weight (Schachter, 1971). The obvious point here is that our informal recollection about our own behavior is often not trustworthy. Patients may be similarly unattentive to caffeine consumption, exercise, anxiety, fingernail biting, etc.

Recording when and where a response occurs produces objective evidence concerning this response that cannot be ignored. The awareness produced by self-monitoring is also important when a person needs to increase the frequency of a behavior. For example, most likely the majority of people who fail to take prescribed medications fail because they simply forget. Asking people to record the frequency of certain desired behaviors helps call their attention to the fact that they are supposed to engage in that behavior.

In addition to prompting awareness, the simple act of recording one's own behavior frequently has some consequent value for the person. When people are attempting to increase some behavior, recording it may become a matter of reinforcement as well as self-monitoring. When people are attempting to decrease some behavior, then monitoring can have some aversive consequence. Clearly, when someone exceeds a particular limit, say, in the number of allowed cigarettes, the recording of that behavior becomes an occasion for self-censure. Simply having a smoker record the frequency of lighting cigarettes often results in a reduction of 25–30% percent of the cigarettes smoked. In addition, recording some behavior, particularly if done before engaging in that behavior, increases the response cost of that behavior; that is, recording increases the amount of effort and/or time required to engage in that behavior and may thus prevent it.

Although self-monitoring alone can produce a change in the target behavior, this effect is a very fragile and transitory one. This effect can be strengthened and prolonged by the addition of environmental restructuring procedures described below.

Environmental Restructuring

A major advantage of an inpatient setting for changing someone's behavior is that one controls stimuli to increase the probability of appropriate behaviors and decrease inappropriate behaviors. Patients can be prompted to do exercises, take medications, and so on. No smoking signs and the absence of ashtrays curtail smoking. The absence of snack foods eliminates eating other than at mealtimes. Implicit in these comments is the assumption that behavior is under stimulus control. Even behaviors seen as being strongly driven often vary considerably from situation to situation. Smokers frequently report that in some situations where smoking is prohibited they seldom even get an urge to smoke. Schachter (1971) and Stunkard (1975) argued strongly that eating is under strong stimulus control. When people do not see food, they are less likely to eat. If they are unaware that it is dinner time, they do not feel as hungry as if they believed it were mealtime.

The first objective, then, of environmental restructuring is to use the information generated by self-monitoring to change stimulus factors in such a way that the probability of desirable responses is increased and that of undesirable responses decreased. The second objective of restructuring one's environment is to change the contingencies or consequences for one's behavior.

Environmental restructuring frequently involves changes in the physical environment. Barker (1968), in a review of psychological ecology, argued persuasively that the simple physical environment has a far greater influence on a person's behavior in that setting than that individual's personality. Similarly, Skinner's (1953) analysis of self-management focused heavily not on consequences per se, but on environmental structuring involving either the physical or psychological environment. It was assumed that the individual could arrange the environment so that the probability of particular responses would increase or decrease. He further assumed that if these changes were successful, there would be environmental consequences to maintain the new behaviors. For example, the story of Odysseus and the Sirens can be seen as an instance of arranging the physical environment to prevent a particular response. At the suggestion of Circe, Odysseus plugged his sailors' ears with wax and then had himself lashed to the mast so that he could hear the Sirens' song without losing his life or his ship.

A recent anecdotal report of a father's efforts to control his children's automobile riding behavior provides a more mundane but perhaps more relevant example of environmental restructuring (Brigham, 1982). The father attempted to influence the trip behaviors of his children (increase positive play and social intercourse while decreasing fighting, screaming, and other abusive actions) by instituting a variety of reinforcement and punishment contingencies, all to no avail. Although familial affection that transcends situational variables is a desirable long-term objective, a realistic assessment of the probability of such behavior under the stimulus situation of a crowded back seat suggests that it is extremely low. The obvious solution (*obvious* is a *post hoc* term; it took many years of trying contingencies before a restructuring approach was taken) was simply to change the adult–child seating patterns. Now the driver and one child sit in the front while the second child and adult sit in the back. Many miles have been covered in relative comfort and peace maintained by small reinforcers in contrast to the small amount of control exerted by contingencies employed in the past. The difference is that the change in the environment eliminated the "accidental" kick or bump, the "friendly" poke, and so on, that led to retaliation and escalated verbal and/or physical violence. This environment was the key to the self-management problem. In it, the probability of disruptive inappropriate responses is increased, even though consequences for those or other behaviors may be programmed. Similarly, the impact of environmental changes on behavior can be seen in the simple instruction to smokers to put away all cigarettes and ashtrays before and after smoking. The manipulation changes the environment by removing stimulus factors that in the past had cued smoking and introduces a delay between the "desire" to smoke and the availability of a cigarette. These small steps consistently result in a 25–30% reduction in the smoking frequency below baseline (Danaher and Lichtenstein, 1978). Certainly additional changes are required before the individual can stop smoking, and the environmental restructuring must be maintained by appropriate contingencies. Nonetheless, small environmental changes can play an important role in the solution of self-control problems.

Thus far the discussion has focused on restructuring the physical environment. How does one restructure the psychological environment? Although a wide variety of procedures might occasionally be used, the core of modification skills consists of the reinforcement, extinction, and shaping of other people's behavior and using commitment to change the probability of particular personal responses. An example of environmental change by reinforcement and extinction is provided by special education students who were taught to change their social and educational environments (Graubard et al., 1974). Special education children often interact with a hostile environment that has labeled them as deviant and subjected them to ridicule and negative comments. A group of special education children were taught some simple reinforcement and extinction techniques. For example, the children were taught to make the "uh huh" ("I understand") response when a teacher carefully explained something to them, and to thank the teacher and praise the teacher's efforts. On the other hand, the students broke eye contact after and were generally unresponsive to the teacher's negative comments. Similar procedures were used with other students in the school. When the special education children used their new social skills, there was an increase in positive comments, approaches, and so on, and a complementary decrease in negative ones by the teachers and "normal" students toward the special education children. The special education students changed their psychosocial environment with reinforcement and extinction and made further positive changes possible. In addition, their changed behavior changed the teacher's environment and that of other students, because the special education children were now a source of social reinforcers. Similar procedures have been utilized in work with juvenile delinquents, couples having marriage problems, and smokers who needed to enlist environmental support for nonsmoking behavior (Brigham, 1982). In summary, dealing with the psychological environment is largely a matter of recognizing that other people's behavior greatly influences one's own and changing the way one interacts with others.

There are other ways of modifying one's psychosocial environment as well. When persons are maintaining records of their own behaviors, these records can be employed as cues for other persons' behavior. Posting, in a public place such as the refrigerator door, records on one's eating, smoking, or medication will elicit comments from others about the patient's progress. These comments can serve as external reinforcements for one's compliance with the self-control regime. Considerable evidence suggests that this procedure is very effective in maintaining motivation to change.

Self-management and other control procedures may be seen as existing on a continuum. In fact it is appropriate at times to consider self-controlling behaviors like any other behavior. Although being in control may be reinforcing in and of itself, self-management behaviors may periodically require support from other sources. When commitment wanes and the effort becomes great, reinforcement from some other person is essential to maintain self-management behaviors. At those times, it may be necessary to move from public posting to a form of contracting. This may be particularly true when people are asked to engage in painful or difficult behaviors. It may also be appropriate, particularly for persons who begin with little commitment, to initiate some behavioral change via other directed procedures and then to shift to self-management procedures for maintenance.

Whenever the physician instructs people to modify their behavior, it is at least an implied contract. People will expect praise and attention from the physician. Anytime the physician fails to keep components of an implied contract, the patient is not likely to keep his or her side of the agreement. Kanfer et al. (1974), for example, reported that when people were asked to engage in some painful behavior, they were quite likely to do so if the other person was attentive and appreciative. They were unlikely to do so when the other person was distracted and engaging in some unrelated task. Such contracts, even implied ones, may have a major influence on the behavior of the patient. A written contract where specific consequences are to be given the patient in return for engaging in some desired behavior or for refraining from undesirable behavior can be useful in producing changes where less concrete procedures have failed.

Research consistently demonstrates that the influence of consequences has a limited temporal range; that is, the value of a consequence increases and decreases as a function of the time to its delivery. If two response–consequence pairs are possible in a situation and one consequence is delivered much sooner than the other, then the first will occur. This is true even though the consequence of the second response may be more important in some sense. In the presence of food the consequence for eating is much more immediate than the consequence for dieting. Similarly, a patient may need to choose between watching television and retrieving and taking antibiotics. Watching television is the more likely response, because the consequence is immediate. If, on the other hand, the patient were able to decide which response to emit when neither consequence was available, he would be more likely to take the antibiotic. As another example, a person trying to lose weight may notice that she always has dessert with lunch. The individual can announce to the lunch companions that she is not having dessert today before they get to the restaurant. Because the dessert is not immediately available, it has less value as a reinforcer, and it is possible for the person to decide that the reduced calories are more important than the taste of the dessert. The statement about dessert will make it very difficult for the individual to order dessert when it is available.

Behaviors that restructure the environment work best if they change the physical as well as psychological environment. A patient in our weight control program was having difficulty with freshly baked cookies. They were available in the student union and every day after lunch she walked by the counter and ended up eating two to four cookies. (They were cheaper in multiples of two.) In analyzing her behavior, it was found that she always ate in one area of the building and then exited in a manner that took her past the cookie counter. She did, however, have a choice of exits, one of which took her out before she got close to the cookie counter. She was given a card to take to lunch with the following written on it: "Do I want any cookies? No, exit through the door on the right. Yes, go straight ahead." She placed the card on her tray and removed it after lunch. The card forced her to make a decision before she was in the presence of the cookies, whether she actually wanted any. The response of leaving the building by the other route made it both physically and psychologically difficult to go back into the building to get cookies. Using this system, in two weeks she had broken the habit and could leave the building through either exit without succumbing to the cookie "urge."

Applications of Self-Management Procedures to Medical Problems

The specific self-management procedures will obviously vary from person to person and from situation to situation. Consequently one must be somewhat flexible in the specific elements that are included in any program. Again, the overriding rule is to do what works. If a set of procedures or elements within those procedures do not appear to be working, modify them. General recommendations can, however, be made for some problems.

Compliance with Medical Regimes

Perhaps the greatest cause of noncompliance is simply forgetting. Many times persons who have been instructed to take medications will not be used to taking medications: If they lack detectable symptoms or are insensitive to or distracted from these symptoms, then they often forget.

Persons who are confined to a wheelchair are instructed to do push-ups on the arms of the chair to eliminate pressure against the skin and prevent skin ulcers. But if they lack feeling in their buttocks and thighs, then they will not experience the physical discomfort that would otherwise prompt them to move. For these kinds of problems some sort of reminder system is needed, at least until the person acquires the habit. Fordyce (1974) referred to such procedures as prosthetic memory.

The simplest sort of prosthetic memory consists of a pencil and paper. Caldwell (1974a) suggested that for persons who have having trouble remembering to take medications, cards should be prepared with appropriate headings on which the patient can record each occurrence of taking the medication. A simple 5-x-7-inch card works nicely for this purpose. If one column indicates the time of day and the number of pills a patient should take, the patient need only make a check mark in the next column each time he or she does so. The patient then engages in a very simple self-monitoring procedure that has all the advantages discussed earlier.

This recording procedure can also serve as a good reminder if the card is placed in some conspicuous place. It is particularly helpful if the card is in a place that the person frequents and where the person is to take the medication. For example, if the patient is to take the medication in the morning, this card could be taped to the mirror in the bathroom. If the patient is to take the medication in the evening, the card could be taped to the headboard of the bed. The physician can help ensure that the person does tape the card in the appropriate place by attaching a bandaid with half the wrapper removed to the card before the patient leaves the office.

Such procedures may be particularly helpful for a patient who will be taking medication in the same place each time. But frequently people must take the medications at several times and consequently different places during any given day. For these situations, the patient could be provided with separate containers for the medication; or it may be easiest to write more than one prescription so that the pharmacist will provide the medication in the appropriate amounts in different containers. These different containers can then be kept in the bathroom, on the counter above the kitchen sink, in a purse or desk, and so forth. Self-recording in such circumstances can be accomplished by taping a piece of paper to the pill container and asking the person to check off each dose taken or note the time each dose is taken.

There will also be times when people will need to engage in some procedure or take medications even more frequently. For these situations a simple timer may be the most effective reminder. These are reasonably inexpensive and could be sold or loaned in the office. Some timers are even small enough that they have been incorporated as part of keychains. While timers may generally be good devices for prosthetic memory, they may also be troublesome. They can go off at inopportune times such as in the middle of a church service. They can also fail and not cue the desired behavior. Particularly when some permanent change in behavior is desired, excessive reliance upon timers may be inappropriate. Such a situation exists when wheelchair patients are required to do push-ups to eliminate, temporarily, pressure on the skin. Under these circumstances, Caldwell (1974b) suggested that the person do the push-ups for the required amount of time (usually 1 second for each minute of sitting, i.e., 1 minute per hour) before the buzzer sounds on the timer. The person can then reset the timer to avoid the buzzing. The buzzer then becomes a reminder that the person has not done something he should have, and possibly a punisher. After repeatedly following this regime and avoiding the buzz of the timer, the person eventually learns to judge the time for himself and to function independently of the timer. Clearly one could avoid the timer going off by performing the required response more often than necessary. This may not create any problem when the required response is chair arm push-ups; it could create problems, however, if the required response is taking medication: The excessive medication could clearly be dangerous. Consequently, the avoidance strategy is not a generally applicable one.

These self-management responses on the part of the patient are not different from other behavior and may require some systematic external support; that is, it may be necessary for the physician to monitor the self-management responses of patients and to reinforce those responses. There are several things that a physician can do to help ensure that patients will in fact follow the prescribed self-management regimes: (1) Put his or her name and address along with a stamp on the reverse side of the recording form and have the patient mail it, (2) promise to review the records personally, (3) have the receptionist or nurse call if the card does not show up on time, and (4) give the patient a free office visit if he or she has complied for a given period of time. It may also be that the patient's compliance will eliminate the need for the next visit. A telephone call from the physician could save that patient the effort of keeping an office appointment and still provide the personal contact to reinforce compliance.

Stopping Smoking

Smoking clearly is a special self-control problem. It is a behavior in which people can engage at almost anytime and in a wide variety of places. Consequently, a person who has smoked for a long perod of time has acquired many cues for that behavior. Seeing someone else smoke, having a cup of coffee, taking a break from work, watching television, driving the car, going to the bathroom, listening to someone else talk in a meeting, and finishing a task all become occasions to smoke.

Smoking also presents a special problem in that the behavior itself may be reinforcing. For a person who has smoked for a long time, smoking a cigarette permits him to avoid the discomfort associated with not smoking; that is, smoking may have physiological reinforcing properties. Consequently, these reinforcers cannot be eliminated by changing the environment. Furthermore, quitting smoking can be quite aversive for the chronic smoker. The variety of discriminative stimuli and the discomfort experienced upon quitting combine to make smoking an extraordinarily difficult behavior to eliminate.

Still there are a number of things that can be done, as has been suggested by Caldwell (1974c). First the smoker should begin by recording each cigarette smoked and noting the situation in which it is smoked. The second step is to make the decision to quit. This should be made in the form of a public commitment response. The person has then both added motivation to stick with the decision and functionally changed his or her environment. The individual could sign a contract announcing the decision to quit smoking, and anyone observing him or her smoking is entitled to a reward of some specified amount. Several copies of this signed contract should be made and posted or distributed. Similarly, the person needs to avoid those situations where smoking previously occurred. The person should sit in the no smoking section of the coffee shop, spend time with nonsmokers, and so on. Additionally, some incompatible alternate behaviors will be helpful, for example, playing with coins or worry beads, doodling, chewing sugarless gum, and taking a deep breath.

One of the problems with quitting is that a person may periodically fail and smoke even a single cigarette. Even one cigarette in a single day can seem like a disaster for the person who gave up two packs a day. Having failed once, they may go back to smoking the entire amount. This problem can be avoided if the person has some legitimate way of smoking without violating the initial contract. The person could be permitted to smoke while standing up in front of a toilet. The bathroom as a legitimate place for smoking has a number of advantages. First, it is available at home, work, and most other places. Second, it requires that the person go to a place in which he or she otherwise does not spend a great deal of time. Furthermore, while the opportunity to smoke is available, the person must expend some effort to avail him- or herself of it. Finally, standing in front of a toilet is not particularly reinforcing.

Another problem with stopping is that the quitter may not feel he is making any progress. The urge to smoke will continue and may seem to get stronger once a person has quit. To counter this problem, the person should be encouraged to count the number of urges to smoke he has but to which he does not give in. During successive days these urges will decline and that decline can be very reinforcing to the person who has been attempting to stop. The decline will even be faster if the person does not comply with the urge.

Obviously if one does continue to smoke in some place such as the bathroom or slowly reduces, the habit will continue, at even a low level. Under these conditions the person may gradually increase smoking and soon return to the original level. Eventually all smoking needs to be eliminated. To do so, the person should periodically practice quitting even in the bathroom. Once the frequency has been reduced to a low level everywhere except in the bathroom, this becomes relatively easy. But again it will be helpful if the person engages in a contract with another person to ensure that he does in fact abstain for a day or two at a time.

Clearly a task as difficult as stopping smoking may require some external support. The kind of procedures followed here may be the same as those selected for reinforcing compliance with medical regimes. Additionally, the chronic smoker may have some other readily available reinforcers. First, many smokers associate with others who would like them to stop smoking. These persons may be able to provide extensive social reinforcement. Furthermore, the chronic smoker could use the money ordinarily spent on smoking for reinforcing events such as movies and clothes. Finally, more information may be needed than it has been possible to present here. An excellent small volume that is written in a systematic but informal manner is *Become an Ex-smoker* by Danaher and Lichtenstein (1978). This book will provide many additional ideas.

Weight Control

Controlling eating poses a problem that is very different from that of stopping smoking. In contrast to smoking, which people can give up entirely, eating is something people must continue doing to some extent. The problem then becomes a matter of controlling specific responses rather than stopping a group of behaviors all together. It is perhaps this feature of weight control that results in people routinely losing and regaining (Stunkard, 1975). Effective weight control procedures then should be ones that contribute not only to weight loss, but also to maintenance of that loss. The focus should be on permanent behavior change rather than upon rapid loss and fad diets.

The weight control program conducted at Washington State University is a modification of those procedures devised by Stuart and Davis (1972) and adopted by Stunkard (1975) and Mahoney and Mahoney (1976). The procedures begin with a screening process. Prior to entering the program persons are told that the program is one that is effective but which requires a great deal of effort on their part. Furthermore, they are informed that the success of the program depends not upon gimmicks and fads, but upon concentrated effort on their part in changing their eating behavior.

The screening also attempts to determine the person's motiviations for losing weight. Periodically persons will attempt to lose weight because they feel that by doing so they will solve other problems such as marital difficulties. These are obviously the wrong solutions to such problems and such persons are referred to other treatment facilities for simultaneous treatment. The screening process can also be used to determine whether the person is living with or frequently associating with persons who may be particularly helpful to them in a weight loss program. Such persons can be very helpful in establishing contracts, modifying their eating behavior to eliminate temptations for the dieter, supporting exercise programs, and so forth.

Finally, particular problem situations for the dieter can be identified in the screening process. Some people will report that they eat primarily later in the day, culminating with a large meal just before bedtime. Others report that continual snacking is the major problem. Most report that they eat when they are bored, happy, sad, nervous, or excited; any emotional response becomes an excuse or an occasion for eating. Most also report that they eat in a variety of places other than in the kitchen: at a desk, in front of the television, and so on. Thus, the screening also helps identify problem situations that should be avoided or changed.

The actual program begins by teaching participants a simple recording system. People are asked to record the number of servings they eat rather than the number of calories per se. A serving is defined as 75 calories, regardless of what kind of food is being eaten. Once a person has learned the serving size of various foods, he or she need not consult calorie books to keep track of the amount consumed. They are able to estimate the number of servings in any given meal, whether they are at home or at a cafeteria. Recording is done before they eat the food, rather than afterward. This at times prevents them from eating some foods or amounts and helps ensure that they do not forget to record their consumption. The record is kept on graph paper, with each square indicating a serving. One line of the paper is used for each day. A bold red line is drawn down the paper to indicate the maximum number of servings the person can allow him- or herself per day. As the number of filled squares increases, the person is able to quickly and visually (rather than numerically) estimate how many servings are left before the limit is reached.

The recording system is based upon food categories; that is, persons use symbols (e.g., M, V, Fr, B) to indicate the major food categories of the servings they consume. This system allows the physician and the client to assess the nutritional balance of their diet. For a number of clients, the major problem category is alcohol (recorded as A). Most overeat in the bread (B) category. Very few are likely to overeat in the fruit (Fr) or milk (Ml) categories.

During the first meeting, the recording system is explained and the person is given a series of forms that they can consult and are asked to memorize. They are asked to indicate what they ate during the previous meal and, as an illustration, this is then recorded on their forms. No limit is placed upon eating during the first week; but the act of recording by itself most often results in clients losing weight during this first week. The importance of the recording system is also stressed by informing the client they will be given a quiz the next week when they return.

If the client has recorded faithfully during the interval between the first and second visit, and if he or she does well on the quiz, then the second step is initiated at the second meeting. The second step consists of instructing people to do a variety of things that will keep them from eating, for example, not buy snack foods; or, if they must buy problem foods for others in the house, store these out of sight and in some place that is off limits to themselves. A high cupboard or closet shelf works well for this. All the foods should be stored in the kitchen and they are restricted to eating only at one place. They are asked to not eat in front of the television or where they can either see or hear the television. The serving dishes are to be left on the stove or counter rather than on the table. If they have an urge to snack, they should leave the kitchen and do something else. Activities that are enjoyable and at least partially incompatible with eating, for example, talking a walk, taking a shower, calling a friend on the phone, or reading a magazine, are recommended. Patients are taught to stir food with a chopstick if they have problems snacking while fixing food or to wear a face mask while cooking if they feel tempted by the smell. To assist clients in carrying out these assignments, they are given a rating scale for indicating the degree to which instructions were followed each day. Our own evaluation and that of Romanczyk (1978) indicate that recording and practicing such stimulus control techniques are the most effective part of the program. Persons who report doing these assignments well are more likely to lose weight than those who do not do them well.

After the clients have mastered this step, they are given assignments designed to alter eating patterns. Clients practice stopping eating by not eating for 2 minutes during the middle of each meal. They are also asked to leave something, even if it is just a crust of bread, on their place. (Clients routinely report that this is the most difficult assignment to carry out.) They are also asked to put the utensil or food down between bites, to chew and swallow the food, and then pick up the food or utensil again. While these techniques appear to be less helpful than the previous ones, they do at times help people keep from taking seconds and it helps reduce the amount that people eat at meals.

Another part of the program asks clients to increase exercise. Frequently clients report that calisthenics are boring and painful. As a consequence, exercises that are enjoyable and which are more likely to be continued are recommended. Playing tennis or handball can be good and enjoyable exercise, and these also involve other individuals, who can provide incentive and reward for exercising. Exercises that can be incorporated as part of a daily routine (e.g., taking the stairs rather than the elevator) are also more likely to be continued than those which required different clothes and scheduling. Clients also record their exercising. Evaluation suggests that exercise may not contribute to losing weight; that is, persons who exercise regularly are not more likely to lose weight than those who do not exercise regularly. However, exercise appears to contribute to the maintenance of weight loss. Those who exercise regularly during the program are more likely to keep the weight off than persons who do not exercise regularly (Peterson and Brigham, 1980).

Another important part of the program is the regular meetings with a clinician. Those persons who meet weekly with a clinician, whether or not they have lost weight during that particular week, are more likely to lose than those who meet irregularly. Because weight control requires some external support, clients are instructed to establish contracts with family members and post a graph of progress at home so that others can compliment their efforts.

This general approach has been fairly effective. Stuart (1967) and Stunkard (1975) reported greater success for such programs than for any other that has been established. Our own evaluation indicates that participants, as a group, lose between 1 and 2 pounds per week. These persons were being seen by medical students and graduate psychology students. Furthermore, the first 1-year follow-up showed that these persons weighed less at the time of the follow-up than when they had finished the training program. While the greater loss at follow-up than at the end of the program is not typical, it should be noted that these procedures are ones that a person can continue for life. They are not crash, fad diet procedures that the person is unable to tolerate for more than a few weeks.

These self-management procedures, sketchily outlined here, are not the only possibilities; rather, self-management procedures may be incorporated into many aspects of medical practice, with minimal amounts of additional professional time. The weight control program requires approximately 20 minutes of contact with the patient per week. Other procedures obviously may require a great deal less.

Some Concluding Suggestions

A variety of techniques for increasing a patient's abilities to deal with important health-related self-control problems have been suggested. Frankly many of these suggestions require more physician input than might normally be possible. An alternative to having the physician be involved in each step of a self-management program would be to have someone on the staff specifically trained to establish and monitor these programs. A nurse could be given special training in behavioral psychology related to self-management. Such a person could then be assigned to work with patients who have problems in these areas.

Also, many health care groups are now hiring psychologists trained in behavioral medicine to be part of the health care team. For example, the Kaiser Permanente Hospitals now have programs for men especially at risk for heart attacks. Although the physician in family or general practice will not need such extensive programs, an arrangement with a good consulting psychologist well trained in behavioral medicine could be of great value to both the physician and his or her patients.

As the area of behavioral medicine or medical psychology continues to develop, the opportunities for cooperative efforts between physicians and psychologists appear numerous. In this chapter only a few of the possible ways that a self-management approach could be used to deal with important medical problems have been discussed. To date the majority of the research on self-management has focused on problems of smoking, eating, and adherence to medical regimes. Other problem behaviors could also be approached from the perspective of self-management. For example, anger control such as for persons who abuse their spouses or for hypertensives may be beneficial. Becker et al. (Chapter 18) have noted the potential for self-management in the treatment of depression.

Particularly those who are familiar with behavioral principles may find that the principles of self-management are not excessively complex. With that realization comes the recognition that these principles may be relatively easily understood by patients and adopted with little resistance. The danger of such a realization is that one may assume that these principles may be applied with less than maximum attention to detail. It has been our consistent experience that nonsystematic application of these principles may do more harm than good. Not only does nonsystematic application often fail, but the patient may come to believe that he or she has failed or cannot change. Under the careful supervision of a skilled clinician these procedures can be very effective and a major benefit to both the physician and patient.

References

Barker, R. G. 1968. Ecological Psychology. Stanford, California: Stanford University Press.

Brigham, T. A. 1982. Self-management: A radical behavioral perspective. In R. Karoly and F. Kanfer, eds.: Self-management and Behavior Change. New York: Pergamon Press.

Caldwell, L. R. 1974a. Behavioral management of self medication regimes. Unpublished manuscript, University of Washington School of Medicine, Seattle, Washington.

Caldwell, L. R. 1974b. Behavior management program for skin care. Unpublished manuscript, University of Washington School of Medicine, Seattle, Washington.

Caldwell, L. R. 1974c. The elimination of smoking. Unpublished manuscript, University of Washington School of Medicine, Seattle, Washington.

Danaher, B., and E. Lichtenstein. 1978. Become an Ex-smoker. Englewood Cliffs, New Jersey: Prentice-Hall.

Fordyce, W. E. 1974. Maintenance of prescribed regimes. Unpublished manuscript, University of Washington School of Medicine, Seattle, Washington.

Graubard, P., H. Rosenberg, and M. Miller. 1974. Student applications of behavior modification to teachers and environments or ecological approaches to social deviancy. In R. Ulrich, T. Stachnick, and J. Mabry, eds.: Control of Human Behavior, Vol. 3. Glenview, Illinois: Scott Foresman.

Kanfer, F. H., C. J. M. Cox, and P. Karoly. 1974. Contracts demand characteristics, and self control. Journal of Personality and Social Psychology 30:605–619.

Mahoney, M. J., and K. Mahoney. 1976. Permanent weight control: A total solution to the dieter's dilemma. New York: W. W. Norton.

Peterson, J. L., and T. A. Brigham. 1980. Women, weight loss and working out: The effects of exercise on weight control. Paper presented at the Association for the Advancement of Behavior Therapy, November 1980, New York:

Romanczyk, R. C. 1978. The behavior treatment of obesity: Treatment interactions. Paper presented at the Midwestern Association of Behavior Analysis, Chicago, Illinois.

Shachter, S. 1971. Some extraordinary facts about obese humans and rats. American Psychologist 26:129–144.

Skinner, B. F. 1953. Science and Human Behavior. New York: MacMillan.

Stimson, G. V. 1974. Obeying doctors orders: A view from the other side. Social Science and Medicine 8:97–104.

Stuart, R. B. 1967. Behavioral control of overeating. Behavior Research and Therapy 5:357–365.

Stuart, R. B., and B. Davis. 1972. Slim Chance in a Fat World: Behavioral Control of Obesity. Champaign, Illinois: Research Press.

Stunkard, A. J. 1975. From explanation to action in psychosomatic medicine: The case of obesity. Psychosomatic Medicine 37:195–236.

II

BEHAVIORAL SCIENCE RESEARCH AND SOME MAJOR MEDICAL PROBLEMS

11

The Relation of Stress
to Health and Illness

William M. Womack, M.D.,* Peter P. Vitaliano, Ph.D.,†
and Roland D. Maiuro, Ph.D.‡

The relation of stress to health and illness has received increased attention by both clinicians and researchers. This relation has been recently underscored by proponents of holistic approaches to medicine who emphasize the importance of not only physical but also emotional and socioenvironmental factors. The purpose of this chapter is to provide an introduction and overview to issues and factors relevant to the relations of stress, health, and illness. To achieve this purpose the following areas are discussed and reviewed: theoretical and conceptual issues related to the definition and phenomenon of stress, measurement techniques, research findings related to health, and current stress management approaches.

Theoretical and Conceptual Issues

In the absence of an operational definition, "stress" can be an ambiguous and vague construct. However, four definitions of stress have been offered that cover the realm in which stress has been conceptualized:

1. Any action or situation that places special physical or psychological demands upon a person.
2. The state manifested by a specific syndrome that consists of all the nonspecifically induced changes within a biological system (Selye, 1956).

*Associate Professor, Department of Psychiatry and Behavioral Sciences, University of Washington School of Medicine, Seattle, Washington.
† Associate Professor, Department of Psychiatry and Behavioral Sciences, University of Washington School of Medicine, Seattle, Washington.
‡ Assistant Professor, Department of Psychiatry and Behavioral Sciences, University of Washington School of Medicine, Seattle, Washington.

3. Any event in which environmental demands, internal demands, or both tax or exceed the adaptive resources of an individual's social system or tissue system (Lazarus and Cohen, 1977).
4. A generic term for the whole area of problems that includes the stimuli-producing stress reactions, the reactions themselves, and the various intervening processes (Lazarus, 1966).

Types of Stressors

Stressors, the things that cause stress, can be physical, such as pain or time pressures; environmental, such as noise and crowding; psychological, such as worrying about past, present, or future events; or social, such as marital discord. Stressors can originate from both inside and outside the individual. Indeed, any life event, whether it be a physical disaster (e.g., an accident or disease) or a daily hassle (e.g., a change in work schedule or time delay), can be viewed as a stressor. Such a generality exists because the degree to which an event is a stressor depends on one's appraisal of that event as threatening, disruptive, or dangerous. In this sense all stressors in part can be viewed as products of cognition and are thus a function of the way one looks at, appraises, and constructs one's relationships with events.

Appraisal often takes the form of a process called "labeling." Labeling may be viewed as an internal dialogue through which one categorizes events, thereby creating a subjective meaning for them. Thus one's internal dialogue creates how one feels and in effect how one will behave toward a particular stressor. In any type of "stressful encounter," environmental demands, cognitive appraisal processes, coping, and emotional responses constantly interact with and affect one another.

Types of Stress Reactions

Responses to stress may be viewed as reactions that generally fall into three categories: (1) physiological, (2) cognitive, and (3) behavioral (Lang, 1969).

Physiological Mechanisms

The body's response to stress is automatic and is often called the "fight–flight response." This response is reflexive and conditions the body so that it is best prepared to either fight or run away. During this response, the body prepares itself by activating the autonomic nervous system and releasing a series of hormones into the blood stream.

Much of the time, the autonomic system operates via visceral reflexes based on impulses from the viscera and some internal sensory receptors.

When these impulses are received by the autonomic system, the appropriate responses to these impulses are transmitted by reflex back to the organs. Autonomic reflexes mobilize the body's resources to deal with stressors. Through this mechanism a person subjected to a mental or physical stressor reacts "automatically" by initiating a complex series of neurophysiological and biochemical changes in his body; these include changes in blood flow, metabolism, and muscle tone.

Two distinct but interdependent parts of the autonomic system are responsible for the regulation of these changes: One is the sympathetic nervous system and the other is the parasympathetic system. Generally the sympathetic system tenses and constricts involuntary muscles such as those of the blood vessel walls and activates the endocrine system. In contrast, the parasympathetic system generally initiates dilation of the body's smooth muscles and induces a state of relaxation. There is one vital distinction between the two systems that is central to an understanding of stress responses: Parasympathetic nervous activity is relatively specific in its influences and selective in its activation of the organs it controls; the sympathetic system, although it too may act selectively, usually acts through a general excitation effect upon neural and glandular functions termed "mass discharge" (Guyton, 1971). Thus, by eliciting a mass discharge response through physiological channels, stress can create a large generalized demand upon the body.

Endocrinological response to stress begins in the hypothalamus in the center of the brain. The hypothalamus stimulates activity in the autonomic nervous system and the pituitary gland. One of the most important of these reactions is the action of the adrenocorticotropic hormone (ACTH) upon the adrenal glands. At the same time that ACTH is acting on the adrenal cortex, the pituitary is also releasing thyrotropic hormone (TTH). This hormone causes the thyroid to secrete thyroxine, which affects the rate at which the body consumes fuel, as well as governs physical growth and sexual and mental development. During stress, metabolism in the tissues is intensely stimulated by thyroxine. When this happens, a person sweats easily and can feel shaky. His heart tends to beat too fast, breathing becomes rapid and unusually deep, and he tires quickly. Thyroxine and adrenaline work together closely to produce many of the same subjective effects. High levels of thyroxine apparently make the system more responsive to adrenaline. Generally adrenaline seems to play a greater role in short-term stress, while thyroxine seems to be present in greater quantities in prolonged stress (McQuade and Aikman, 1974).

The adrenals are only one part of a very complex endocrine system, but their significance in terms of understanding the relation between stress and psychosomatic disease is great. The adrenals have two functionally distinct parts: (1) the outer and larger part, the adrenal cortex and (2) the inner part, the medulla. In the initial stages of the stress response it is the medulla that is called into action by stress signals relayed through sympathetic nervous stimuli. In response to these stimuli, the medulla secretes adrenaline and noradrenaline. Under stress, adrenaline enters the bloodstream and is distributed throughout the body. All of us are familiar with the feeling of a sudden flush of excitation or an "adrenaline rush." This occurs when the adrenal medulla releases its stress hormones and causes the entire body to respond to the jolt in a tremendous surge of energy. Such a reaction sometimes enables people to perform feats of physical strength that they would not normally be able to do, such as when a wife lifts an automobile to save her trapped husband. The whole system enters a state of hyperactivation in which the heart races, body temperature rises, and oxygen consumption increases (Fig. 1).

Human stress stimulates an essential physiological process that enables individuals to response to the multitude of challenges confronted each day. It is one of the body's most sensitive and vital survival systems. There is a basic problem, however, in the way human beings are designed to respond to stress. Physiologically, we are equipped with much the same systems as animals have to cope with stress, but there is an added complication in human reactivity. Information perceived through the higher awareness centers also generates a physical stress response. This information is of a psychological and emotional nature, based upon the individual's perception of events in the environment around him. Basically, when human beings are subjected to major stress, they are aroused to a fight or flight reaction in the same way as animals; but the problem is that an animal can deal with a threat through fight or flight, but people often cannot. In civilized encounters much of the stress experienced cannot be dealt with by either fighting or running away, although our initial inclination certainly may be to do one or the other. When the negative psychological state persists, the physiological stress response also continues. It is under these circumstances, when a stress response is prolonged and unabated, that the biochemical changes associated with stress become potentially detrimental to health.

Selye's General Adaptation Syndrome

Foremost among researchers of the physiology of stress is Hans Selye, an endocrinologist who is the director of the Institute on Experimental Medicine and Surgery at the University of Montreal. In 1956 Selye published *The Stress of Life*, which remains a classic in the field. His research on the adrenal glands and their relation with the pituitary and other physiological processes laid the groundwork for a great deal of research on stress. Selye is also responsible for the introduction of stress into the life sciences as a systematic concept. Selye defined stress as "the state manifested by a specific syndrome which consists of all the

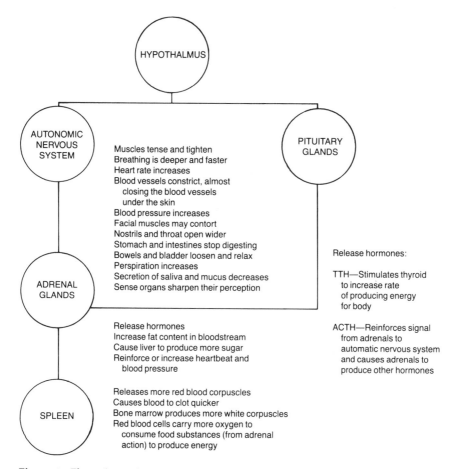

Figure 1. Flow chart of body response to stress.

nonspecifically induced changes within a biologic system" (Selye, 1956). In other words, stress is manifested as a specific configuration of physiological processes rather than as the processes themselves. This specific series of processes Selye termed general adaptation syndrome (GAS) (Fig. 2). Activation of the GAS may result from any number of different stimuli and is therefore "nonspecifically induced."

Selye's stress model places heavy emphasis on the role of the pituitary hormone ACTH. Recently, researchers have tended to distinguish between two kinds of stress and their respective effects upon the body. The first is acute stress, in which the threat is immediate and the need to respond is instantaneous; the second is chronic stress, which is prolonged

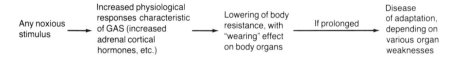

Figure 2. Selye's general adaptation syndrome model.

and unabated. Most current investigative work seems to indicate that in acute stress it is the adrenaline and noradrenaline that are called into play. In chronic stress the role and presence in the blood of corticoids from the adrenal cortex increase and assume more importance.

According to Selye, GAS passes through three phases: (1) alarm, (2) resistance, and (3) exhaustion (Fig. 3). The alarm phase is the first and most dramatic response to a stressor. At that point the body's entire stress mechanism is mobilized and the stressor has a generalized effect on psychophysiological functioning. During the alarm stage, adrenal cortical secretions rise sharply. One of the primary tasks of the GAS is to delegate responsibility for dealing with the stressor to the organ or system best capable of handling it, seeking out and calling into action the most appropriate channel of defense. At this point the resistance phase is initiated. During this period, adrenocortical secretions decrease and coping with the stressor becomes the specific job of the particular system(s) best suited to the task. Resistance to the stressor is high during this phase, but because of the effects of the GAS and the fact that resources are diverted away from other areas, general resistance to disease may be low, but the stressor becomes worn out and breaks down. Once again adrenocortical secretions rise and the burden is shifted away from the worn out system and again taken on by the nonspecific response characteristic of the alarm phase. In effect, this entire process functions to maximize the body's ability to resist the stressor. This three-phase response does not inevitably lead to psychosomatic illness, and stress

Figure 3. The stress syndrome: (1) an alarm reaction, (2) a stage of resistance, and (3) a stage of exhaustion.

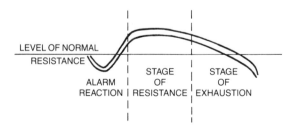

reactivity should not be equated with damage or pathology. Prolonged stress, however, will wear out the body and lower resistance. When the body fails to adapt or overcome stress, diseases of adaptation are frequently the result. What Selye called diseases of adaptation are simply ordinary diseases that develop as a consequence of unabated GAS activity. Such disorders cannot be attributed to stress alone, but to the fact that the body's attempt to adapt to stress may cause physiological conditions that precipitate disorders or predispose an individual toward pathology.

Cognitive–Behavioral Mechanisms

For an experience to be stressful, it must be cognitively perceived as potentially harmful, threatening, or unpleasant to the individual involved. Lazarus (1966) has termed this perceptual process "appraisal." The appraisal of a stressful event has been discussed in terms of its (1) psychological meaning/relevance (Basowitz et al., 1955; Pepitone, 1967), (2) potential dangerousness (Lazarus, 1966), and (3) salience and controllability (Stokols, 1979).

In their classic study of paratrooper training, Basowitz et al. (1955) found that individuals varied considerably in the amounts of stress they experienced and that people differed in their reactions to stress, depending upon how psychologically meaningful the event was for them. Basowitz et al. suggested that we need to regard stress as a continuum of events, from those that evoke anxiety in everyone to those which are meaningful to just a few. Similarly, Pepitone (1967) proposed that the relevance of a situation determines the degree of distress it evokes. For example, in achievement situations the development of stress may depend on the consequences of success or failure for the person. Appraisal is a key component in Lazarus' trans*actional* model of stress. In this model appraisal is influenced by the combination of a person's beliefs, expectations, learning, past experiences, and responsibility. These factors affect the cues that are recognized and the ways in which they are used in evaluating the potential harm of a situation. Stokols (1979) has proposed that stress can best be understood in terms of the salience/importance of the stressor to the person and the extent to which the stressful event can be controlled. Controllability refers to the person's ability to respond effectively to the stress. Stokols' model predicts that as controllability decreases, stress increases and will be highest when control is low and salience high.

The relation between control over an aversive event and the amount of distress the event produces have been studied in terms of a person's avoidance behavior. Avoidance strategies of control lead one to ignore, deny, disassociate, or distract oneself from an event. Nonavoidance strategies focus on the event through heightened sensitivity, rumination, and attempts to control physiological or cognitive reactions. The possible differential effects of such cognitive/behavioral styles are well illustrated in Janis' (1958) basic study of the coping strategies of patients awaiting surgery. Janis found that patients who adopted the avoidance strategy experienced less preoperative anxiety but had less favorable postoperative attitudes. In contrast, patients who adopted a nonavoidance strategy experienced more preoperative anxiety but had more favorable post-operative attitudes. Janis' findings have since been replicated and ampli-fied by the work of other investigators (Andrew, 1970; Kendall et al., 1979) and indicate that patients' cognitions can significantly affect the duration of hospitalization, the amount of medication used, and the overall adjustment to surgical interventions.

The individual development of a person prior to exposure to a potential stressor is an important factor in determining whether or not an event functions as a stressor. Such characteristics as a person's personality, abilities, and learning/experiences (Mechanic, 1962), have been posited as important individual factors. Personality may be viewed as the cognitive behavioral style of perceiving or responding characteristic of an individual, as such personality clearly affects the way a person handles stress. Stress experiences early in life may lead to the adoption of certain methods of coping with problems. Certain psychological and behavioral defenses are then integrated into the personality and determine the way an individual attempts to manage stress throughout his life. One should note that some researchers have focused on coping styles as personality "traits" (Haan, 1963, 1965, 1977), while others have argued that they are also "states" of behavior (Lazarus, 1966), that is, more affected by the type of stressor (i.e., health problems versus work problems) than the individual's personality. It would appear that coping styles are the result of multiple inputs, including the environmental event (stressor), the cognitive processes, and the behavioral repertoire. Moreover, these inputs function in an inter-actional and dynamic fashion (see Fig. 4).

Figure 4. Interrelations of stressors, cognitive processes, and behavioral reac-tions.

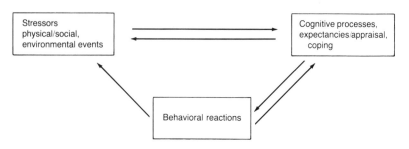

A Transactional Model of Stress

It is important to keep in mind that the experience of stress is a phenomenon derived from the interaction of environmental stressors, physiological processes, cognitive processes, and behavioral mechanisms. Lazarus and Cohen (1976) have attempted to develop a heuristic model to illustrate this dynamic interplay that integrates the psychological, physiological, and social components of stress and distress. The model consists of (1) inputs (or precedents), (2) physiological, psychological, and social processes and reactions (mediators) concerned with emotions and coping, and (3) outcomes. Inputs may be grouped into environmental stressors and individual characteristics. Examples of environmental stressors are life changes (e.g., death of a spouse, loss of a job) and chronic daily hassles (e.g., finances, work, health, family problems). While these may be less dramatic than life changes, their chronicity may exact a price in emotional distress and enervation. Finally, the social and institutional network in which a person lives also produces environmental stressors.

Figure 5 illustrates the transactional model of stress as adapted from Lazarus and Launier (1978) and Novaco (1981). In this model one can appreciate the complexity of the phenomenon of "stress," that is, several internal and external components acting together to yield either adaptive or maladaptive reactions. In particular, cognitive styles present in the

Figure 5. Interrelations of cognitive processes, stressors, psychophysiological mediators, resources,and reactions. Adapted from Lazarus and Launier (1978) and Novaco (1981).

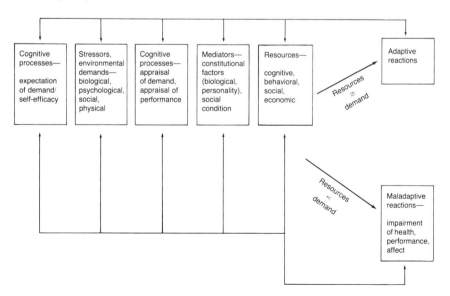

individual prior to exposure to a stressor determine how the individual views the stressor. Such expectations result from the person's psychosocial development. Locus of control (Rotter, 1966) is one kind of generalized expectancy. Locus of control is a bipolar concept, with internal control referring to the expectation that positive and/or negative events are a consequence of one's behavior and under personal control. External control refers to the perception that events are beyond one's control. Internal locus of control appears to be correlated with greater psychological adjustment in response to stress.

Cognitive processes were discussed above as important factors in determining the way in which an individual appraises a stressor once it occurs. Constitutional factors (i.e., personality, heredity), however, can also mediate the relation between a stressor and distress. For example, the type A personality (Friedman and Roseman, 1974) has been implicated as one type of behavior that can exacerbate a stressful situation. In contrast to the type B behavior, which is free of a frantic sense of urgency and which allows time for quiet contemplation, type A behavior is characterized by an obsessive, competitive drive, fierce impatience, and little time for leisure.

Resources such as one's social supports and coping behavior can also modify the degree to which a stressor is damaging. Data from naturalistic and correlational studies of animal and human subjects have suggested that social support can mediate the association between stressors and distress (for reviews, see Cassell, 1976; Cobb, 1976; Dean and Lin, 1977; Heller, 1979). In particular, it has been noted that adequate social support has prophylactic properties, whereas weak social support is a risk factor for illness (Henderson, 1977).

There is evidence that the role of a supportive social network for a particular individual interacts with such factors as the subject's cognitive styles and behavioral responses (Carson, 1969; Leary, 1957; Sullivan, 1953). Pearlin and Schooler (1978) have suggested that coping styles significantly influence a subject's ability to use available resources. Recently, Folkman and Lazarus (1980) have shown that the way in which an individual copes (solving the problem versus wishful thinking) depends on how the stressor is appraised and on the particular type of stressor (i.e., work versus a health problem).

The arrows in Fig. 5 illustrate the dynamic feedback loops linking the various components that result in adaptive or maladaptive responses to a stressor. In particular, the model indicates that when resources are greater than or equal to the demands presented by a stressor, adaptive responses occurs. In contrast, if resources are less than demands, such maladaptive responses as impairments in health, performance, or affect can result. In summary, the reciprocity between the components further determines the stages that define a stressful experience. The successful physician will assess each, as well as their interactions, and take those into account in planning treatment.

Measurement Techniques

In order to discuss how researchers have attempted to measure stress, one needs to distinguish stressors from stress. While the term *stress* refers to a hypothetical construct, the term *stressor* refers to the external stimulus that impinges on the organism. Christensen (1981) has provided a comprehensive categorization of stressors that includes (1) environment (i.e., crowding, social isolation, noise, temperature extremes, pollution, food/water deprivation, traffic, crime), (2) social status (i.e., racism, sexism, age discrimination), (3) personal handicaps (i.e., physical/mental disabilities), (4) economic matters (i.e., inflation, unemployment, poverty), (5) natural disasters (i.e., hurricanes, earthquakes, droughts, volcanic eruptions), (6) technological catastrophies (i.e., airplane/nuclear accidents), and (7) war (e.g., actual and anticipated).

In addition to these stressors, more ordinary life changes (i.e., change of job, illness, change in sleeping habits, vacation) can also induce distress. Both everyday life changes and extraordinary events have been the major types of stressors studied in the past 25 years. We shall provide a brief history of the measurement tools developed and some methodological issues surrounding the use of these scales.

In the past 25 years a number of researchers at the University of Washington, Seattle, Washington, have developed measures to examine life change stress. The schedule of recent experience (SRE) (Hawkins et al., 1957) was the first of several life change scales to measure changes in family, home, work, finances, and so on. In 1964 Holmes and Rahe (1967) developed the social readjustment rating scale (SRRS), which was an important advance over the SRE because it included 43 life events (see Table 1) along with a method of quantifying life change units (LCU) according to the amount of readjustment they require in the average person's life. Since then, two other revisions, the schedule of recent events (SRE) and the recent life change questionnaire (RLCQ) (Rahe, 1975) were developed. In each scale, scoring is done by summing the LCU values for all items checked (Holmes and Masuda, 1974).

One should note that the SRE has been criticized because its norms (LCUs) were developed on a specific urban population. The items are too restricted, they do not specify the directionality of change in some events, and they are confounded with illness outcome (29 of the 43 life events on the SRRS are often the symptoms of consequences of illness). Furthermore, the SRE does not consider individual differences in the perception of stress. Finally, these measures alone do not take into account the person's resources for coping.

Table 1. The Social Readjustment Rating Scale[a]

Life event	Mean value
1. Death of spouse	100
2. Divorce	73
3. Marital separation	65
4. Jail term	63
5. Death of close family member	63
6. Personal injury or illness	53
7. Marriage	50
8. Fired at work	47
9. Marital reconciliation	45
10. Retirement	45
11. Change in health of family member	44
12. Pregnancy	40
13. Sex difficulties	39
14. Gain of new family member	39
15. Business readjustment	39
16. Change in financial state	38
17. Death of close friend	37
18. Change to different line of work	36
19. Change in number of arguments with spouse	35
20. Mortgage or loan for major purchase (home, etc.)	31
21. Foreclosure of mortgage or loan	30
22. Change in responsibilities at work	29
23. Son or daughter leaving home	29
24. Trouble with inlaws	29
25. Outstanding personal achievement	28
26. Wife begins or stops work	26
27. Beginning or end of school	26
28. Change in living conditions	25
29. Revision of personal habits	24
30. Trouble with boss	23
31. Change in work hours or conditions	20
32. Change in residence	20
33. Change in schools	20
34. Change in recreation	19
35. Change in church activities	19
36. Change in social activities	18
37. Mortgage or loan for lesser purchase (car, TV, etc.)	17
38. Change in sleeping habits	16
39. Change in number of family get-togethers	15
40. Change in eating habits	15
41. Vacation	13
42. Christmas	12
43. Minor violations of the law	11

[a]See Holmes and Rahe (1967) for complete wording of the items.

Because of these criticisms, several researchers have attempted to develop alternative measures (Cochrane and Robertson, 1973; Dohrenwend et al., 1978; Hurst et al., 1978, Paykel et al., 1971). In general, however, the SRE has been used in the vast majority of studies because, in spite of its limitations, it is a valid scale if one wishes to gain a general estimate of the amount of stress an individual has experienced within a given time period (Christensen, 1981).

Stress and Illness: Research Findings

Stress and life change have been studied in relation to both the onset and exacerbation of a large number of disorders. These disorders have ranged from minor illnesses to life-threatening conditions such as cancer and cardiovascular disease. The typical research design has been to examine the personal history of a select patient sample in relation to the onset and course of the illness. In many studies, personality variables have been assessed and stressors quantified with a life events rating scale such as that developed by Holmes and Rahe (1967).

In an early series of studies investigating the onset and course of a variety of minor illnesses in a large military sample, Rahe and his associates found a direct and positive relation between life change scores and the incidence of health problems (Rahe, 1968, 1969a,b; 1972; Rahe and Arthur, 1968). Kimball (1971) observed a similar pattern in a patient sample suffering from diabetes mellitus. A study of 41 postoperative patients followed for 4 years after surgery for duodenal ulcer revealed a peak of life change stressors during the year preceding the required surgery. Moreover, patients with higher postoperative exposure to stress continued to have significantly more residual ulcer symptoms than patients with lower life events scores (Stevenson et al., 1976).

Stress and Cardiovascular Disease

The relation between stress and cardiovascular disease has been extensively studied. The most comprehensive work in the area has been conducted by the cardiologists Friedman and Rosenman within a paradigm that has been called "type A research" (Friedman and Rosenman, 1974). As a result of years of observation, these researchers have identified a coronary-prone profile that has been described as "a characteristic action–emotion complex which is exhibited by those individuals who are engaged in a relatively *chronic struggle* to obtain an unlimited number of *poorly defined* things from their environment in the *shortest period of time* and, if necessary, against the opposing efforts of other things in this same environment" (Friedman, 1969). Unlike his "type B" counterpart, who appears less hurried, more reflective, and more leisurely paced, the type A individual has been observed to interact with the environment with (1) a relatively extreme degree of competitiveness and aggressiveness around achievement issues, (2) an exaggerated sense of time urgency, and (3) overinvolvement in his job and professional responsibilities, often to the neglect of other aspects of his life (Zyzanski and Jenkins, 1970).

In their initial research on type A and coronary heart disease, Friedman et al. (1958) observed a definite link between type A work attitudes and habits and abnormal changes in serum cholesterol and blood clotting time. Further study of these individuals indicated that actual coronary artery disease was seven times more prevalent in type A individuals than in type B persons, and that this finding could not be explained by differences in exercise, cigarette smoking, or drinking or eating habits. More recent research has further confirmed and refined the early work of Friedman and his associates and documented a relation between the strength of the type A action complex and the degree of arteriosclerosis as determined by coronary angiography (Jenkins, 1975), the incidence of both angina pectoris and myocardial infarction, as well as the occurrence of reinfarction in people who already have coronary disease (Jenkins, 1976).

Stress and Cancer

The role of stress in the development of cancer is a controversial but fascinating subject of research. From a purely biological perspective, carcinogenesis occurs as a result of a mutation that overcomes or obviates the normal resistance mechanisms of the body. In contrast, a stress illness model would postulate a different course of action whereby stressors first affect a pathological lowering of resistance. The lowered resistance then permits the action of a carcinogen that ordinarily would not produce a cancerous growth, as in the case of transplant immunosuppresant complications.

At this point there is ample evidence that psychosocial and environmental stressors induce immunological compromise that may in turn affect the pathogenesis of tumor growth. An excellent annotated bibliography of this research up to 1976 has been compiled by Achterberg et al. in *Stress, Psychological Factors, and Cancer* (1976). Other research relating to this area has been reported by Monjan and Collector (1977), and Riley (1975) and may be summarized as follows (Skylar and Anisman, 1981):

1. Stress under specified conditions will enhance tumor development and metastases in animals. Life stress appears to be related to neoplasia in humans. In both instances, the inability to cope adequately with stress appears to be an essential element in predicting tumor genesis.

2. Little information is available concerning the effects of stress on carcinogen-induced tumors.
3. Stress may influence the progress of the neoplasm in humans. Under less than ideal conditions, created by the inability to cope with acute stress, the organism's natural defenses might be inadequate to prevent cell proliferation and hence tumor progress.
4. Stress may influence the final stages of human neoplastic disease. There is data showing enhanced tumor growth and metastases following surgery that seems to not be specifically related to the release of tissue cells into the circulation. There is some suggestion from animal studies that this effect is due primarily to immuno-suppression stemming from the stressful nature of treatment.
5. To date, most studies have focused on either early life stress or life stress preceding cancer diagnosis. Cancer may, however, be related to complex interactions involving early life experience, trauma experienced in adulthood, and the presence or absence of social support systems.
6. Stress is an environmental event with profound effects on physio-logical functioning and may influence the course of neoplastic disease. Because of the intricate relation between the neurochemical, hormonal, and immune systems, disruption of any of these processes, as a result of a potential exhaustion of resources that makes the organism less capable of efficiently contending with malignant cells, could increase the probability of cancer cell proliferation.

Stress and Mental Illness

Stress has also been implicated in the clinical onset of a variety of mental or psychiatric ailments (Rahe, 1969b). In a series of studies, Paykel et al. (1969), Paykel and Tanner (1975), and Jacobs et al. (1974) examined large numbers of depressed patients, using clinical and life event scaling measures. Compared with a sample of 900 normals, the depressed patients reported over three times the number of life events in the 6-month period preceding onset of their disorder. Differences were most notable in terms of "exit events," with patients reporting significantly more losses (e.g., a death in the family, separation) than normals. There were also significant differences in a variety of other socially undesirable or negative events, such as arguments with one's spouse, physical illness, and a variety of unexpected work changes. As would be predicted, depressives requiring inpatient hospitalization evidenced even higher life events scores than outpatients, with suicidal patients exhibiting the highest level of all. Follow-up assessment of patients who experienced early relapse after recovery also indicated a positive correlation between relapse and the number of stressors in the patient's environment (Paykel and Tanner, 1975).

Life change events have also been linked to a variety of anxiety-based disorders (Cooper and Sylph, 1973), as well as severely incapacitating disorders such as schizophrenia. In the case of psychotic disorders such as schizophrenia, such events appear to play more of a part in precipitation than a formative role in relation to the symptom picture of other health disorders. The effect of stress events upon mental illness appears to be mediated by a variety of factors related to cognitive–perceptual styles, social supports, psychological defenses, and coping resources (Rahe and Arthur, 1978).

Stress Management

Given the realistic limitations involved in controlling constitutional factors and social conditions, much of the work in the area of prevention and rehabilitation has focused on developing personal, ecological, and cognitive behavioral approaches to stress management. As a result of this focus, two primary ways of managing or modifying the impact of stress have emerged: The first involves strategies to decrease or change the environmental input of stressors, and the second involves strategies to increase or strengthen the resources an individual possesses for dealing with the stressors.

The most commonly used method to decrease stressor input is purely environmental and simply involves changing the life space or personal ecology of the individual. An example of this approach includes the age-old advice to "take a vacation" and thus experience a time out from ongoing troubles and pressures. Such an approach is, of course, temporary and is designed to allow the person to renew himself or recover from a demanding schedule. In some cases, a more permanent adjustment is necessary whereby the individual makes a more long-term change in his environment. Changes in job description, employment setting, social circles, and even residence are examples of this type of approach and they are often indicated when a person is, for some reason, unable to recover sufficiently to return to the old environment or needs to change environments for positive growth reasons.

However, making a change in one's environment is often difficult and not always feasible or desirable. In such cases, the second approach to stress management is worth considering and consists of a variety of techniques designed to improve a person's ability to live with existing environmental stressors.

During the past 10–15 years, a considerable amount of clinical research has been devoted to the development and evaluation of psychologically based cognitive and behavioral coping techniques (Meichenbaum, 1974;

Kendall and Hollon 1979). Cognitive techniques are designed to change the way the individual thinks about, interprets, or appraises the stress-inducing stimuli. Simply put, if a person continuously thinks of problem situations in negative, exaggerated, unchangeable, and overwhelming terms, the stressors are likely to have a frustrating and draining effect. "Cognitive restructuring" techniques are frequently used by mental health professionals to help people relabel or redefine the stressors into more positive, realistic, and changeable terms so that they can be managed more effectively. Thus it is important to analyze a person's expectations or self-statements when he or she is faced with a stressful situation so as to determine whether it is helping or hurting functioning.

A number of behavioral skills have been shown to be effective in reducing anxiety and stress as well as in facilitating optimal performance. One of the most useful skills is that of personal assertiveness (Alberti and Emmons, 1974; Linehan, 1979). Once acquired, assertiveness skills allow persons to directly express their needs and wants in a firm but diplomatic fashion and also protect themselves from excessive or unreasonable demands. By behaving assertively, one can minimize the buildup of resentments that frequently damage social and vocational relationships and threaten personal well-being. Effective communication and negotiation skills can further refine an individual's ability to relate smoothly with others and solve problems without assuming a rigid "win–lose" attitude characteristic of stressful encounters (Alberti and Emmons, 1974; Eisler and Hersen, 1973). Goal setting and time management skills can also be useful for reducing stress, particularly in work-related or business settings, where ongoing pressures and demands are virtually a way of life. On a less technical level, behavioral attitudes such as physical exercise and the scheduling of pleasurable events have also been shown to help reduce tension by channeling excess arousal and lending a sense of balance and perspective to ongoing events.

In addition to the above strategies, there are a variety of cognitive–behavioral stress management procedures that fall into the category of relaxation techniques. Progressive muscle relaxation is probably the most commonly used and thoroughly studied of these techniques and involves body awareness training and the gradual release of tension from the major and minor muscle groups (Jacobson, 1938; Bernstein and Borkovec, 1973). Once acquired, this skill can be used to maintatin generally low levels of physiological activity throughout the day or as a self-control technique in the face of an active or immediate stressor (Goldfried and Trier, 1974). Progressive muscle relaxation techniques have been shown to reliably lower autonomic activity in the form of electromylographic, galvanic skin response, blood pressure, and heart rate indices, and have been successfully applied to a wide range of stress-related problems, including common psychosomatic disorders (Alexander, 1972), headaches (Chesney and Shelton, 1976), insomnia (Pendleton and Tasto, 1976), and hypertension (Graham et al., 1977). Autogenic training (Luthe, 1962) and meditation (Narango and Ornstein, 1971) represent variants of relaxation procedures that have similar effects but which also include self-verbalization, visual imagery, and philosophical components. All three relaxation methods have been shown to be effective in producing a state of lowered arousal and there may be some degree of specificity in terms of which technique a particular individual will find most appealing and beneficial. Those who tend to experience stress responses primarily in their autonomic nevous system in the form of muscle tension, stomach cramps, or palpitations may benefit most from progressive muscle relaxation or autogenic training. People who are prone to obsessively rehash the day's events or drudge up old traumatic experiences may get better results with some form of meditative or hypnotic techniques with cognitive elements.

Biofeedback techniques represent yet another and decidedly more technical approach to stress management. Unlike the previously discussed techniques, these procedures generally require the use of specialized electronic equipment to help the individual "shape up" a particular physiological pattern by repeated practice, successive approximations, and immediate feedback through auditory, visual, or tactile cues.

Summary and Conclusions

This chapter has attempted to examine the relation of stress and illnes through biological, psychological, and social mechanisms. One way of integrating the material presented in this chapter is to use an explanatory model of distress (Albee, 1977). In this model, illness depends on exposure to a stressor, vulnerability to stress, and psychological (i.e., coping) and social adaptation (i.e., social supports), expressed as the formula

$$\text{Distress} = \frac{\text{Exposure to a stressor} + \text{vulnerability}}{\text{Psychological and social adaptation}}$$

This model is not mathematical, since the variables do not contain coefficients that describe their relative importance in predicting distress/illness. Moreover, the variables are not independent; that is, vulnerability and resources are themselves interrelated. The model does, however, offer a structure for discussing the interrelations of variables as they relate to distress/illness. For example, if the amount of stress and psychological/social adaptation is held constant, a person who is vulnerable should experience more distress than one who is not vulnerable. As noted in this chapter, examples of vulnerability are sensitivity to autonomic nervous system arousal, genetic composition, age, socioeconomic status, and personality. The techniques of stress management suggested in this chapter represent one possible system that can be used to influence coping and thereby modify the relations of stress, vulnerability, and illness.

References

Achterberg, J., O. C. Simonton, and S. Matthews-Simonton. 1976. Stress, Psychological Factors, and Cancer. Forth Worth, Texas: New Medicine Press.

Albee, G. 1977. Strategies of Primary Prevention. Paper presented at Primary Prevention Conference, National Council of Mental Health Centers, Tucson, Arizona, October 1977.

Alberti, R. E., and M. L. Emmons. 1974. Your Perfect Right. San Luis Obispo, California: Impact.

Alexander, A. B. 1972. Systematic Relaxation and flow rates in asthmatic children: Relationship to emotional precipitants and anxiety. Journal of Psychosomatic Research 16:405–410.

Andrew, J. M. 1970. Recovery from surgery with and without preparatory instruction, for three coping styles. Journal of Personality and Social Psychology 15:223–226.

Basowitz, H., H. Persky, S. J. Korchin, and R. R. Grinker. 1955. Anxiety and Stress. New York: McGraw-Hill.

Bernstein, D. A., and T. D. Borkovec. 1973. Progressive Relaxation Training: A Manual for Helping Professionals. Champaign, Illinois: Research Press.

Carson, R. I. 1969. Interaction Concepts of Personality. Chicago, Illinois: Aldine-Atherton.

Cassell, J. 1976. The contribution of the social environment to host-resistance. American Journal of Epidemiology 104:107–123.

Chesney, M. A., and Shelton, J. L. 1976. A comparison of muscle relaxation and electromyogram biofeedback treatments for muscle contraction headache. Journal of Behavior Therapy and Experimental Psychiatry 7:221–225.

Christensen, J. F. 1981. Assessment of Stress: Environmental, intrapersonal, and outcome issues. In P. McReynolds, ed.: Advances in Psychological Assessment. San Francisco, California: Jossey-Bass, pp. 62–123.

Cobb, S. B. 1976. Social support as a moderator of life stress. Psychosomatic Medicine 38:300–314.

Cochrane, R., and A. Robertson. 1973. The life events inventory: A measure of the relative severity of psycho-social stressors. Journal of Psychosomatic Research 17:135–139.

Cooper, B., and J. Sylph. 1973. Life events and the onset of neurotic illness: An investigation in general practice. Psychological Medicine 3:421–435.

Dean, S., and N. Lin. 1977. The stress-buffering role of social support. Journal of Nervous and Mental Disease 165:403–417.

Dohrenwend, B. S., L. Krasnoff, A. R. Askenasy, and B. P. Dohrenwend. 1978. Exemplification of a method for scaling life events: The PERI life events scale. Journal of Health and Social Behavior 19:205–229.

Douglass, M. E. 1977. Stress and personal performance. Personnel Administrator, August, pp. 60–63.

Eisler, R. M., and M. Hersen. 1973. Behavioral techniques in family oriented crisis interventions. Archives of General Psychiatry 28:111–116.

Folkman, S., and R. S. Lazarus. 1980. Coping in an adequately functioning middle-aged population. Journal of Health and Social Behavior 19:219–239.

Friedman, M. 1969. Pathogenesis of Coronary Artery Disease. New York: McGraw-Hill.

Friedman, M., and R. H. Rosenman. 1974. Type A Behavior and Your Heart. New York: A. A. Knopf.

Friedman, M., R. H. Rosenman, and V. Carroll. 1958. Changes in serum cholesterol and blood clotting time in men subjected to cyclic variation of occupation stress. Circulation 17:852–861.

Goldfried, M. R., and C. S. Trier. 1974. Effectiveness of relaxation as an active coping skill. Journal of Abnormal Psychology 83:348–355.

Graham, L. E., I. Beiman, and A. R. Ciminero. 1977. The generality of the therapeutic effects of progressive relaxation training for essential hypertension. Journal of Behavior Therapy and Experimental Psychiatry 8:161–164.

Guyton, A. C. 1971. Textbook of Medical Physiology, 4th ed. Philadelphia, Pennsylvania: W. B. Saunders.

Haan, N. 1963. Proposed model of ego functioning: Coping and defense mechanisms in relationship to IQ change. Psychological Monographs 77:1–23.

Haan, N. 1965. Coping and defense mechanisms related to personality inventories. Journal of Consulting Psychology 29:373–378.

Haan, N. 1977. Coping and Defending. New York: Academic Press.

Hawkins, N. G., R. Davies, and T. H. Holmes. 1957. Evidence of psychosocial factors in the development of pulmonary tuberculosis. American Review of Tuberculosis and Pulmonary Disease 75:768–780.

Heller, K. 1979. The effects of social support: Prevention and treatment implications in maximizing treatment gains: Transfer enhancement. In A. P. Goldstein, and F. H. Kanfer, eds.: Psychotherapy. New York: Academic Press, pp. 353–382.

Henderson, S. 1977. The social network, support and neurosis: the function of attachment in adult life. British Journal of Psychiatry 131:185–191.

Holmes, T. H., and M. Masuda. 1974. Life change and illness susceptibility. In B. S. Dohrenwend and B. P. Dohrenwend, eds.: Stressful Life Events: Their Nature and Effects. New York: Wiley, pp. 45–72.

Holmes, T. H., and R. H. Rahe. 1967. The social readjustment rating scale. Journal of Psychosomatic Research 11:213–218.

Hurst, M. W., C. D. Jenkins, and R. M. Rose. 1978. The assessment of life change stress: A comparative and methodological inquiry. Psychosomatic Medicine 40:126–141.

Jacobs, S. C., B. A. Prusoff, and E. S. Paykel. 1974. Recent life events in schizophrenia and depression. Psychological Medicine 4:444–453.

Jacobson, E. 1938. Progressive Relaxation. Chicago, Illinois: University of Chicago Press.

Janis, I. 1958. Psychological Stress. New York: Wiley.

Jenkins, C. D. 1975. The coronary-prone personality. *In* W. D. Gentry and R. B. Williams, eds.: Psychological Aspects of Myocardial Infarction and Coronary Care. St. Louis, Missouri: C. V. Mosby, pp. 5–30.

Jenkins, C. D. 1976. Recent evidence supporting psychologic and social risk factors for coronary disease. New England Journal of Medicine 294:987–994.

Kendall, P.C., and S. D. Hollon. 1979. Cognitive–Behavioral Interventions. New York: Academic Press.

Kendall, P. C., L. Williams, T. Pechacek, L. Graham, C. Shisslak, and N. Herzoff. 1979. Cognitive–behavioral and patient education interventions in cardiac catherization procedures: The Palo Alto Medical Psychology Project. Journal of Consulting and Clinical Psychology 47:49–58.

Kimball, C. P. 1971. Emotional and psychosocial aspects of diabetes mellitus. Medical Clinics of North America 55:1007–1018.

Lang, P. J. 1969. The mechanics of desensitization and the laboratory study of human fear. *In* C. M. Franks, eds.: Behavior Therapy—Appraisal and Status. New York: McGraw-Hill, pp. 160–191.

Lazarus, R. S. 1966. Psychological Stress and the Coping Process. New York: McGraw-Hill.

Lazarus, R. S., and J. B. Cohen. 1976. Study of Stress and Coping in Aging. Paper presented at the 5th WHO Conference on Society, Stress and Disease: Aging and Old Age, Stockholm, Sweden, June 1976.

Lazarus, R. S., and J. C. Cohen. 1977. Environmental stress. *In* I. Altman and J. F. Wohlwill, eds.: Human Behavior and Environment, Vol. 2. New York: Plenum Press.

Lazarus, R. S., and R. Launier. 1978. Stress-related transaction between person and environment. *In* L. A. Pervin and M. Lewis, eds.: Perspectives in Interactional Psychology. New York: Plenum Press, pp. 287–327.

Leary, T. 1957. Interpersonal Diagnosis of Personality. New York: Ronald Press.

Linehan, M. M. 1979. Structured cognitive–behavioral treatment of assertion problems. *In* P. C. Kendall and S. D. Hollon, eds.: Cognitive–Behavioral Interventions. New York: Academic Press, pp. 205–240.

Luthe, W. 1962. Method, research and application of autogenic training. American Journal of Clinical Hypnosis 5:17–23.

McQuade, W., and A. Aikman. 1974. Stress. New York: E. P. Dutton.

Mechanic, D. 1962. Students Under Stress. New York: The Free Press of Glencoe.

Meichenbaum, D. 1974. Cognitive Behavior Modification. Morristown, New Jersey: General Learning Press.

Monjan, A. A. and M. I. Collector. 1977. Stress induced modulation of the immune response. Science 196:307.

Naranjo, C., and R. E. Ornstein. 1971. On the Psychology of Meditation. New York: Viking Press.

Novaco, R. 1981. The cognitive regulation of anger and stress. *In* P. C. Kendall and S. D. Hallon, eds.: Cognitive–Behavioral Interventions—Theory, Research and Procedures. New York: Academic Press, pp. 241–285.

Paykel, E. S., and J. Tanner. 1975. Life events, depressive relapse and maintenance treatment. Psychological Medicine.

Paykel, E. S., J. K. Meyers, M. V. Dienelt, G. L. Klerman, J. J. Lindenthal, and M. P. Pepper. Archives of General Psychiatry 21:753–760.

Paykel, E. S., B. A. Prusoff, and E. H. Uhlenhuth. 1971. Scaling of life events. Archives of General Psychiatry 25:340–347.

Pearlin, L. I., and C. Schooler. 1978. The structure of coping. Journal of Health and Social Behavior 19:2–21.

Pendleton, L. R., and D. L. Tasto. 1976. Effects of metronome-conditioned relaxation, metronome-induced relaxation and progressive muscle relaxation in insomnia. Behavior Research and Therapy 14:165–166.

Pepitone, A. 1967. Self, social environment, and stress. In M. H. Appley and R. Trumbull, eds.: Psychological Stress. New York: Appleton-Century-Crofts, pp. 182–208.

Rahe, R. H. 1968. Life change measurement as a predictor of illness. Proceedings of the Royal Society of Medicine 61:1124–1126.

Rahe, R. H. 1969a. Multi cultural correlations of life change scaling, America, Japan, Denmark and Sweden. Journal of Psychosomatic Research 13:191–195.

Rahe, R. H. 1969b. Life crises and health change. In P. R. A. May and J. K. Wittenborn, eds.: Psychotropic Drug Responses, Advances in Prediction. Springfield, Illinois: Charles C. Thomas. 92–125.

Rahe, R. H. 1972. Subjects' recent life change and their near future illness susceptibility. Advances in Psychosomatic Medicine 8:2–19.

Rahe, R. H. 1975. Update to Life Change Researchers. Unpublished manuscript, U.S. Navy, Medical Unit, GUAM.

Rahe, R. H., and R. J. Arthur. 1968. Life change patterns surrounding illness experience. Journal of Psychosomatic Research 11:341–345.

Rahe, R. H., and R. J. Arthur. 1978. Life change and illness studies: Past history and future directions. Journal of Human Stress 4:3–15.

Riley, V. 1975. Mouse mammary tumors: Alteration of incidence as apparent function of stress. Science 189:465–467.

Rotter, J. 1966. Generalized expectancies of internal versus external control of reinforcement. Psychological Monographs 80 (whole No. 609), pp. 1–28.

Selye, H. 1956. The Stress of Life. New York: McGraw-Hill.

Skylar, L. S., and H. Anisman. 1981. Stress and cancer. Psychological Bulletin 89:369–406.

Stevenson, D. K., D. C. Nabsith, M. Masuda, and T. H. Holmes. 1976. Life change and the post operative course of duodenal ulcer patients. Unpublished manuscript, Department of Psychiatry, University of Washington School of Medicine, Seattle, Washington. 19–28.

Stokols, D. 1979. A congruence analysis of human stress. In I. Sarason and C. Spielberger, eds.: Stress and Anxiety, Vol. 6. New York: Hemisphere.

Sullivan, H. S. 1953. The Interpersonal Theory of Psychiatry. New York: W. W. Norton.

Zyzanski, S., and C. D. Jenkins, 1970. Basic dimensions within the coronary-prone behavior pattern. Journal of Chronic Diseases 22:781–795.

12

Psychological Aspects
of Hypertension

George N. Aagaard, M. D.*

There are many reasons to believe that psychological aspects of the individual and his environment may be important in high blood pressure in humans. Physicians who care for hypertensive patients are impressed with the frequency with which the development or aggravation of a problem in the domestic, occupational, or social life of a patient is associated with an increase in blood pressure. Studies conducted with experimental animals and with humans demonstrate that blood pressure is increased by a variety of stimuli. In humans blood pressure may be increased by stress, and the incidence of complications of hypertension, such as stroke and myocardial infarction, may be influenced by psychosocial factors.

Unfortunately, many problems confront us in our understanding of psychosocial factors in hypertension. It is impossible to equate short-term influences on blood pressure with hypertension outcomes, which are observed only after decades. Studies on humans do not permit rigid control of all those aspects of the environment that may influence blood pressure. The same event may have a vastly different meaning to different people, and hence have a difference influence on blood pressure. For example, the death of a parent may liberate one child from a hated, domineering influence, but cause a great sense of guilt in a sibling who had left home.

Following a brief review of the prevalence, significance, and causes of high blood pressure, considerable attention will be devoted to the application of psychological–behavioral methods to the management of human hypertension.

---

*Professor of Medicine and Pharmacology, Division of Clinical Pharmacology, University of Washington School of Medicine, Seattle, Washington.

The Prevalence and Significance of High Blood Pressure

In most of the Western world, systolic and diastolic pressures rise with age in both males and females. Mortality increases and life expectancy decreases with both systolic and disastolic pressure independently. The blood pressure level at which increased mortality is apparent for a population of men of age 30–39 years is 128–137 mmHg systolic and 83–92 mmHg diastolic (Metropolitan Life Insurance Company, 1961). Increased blood pressure is a major risk factor in coronary heart disease and stroke, two of the United States' most important health problems.

Causes of High Blood Pressure

In 5–10% of patients with high blood pressure, a specific cause can be recognized. The most important ones are kidney disease; lesions of the renal arteries, causing renal ischemia; aldosterone-producing adenomas of the adrenal cortex, and pheochromocytomas, tumors of the adrenal medulla. In 90–95% of hypertensive patients, no specific cause can be found. These are diagnosed as essential hypertension.

It is important to distinguish between initiating and sustaining causes of hypertension. A psychological stress may initiate increased blood pressure in a person with a genetic background of essential hypertension and have no effect in someone who has a negative family history. In the prehypertensive but genetically vulnerable person, the stress sets in motion hormonal and physiological changes that may differ in type, degree, and duration from the response in a normotensive. The result is elevated blood pressure. The cause of hypertension is not just the stress or stimulus, but also the as yet unknown factors that produce and sustain exaggerated blood pressure responses in hypertensive individuals.

Pathophysiology of Essential Hypertension

Blood pressure is an expression of many influences, including the structure, function, and control of cardiac and vascular smooth muscle, renal function, the renin–angiotensin–aldosterone system, catecholamine synthesis and release, corticohypothalamic–bulbar–neurohomonal influences, baroreceptor reflex mechanisms, and control of plasma volume. The regulation of these and other factors to provide optimal perfusion to all tissues is obviously complex. According to the "mosaic theory" (Page, 1949), essential hypertension is a disease of regulation in which the relations between these factors are disturbed.

Hemodynamic and hormonal mechanisms operating in hypertension may vary with the age of the hypertensive patient and with the duration of hypertension. Young patients with newly established hypertension are likely to have an increased cardiac output with normal peripheral resistance, whereas patients with long-established hypertension usually have a normal cardiac output and increased peripheral resistance. Low renin hypertension is much more common in older hypertensives.

Abundant evidence suggests that the brain and the sympathetic nervous system are involved in blood pressure control. It is apparent that the brain has ample influence on the sympathetic nervous system and endocrine system. The brain controls the intensity of traffic through the sympathetic nervous system. The manner in which an external or internal event is perceived by the cerebral cortex determines the extent to which the sympathetic nervous system responds. The hypothalamus, vasomotor center, baroreceptors, nucleus tractus solitarius, and the peripheral sympathetics process and intergrate signals that originate in the brain and ultimately influence blood pressure.

Evidence of increased sympathetic nervous system drive is present in some but not all hypertensives. It is most likely in labile hypertension and in established hypertension in younger people. Approximately one-third to one-half of essential hypertensives have a significantly increased level of plasma catecholamines (Engelman et al., 1970). Studies in which large doses of adrenergic receptor-blocking drugs are given also suggest that hypertensives have excess sympathetic tone (Julius et al., 1971). The response to atropine suggests a deficiency of parasympathetic tone as well.

In a study of young hypertensives, Esler et al. (1977) found that heart rate and cardiac output were higher in subjects with high plasma renin activity than in young hypertensives with normal renin. The high-renin subjects also had higher plasma norepinephrine than normal-renin hypertensives and normotensives. In addition to this evidence for increased sympathetic nervous system activity, Esler et al. found less reflex slowing of the heart rate when blood pressure was raised by administration of norepinephrine. This the authors regarded as evidence of reduced parasympathetic tone.

Evidence of increased sympathetic nervous system activity has also been found in young normotensives with hypertensive parents (Falkner et al., 1979). The stress of mental arithmetic caused an increase in blood pressure and plasma chatecholamines that was greater than in normals whose parents were normotensive. Thus increased reactivity of blood pressure and catcholamine release appear to be present in the children of hypertensive parents, whereas resting blood pressure is normal.

The increase in plasma catecholamines may be due to increased production and/or release or to impaired degradation. Nestel (1969) found increased urine catecholamines in hypertensive subjects who did 40 minutes of mental work; this suggested increased release of catecholamines. FitzGerald et al. (1981), on the other hand, found that release of catecholamines was not changed, but that degradation of circulating catecholamines was impaired.

Brod et al. (1959) found that mental work in hypertensive subjects caused an increase in cardiac output, an increased blood flow to the muscles of the extremities and to the brain, and usually a decrease in blood flow to the splanchnic and renal circulations. They also found that the increased blood flow to the muscles was shunted to the right heart by increased venous tone. The effect on total peripheral resistance was quite variable, ranging from increased to decreased.

In general, blood pressure will increase with mental and physical activity and the amount of the increase will relate positively to the intensity of the activity. In populations during a disaster and military personnel during a heavy bombardment, an increased prevalence of hypertension has been observed (Ruskin et al., 1948; Graham, 1945). Even mild mental activity, such as in going from a passive state to an alert observing state, is associated with evidence of increased sympathetic nervous system activity, that is, increased heart rate and blood pressure. The amount of mental workload, the amount of information processed per unit of time, is directly related to the degree of blood pressure increase (Ettema, 1969).

A painful stimulus such as an electric shock or cold water will cause a blood pressure increase. The response will be influenced by the meaning to the individual of the stimulus in the light of previous experience and training. The arousal of emotion also will increase blood pressure. This is true for pleasant as well as painful emotions, with joy causing as large a blood pressure increase as fear. The intensity of the emotional response appears to be directly related to the magnitude of the blood pressure increase. The extent of engagement–involvement in an interview setting has been rated according to the directness, intensity, and immediacy of the interaction between the subject and the interviewer and the rate at which words were spoken. The intensity of involvement and blood pressure response are positively related (Williams et al., 1972; Innes et al., 1959).

In general, the blood pressure increase to mental activity, pain, or emotional arousal in hypertensives will be greater in degree and duration than in normotensives (Shapiro, 1961). The responses of normotensive children of hypertensive parents will be greater than the normotensive children of normotensive parents (Falkner et al., 1979).

The attitude of subjects may influence the response even to a painful stimulus. Obrist et al. (1978) have shown that subjects responded with greater blood pressure increases when they had some hope of preventing an electric shock by their performance at a task than when there was no way to avoid the shock. When they gave up and accepted the inevitable, blood pressure response was less then when they strived to avoid the shock.

It is difficult to design, conduct, and interpret studies that relate the specific thematic content of thoughts to blood pressure change. Thoughts of the possibility of personal failure, of loss of status, of no longer being useful or needed, and of the failure of others to meet standards were more likely to precede increases in blood pressure than decreases in blood pressure (Adler et al., 1976–1977). McCanne and Iennarella (1980) found that relaxing thoughts were associated with a decrease in heart rate, while anxious thoughts were associated with increased heart rate.

Frustration and its relief by physical or verbal expression of agressive feelings were studied by Hokanson and Burgess (1962). The increase in systolic pressure and heart rate that was associated with frustrating circumstances in the laboratory was reduced when aggression was expressed against the frustrator, but not when expressed against someone other than the frustrator. The status of the frustrator appeared to influence the degree of blood pressure reduction that occurred. Aggression expressed against a low-status frustrator lowered blood pressure, whereas there was no decrease when the frustrator was of high status. Feelings of guilt or anxiety related to the status of the frustrator may have been of significance in these results. Gambaro and Rabin (1969) found that low-guilt subjects had a significant decrease in diastolic pressure when they expressed anger against a frustrator, whereas high-guilt subjects showed an increase.

The degree of cardiovascular response to a stressful stimulus is influenced by psychological characteristics. Gastorf (1981) found that type A coronary-prone subjects had a greater blood pressure response than type B subjects when they were given an easy task that had been presented as a difficult task. Type A subjects prepared themselves and responded excessively when anticipating a difficult task even though the task was easy, whereas type B subjects responded appropriately to the difficulty of the task and were not influenced by the label that was given prior to the stress. Type A subjects expended excess cardiovascular energy because of their anticipation of difficulty, which probably is an expression of anxiety and a need to perform well.

The occurrence and outcome of complications of hypertension appear to be related to psychosocial noxious stimuli. Reiser et al. (1951) found close chronological correlations between the precipitation of the malignant phase of hypertension and the occurrence of emotionally charged situations. Adler et al. (1971) retrospectively studied 32 men who had ischemic strokes. In all of them, the stroke occurred during a period of sustained or intermittent and often severe emotional disturbance. Often this had been going on for some time and had been intensified shortly before the stroke occurred.

Conversely, the presence of positive psychosocial features may have a favorable influence on the development of angina pectoris, a manifestation of coronary heart disease. Hypertension is widely recognized as a major risk factor for coronary heart disease. Medalie and Goldbourt (1976) studied men with high risk factor scores. They found a lower incidence of angina pectoris in men who had a wife who was loving and emotionally supportive.

Kasl and Cobb (1970) studied a group of men employed in a plant that was scheduled to be closed. They found increased blood pressure during anticipation of job loss, the period of unemployment, and probationary reemployment. The rise in blood pressure was correlated with the subjective rating of felt stress associated with employment status. Blood pressures were reduced significantly when new jobs were started. Subjects judged to have high ego resilience showed a greater decrease in blood pressure when on the new job. The perception of the subjects regarding the significance and duration of unemployment appeared to be important in determining the rise of blood pressure before and during job loss and the rate and degree of blood pressure reduction with rehiring.

Socioeconomic circumstances have a significant impact on mortality from hypertension (Jenkins et al., 1979). Census tract areas characterized by low occupational status, a low median education, widespread poverty (low income level), a high incidence of broken families, substandard housing, and a high percentage of disabled and handicapped persons had an increase in deaths from hypertension and all hypertension-associated mortality. Low education and low occupational status appeared to be the most powerful predictors of excess hypertensive mortality.

An interesting study involving 22,000 persons, 98% of them subscribers to a prepaid plan for health care, examined blood pressure and social class for blacks and whites (Syme et al., 1974). For blacks and whites, blood pressures were higher in lower social classes. For all social classes, blood pressures were higher for blacks. The results were not changed when a special effort was made to eliminate the effect that social class might have on the availability of health care.

Harburg et al. (1973) studied the importance of socioeconomic factors and associated anger–guilt feelings in hypertension. They classified urban areas as high- or low-stress areas according to such variables as income, years of education, unemployment, adult and juvenile crime rates, and marital instability. They found that high-stress areas had higher systolic and diastolic pressures for both blacks and whites than low-stress areas. The level of blood pressure in blacks was also correlated with the darkness of skin. The authors studied hostile and guilt feelings and found that suppressed hostility, and guilt feelings if anger was expressed, was related to high blood pressure levels and a high prevalance of hypertension in both blacks in high-stress areas and whites in low-stress areas.

It is difficult to determine the effect of race on the prevalence and course of hypertension. In the United States, hypertension is more prevalent in blacks than in whites and more rapidly progressive to secondary change and stroke. However, socioeconomic influences, diet, accessibility to health care, and the level of education may explain some of this racial difference. Genetic factors may also contribute.

Societal changes associated with migration are related to increases in blood pressure (Beaglehole et al., 1977). Polynesians who retained their traditional life-style had the lowest mean blood pressure; those who migrated to New Zealand had higher pressures and blood pressure was related to the degree of interaction with the New Zealand life-style. However, the amount of variance of blood pressure that was explained by the degree of interaction with New Zealand society was small compared to that explained by measures of obesity.

On the other hand, McGarvey and Baker (1979) found that only Samoan migrants who had originated from more traditional areas of Samoa had higher blood pressures in Oahu than Samoans who remained at home. That report, together with another by Hanna and Baker (1979), shows that the most urbanized migrant Samoans, those who lived in Honolulu, had lower blood pressures than those who lived in more rural Oahu settings.

Studies of migrants are extremely difficult to interpret and compare. Much depends upon the attitudes of the migrants to the move, the amount of time in the new setting, the degree of family disruption, the dietary change, housing conditions, and employment status.

Personality

Much attention has been given to the personality of patients with essential hypertension. Several early studies have suggested that hypertensives have difficulty expressing hostility (Alexander, 1939). Other studies have found that hypertensives are more anxious than normals (Moses et al., 1956). Harris and Singer (1968) found that hypertensives perceived hostility in their environment more than normals and that this tendency was apparent in young women before hypertension was established or persistent. However, Sapira et al. (1971) found that hypertensives were less likely than normals to be offended by inappropriate conduct portrayed on a motion picture film. Presumably they were protecting themselves from noxious stimuli.

Studies of personality characteristics and blood pressure level require careful evaluation. A major problem is the time relation between the performance of the psychological studies and the diagnosis of high blood pressure (Mann, 1977a,b). Early studies of personality and hypertension often dealt with patients with long-standing and severe hypertension. Ample justification for anxiety and hostility was present in the health care milieu of the studies.

Ideally, psychological observations should be made on hypertensive subjects before they are aware of blood pressure elevation. Few studies meet this condition. The possible effects of drug and diet therapy on psychological measures can also limit the validity of results. Although several antihypertensive drugs cause feelings of fatigue, lassitude, and depression, little is known concerning their effects on personality test scores and tests of cognitive functions.

The evidence available from more recently completed studies suggests that hypertensives are not different from normals in personality characteristics or mental well-being (Goldberg et al., 1980). Anxiety, hostility, and neurotic behavior appear to be have the same prevalence among hypertensive and normotensive individuals.

Psychosocial–Behavioral Measures in the Management of Hypertension

Much has been written on the effects of various psychosocial and behavioral measures on blood pressure and on hypertension and its complications. Many studies suffer from faults of design that make interpretation difficult. It is essential to have a sufficient number of blood pressure readings under standardized conditions over a significant baseline period to establish a pretreatment level. Random assignment of appropriately matched subjects to a control group and/or to alternate treatment conditions is usually desirable. In most studies it is essential that the individuals who are recording blood pressure and making other evaluations are blind to the treatment group assignment of the subjects.

The need for a control group in hypertension research is illustrated by the profound effect of placebo treatment on blood pressure. Goldring et al. (1956) found that exposure to a harmless "electronic gun" had a significant blood pressure-lowering effect on many patients with moderate to severe hypertension. A portion of the placebo effect is undoubtedly due to the confidence the patient has in the physician and the reassurance received. Also, operating may be the fulfillment of a basic need of humans as social beings for meaningful contact with another human.

That a strong social support system may influence the course of hypertension has been suggested but not proved by the results of the Hypertension Detection and Follow-Up Program (HDFP) Cooperative Group (1979). In that study a large number of subjects with mild hypertension (diastolic 90–104 mmHg) were randomly assigned to a special care (SC) or regular care (RC) treatment group. The majority of subjects in both groups received antihypertensive drugs, more in SC than in RC. The RC subjects received care as available in the offices of community physicians or in the clinics of community hospitals. The SC subjects, on the other hand, were involved in a program especially designed to encourage them to continue treatment for the 5-year study period. A secretary-clerk called to remind subjects of the clinic appointment. A van driver was available to transport them to and from the clinic. A babysitter was provided if needed. Arrangements were made, if necessary, to get excuses from work so that there would be no loss of pay when attending the clinic. A physician was available 24 hours a day for any problem that might be related to hypertension. A group of 10–15 trained people at each special care center functioned as a team whose responsibility was to serve SC subjects without cost. This was truly social and psychological support. Diastolic pressure was reduced more in SC than in RC subjects, but the differences were small. The average diastolic was 5.5mmHg lower in SC than in RC subjects in year 1, and 4.4mmHg lower in year 5.

The end point of the HDFP was the number of deaths during the 5-year period. The data show 20.3% fewer deaths in the SC than in RC subjects. Deaths from myocardial infarction and strokes were reduced by 46 and 45% in SC subjects.

The HDFP Cooperative Group (1979) results are in sharp contrast to those of the Veterans Administration (VA) Cooperative Study Group on Antihypertensive Agents (1970) and the U.S. Public Health Service (USPHS) Hospitals Cooperative Study Group (1977) of mild hypertension. In these studies, which were double blind and placebo controlled, both drug and placebo subjects received identical supportive care. These studies, like the HDFP, were long term. The VA study was conducted over a period of 5 years, with an average follow-up of 3.3 years, while the USPHS study was 10 years, with an average follow-up of 8 years. The difference in diastolic pressures between active drug treatment and placebo groups was 18.6 mmHg in the VA study and 10 mmHg in the USPHS study. In these studies, there was no significant difference in morbidity and mortality between active drug treatment subjects and controls.

Thus the VA and USPHS studies that compared drug treatment with placebo showed significant differences in blood pressure between groups, but identical social and psychological support for both groups, and no differences in morbidity or mortality. The HDFP had a majority of both SC and RC subjects receiving drugs, small differences in blood pressure, large differences in social and psychological support, and a significant reduction in overall mortality and in deaths due to stroke and myocardial infarction in SC. The comparative results of these studies strongly suggest that social and psychological support will influence the frequency of deaths from two of the major complications of hypertension. However, it was not possible to define a particular aspect of management that was responsible. The SC subjects were caught up in and became a part of a team effort that gave friendship, reassurance, and meaningful relationships with clinic staff, as well as with other study participants. These and other positive features of the health care system could have contributed to favorable results.

Interest in the effect of psychological and behavioral techniques on blood pressure was stimulated by the demonstration by Shapiro et al. (1970) that blood pressure and heart rate in humans could be influenced by operant conditioning. This led to a large number of studies on the treatment of hypertension with relaxation, meditation, biofeedback, hypnosis, and other behavioral techniques.

Several studies have showed that diastolic and systolic pressures can be reduced in the short term through meditation, muscular relaxation, and feedback of blood pressure, electromyographic, or skin conduction data (Datey et al., 1969; Benson et al., 1974; Blanchard et al., 1975; Stone and DeLeo, 1976). In general, these different techniques appear to cause similar blood pressure reductions.

Less convincing, however, are the results of long-term use of meditation, muscular relaxation, and biofeedback. Patel and North (1975) has reported significant blood pressure reduction from a combination of meditation and biofeedback in studies of as long as 1 year in duration. In some of Patel's studies, other techniques were used in addition to help subjects relax and prevent excess response to stress.

Other long-term studies have shown little or no difference between blood pressure achieved by subjects practicing these techniques and that of control subjects (Surwit et al., 1978; Frankel et al., 1978). In our study of meditation and muscular relaxation, these techniques did not add to the blood pressure-lowering effect of a program of weight reduction, dietary salt restriction, and daily exercise in subjects followed for 1 year (Aagaard and Doerr, 1974).

The lack of long-term results from the use of meditation, muscular relaxation, and biofeedback may be because these techniques alone do not sufficiently change the hypertensive's perception of or cognitive response to stress. Perhaps more importantly, these techniques probably do not help patients to examine and change, when desirable, their attitudes, feelings, and goals and their ways of responding to life.

It is logical, nonetheless, to attempt to help hypertensives to develop and maintain a life-style with a minimum of anger, anxiety, and hurry and a maximum of contentment, confidence, and deliberateness. It is important for patients to become aware of negative feelings of anger, anxiety, and time pressure, and to recognize their internal and external causes. It is also important to help patients appreciate a lack or deficiency of pleasant and enjoyable feelings and to take steps to improve this situation.

In working with hypertensives, it should be emphasized at the outset and throughout the course of treatment that the therapist is attempting to help the patient to become as serene and contented and as free from anxiety, anger, and hurry as possible. This does not mean that the hypertensive is more anxious, angry, or hurried than the normotensive, but that these emotions tend to increase blood pressure and, therefore, it is desired to prevent their arousal or reduce their intensity and duration. Similarly, the treatment program does not signify that the hypertensive is less contented, serene, or calm than the normotensive, but that the goal is to help the patient achieve and maintain a state of maximum serenity and contentment because this will help lower blood pressure.

The recognition of negative feelings may be difficult, especially if these feelings are frequently evoked and moderate in degree. Patients must learn that worry, concern, and apprehension are forms of anxiety, and that frustration, annoyance, and resentment are forms of anger. The goal is to recognize these negative feelings when they occur, to cope quickly and effectively with the circumstances that caused their arousal, and to work to prevent their arousal in the future.

It is possible that techniques that provide periods of quiet passivity like meditation, relaxation, and biofeedback may help patients become aware of negative feelings of anger, anxiety, and hurry. With awareness may come the possibility of recognizing the causal circumstances.

Since earlier studies have suggested that hypertensives have limited ability to express hostility, courses in assertiveness have been offered in an effort to help hypertensives. In a study involving a small number of subjects, such training appeared to negate the blood pressure-lowering effect of weight reduction, dietary salt restriction, and exercise (Aagaard and Doerr, 1974). It may be better to help hypertensives prevent the arousal of anger than to teach them how to express it more effectively.

On the positive side, it may be possible to help patients become more deliberate, speak more slowly, schedule activities more loosely, and arrive at appointments ahead of schedule. With a deliberate pace, it becomes possible to experience life more fully and in some instances to enjoy occupational, social, and recreational activities instead of hurrying through them with grim determination. Patients can be urged to take time to enjoy more fully the senses of smell, taste, hearing, vision, and touch in everyday life and in unusual circumstances.

Confidence and self-esteem may be increased by recalling past successes. Imagery may be used to relive happy and memorable events. Cognition can be utilized positively in setting realistic goals for one's self. Cognition can also be utilized in limiting expectations of others. Interpersonal relationships can be reviewed. The patient may wish to strengthen old relationships and expand some social network through new contacts and activities.

A therapeutic program that includes some of the measures described above must be tailored to the needs, circumstances, interests, and capabilities of the individual patient and may have to be of long duration. Decreases in negative behavior and increases in positive behavior may develop slowly. Nevertheless, hypertensives can change. They can enjoy the challenge of learning to change and grow in the same way they enjoy

participating in a well-contested game or solving an interesting and
difficult puzzle.

References

Aagaard, G. N., and H. O. Doerr. 1974. Effect of progressive muscular relaxation
and meditation in mild to borderline hypertension. Unpublished Study,
Departments of Medicine and Psychiatry and Behavioral Sciences, University of
Washington, Seattle, Washington.

Adler, R., K. MacRitchie, and G. L. Engel. 1971. Psychologic processes and ischemic
stroke (occlusive cerebrovascular disease). Psychosomatic Medicine 33:1.

Adler, R., J. M. Herrmann, N. Schäfer, T. Schmidt, O. W. Schonecke, and
T. von Uexkull. 1976–1977. A context study of psychological conditions prior to
shifts in blood pressure. Psychotherapy and Psychosomatics 27:198.

Alexander, F. 1939. Emotional factors in essential hypertension. Psychosomatic
Medicine 1:173.

Beaglehole, R., C. E. Salmond, A. Hooper, J. Huntsman, J. M. Stanhope, J. C. Cassel,
and I. A. M. Prior. 1977. Blood presure and social interaction in Tokelauan
migrants in New Zealand. Journal of Chronic Diseases 30:803.

Benson, H., B. A. Rosner, B. R. Marzetta, and H. M. Klemchuk. 1974. Decreased
blood-pressure in pharmacologically treated hypertensive patients who regularly elicited the relaxation response. Lancet 1:289.

Blanchard, E. B., L. D. Young, and M. R. Haynes. 1975. Technique innovations. A
simple feedback system for the treatment of elevated blood pressure. Behavior
Therapy 6:241.

Brod, J., V. Fencl, Z. Hejl, and J. Jirka. 1959. Circulatory changes underlying blood
pressure elevation during acute emotional stress (mental arithmetic) in normotensive and hypertensive subjects. Clinical Science 18:269.

Datey, K. K., S. N. Deshmukh, C. P. Dalvi, and S. L. Vinekar. 1969. Shavasan: A
yogic exercise in the management of hypertension. Angiology 20:325.

Engleman, K., B. Portnoy, and A. Sjoerdsma. 1970. Plasma catecholamine
concentrations in patients with hypertension. Circulation Research 26 and 27,
Suppl. 1:1–141.

Esler, M., S. Julius, A. Zweifler, O. Randall, E. Harburg, H. Gardiner, and
V. DeQuattro. 1977. Mild high-renin essential hypertension. Neurogenic human
hypertension? New England Journal of Medicine 296:405.

Ettema, J. H. 1969. Blood pressure changes during mental load experiments in man.
Psychotherapy and Psychosomatics 17:191.

Falkner, B., G. Onesti, E. T. Angelakos, M. Fernandes, and C. Langman. 1979.
Cardiovascular response to mental stress in normal adolescents with hypertensive parents. Hemodynamics and mental stress in adolescents. Hypertension
1:23.

Fitzgerald, G. A., V. Hossman, and C. T. Dollery, 1981. Norepinephrine release in
essential hypertension. Clinical Pharmacology and Therapeutics 30:164.

Frankel, B. L., D. J. Patel, D. Horwitz, W. T. Friedewald, and K. R. Gaarder. 1978.
Treatment of hypertension with biofeedback and relaxation techniques.
Psychosomatic Medicine 40:276.

Gambaro, S., and A. I. Rabin. 1969. Diastolic blood pressure responses following direct and displaced aggression after anger arousal in high- and low-guilt subjects. Journal of Personality and Social Psychology 12:87.

Gastorf, J. W. 1981. Physiologic reaction of type A's to objective and subjective challenge. Journal of Human Stress 7:16.

Goldberg, E. L., G. W. Comstock, and C. G. Graves. 1980. Psychosocial factors and blood pressure. Psychological medicine 10:243.

Goldring, W., H. Chasis, G. E. Schreiner, and H. W. Smith. 1956. Reassurance in the management of benign hypertensive disease. Circulation 14:260.

Graham, J. D. P. 1945. High blood-pressure after battle. Lancet 1:239.

Hanna, J. M., and P. T. Baker. 1979. Biocultural correlates to the blood pressure of Samoan migrants in Hawaii. Human Biology 51:481.

Harburg, E., J. C. Erfurt, L. S. Hauenstein, C. Chape, W. J. Schull, and M. A. Schork. 1973. Social–ecological stress, supressed hostility, skin color and black–white male blood pressure. Psychosomatic Medicine 35:276.

Harris, R. E., and M. T. Singer. 1968. Interaction of personality and stress in the pathogenesis of essential hypertension. In J. Edwin Wood, ed.: Hypertension, Vol. 16. Neural Control of Arterial Pressure, Proceedings of the Council for High Blood Pressure Research, Cleveland, 1967. New York: AHA; p. 104.

Hokanson, J. E., and M. Burgess. 1962. Effects of status, type of frustration, and aggression on vascular processes. Journal of Abnormal and Social Psychology 65:232.

Hypertension Detection and Follow-up Program Cooperative Group. 1979. Five-year findings of the hypertension detection and follow-up program. 1. Reduction in mortality of persons with high blood pressure, including mild hypertension. Journal of the American Medical Association 242:2562.

Innes, G., W. M. Millar and M. Valentine. 1959. Emotion and blood-pressure. Journal of Mental Science 105:840.

Jenkins, C. D., R. W. Tuthill, S. I. Tannenbaum, and C. Kirby. 1979. Social stressors and excess mortality from hypertensive diseases. Journal of Human Stress 5:29.

Julius, S., A. V. Pascual, and R. London. 1971. Role of parasympathetic inhibition in the hyperkinetic type of borderline hypertension. Circulation 44:413.

Kasl, S., and S. Cobb. 1970. Blood pressure changes in men undergoing job loss: A preliminary report. Psychosomatic Medicine 32:19.

McCanne, T. R., and R. S. Iennarella. 1980. Cognitive and somatic events associated with discriminative changes in heart rate. Psychophysiology 17:18.

McGarvey, S. T., and P. T. Baker. 1979. The effects of modernization and migration on Samoan blood pressures. Human Biology 51:461.

Mann, A. H. 1977a. The psychological effect of a screening programme and clinical trial for hypertension upon the participants. Psychological Medicine 7:431.

Mann, A. H. 1977b. Psychiatric morbidity and hostility in hypertension. Psychological Medicine 7:653.

Medalie, J. H., and U. Goldbourt. 1976. Angina pectoris among 10,000 men. II. Psychosocial and other risk factors as evidenced by a multivariate analysis of a five year incidence study. American Journal of Medicine 60:910.

Metropolitan Life Insurance Company. 1961. Statistical Bulletin. Mortality of men with above-average blood pressure. By age at issue, ages 30–59. Men accepted for ordinary life insurance in 1935–53. Traced to policy anniversary in 1954. *In* G. Pickering, ed.: High Blood Pressure. New York: Grune and Stratton; p. 368.

Moses, L., G. E. Daniels, and J. L. Nickerson. 1956. Psychogenic factors in essential hypertension. Methodology and preliminary report. Psychosomatic Medicine 18:471.

Nestel, P. J. 1969. Blood-pressure and catecholamine excretion after mental stress in labile hypertension. Lancet 1:692.

Obrist, P. A., C. J. Gaebelein, E. S. Teller, A. W. Langer, A. Grignolo, K. C. Light, and J. A. McCubbin. 1978. The relationship among heart rate, carotid dP/dt, and blood pressure in humans as a function of the type of stress. Psychophysiology 15:102.

Page, I. H. 1949. Pathogenesis of arterial hypertension. Journal of the American Medicine Association 140:451.

Patel, C., and W. R. S. North. 1975. Randomised controlled trail of yoga and biofeedback in management of hypertension. Lancet 2:93.

Reiser, M. F., M. Rosenbaum, and E. B. Ferris. 1951. Psychologic mechanisms in malignant hypertension. Psyschosomatic Medicine 13:147.

Ruskin, A., O. W. Beard, and R. L. Schaffer. 1948. Blast hypertension. Elevated arterial pressures in the victims of the Texas City disaster. American Journal of Medicine 4:228.

Sapira, J. D., E. T. Scheib, R. Moriarty, and A. P. Shapiro. 1971. Differences in perception between hypertensive and normotensive populations. Psychosomatic Medicine 33:239.

Shapiro, A. P. 1961. An experimental study of comparative responses of blood pressure to different noxious stimuli. Journal of Chronic Disease 13:293.

Shapiro, D., B. Tursky, and G. E. Schwartz. 1970. Control of blood pressure in man by operant conditioning. Circulation Research 26 and 27, Supplement 1:1–27.

Stone, R. A., and J. DeLeo. 1976. Psychotherapeutic control of hypertension. New England Journal of Medicine 294:80.

Surwit, R. S., D. Shapiro, and M. I. Good. 1978. Comparison of cardiovascular biofeedback, neuromuscular biofeedback and meditation in the treatment of borderline essential hypertension. Journal of Consulting and Clinical Psychology 46:252.

Syme, S. L., T. W. Oakes, G. D. Friedman, R. Feldman, A. B. Siegelaub, and M. Collen. 1974. Social class and racial differences in blood pressure. American Journal of Public Health 64:619.

United States Public Health Service Hospitals Cooperative Study Group. 1977. Treatment of mild hypertension. Results of a ten-year intervention trial. Circulation Research 40, Supplement 1:1–98.

Veterans Administration Cooperative Study Group on Antihypertensive Agents. 1970. Effects of treatment on morbidity in hypertension. II. Results in patients with diastolic blood pressure averaging 90 through 114 mm Hg. Journal of the American Medical Association 213:1143.

Williams, R. B., Jr., C. P. Kimball, and H. N. Williard. 1972. The influence of interpersonal interaction on diastolic blood pressure. Psychosomatic Medicine 34:194.

13

Biobehavioral Interactions and Hypertension

Orville A. Smith, Ph.D.*

Although there are no sharp dividing lines between normal blood pressure and what is labeled hypertension, most physicians would agree that a systolic blood pressure of 150 with a diastolic pressure of 100 or over is life threatening. These arbitrary blood pressure levels make up a significant fraction of the normal distribution or bell-shaped curve for blood pressure in the population as a whole. This means that hypertension will help kill 250,000 Americans each year. This turns out to be five times the number that will be killed in automobile accidents or one out of eight people who will die from anything at all. Put another way, the chances are one in ten that any randomly chosen American can be labeled as being hypertensive. Translated into absolute numbers, approximately 23 million Americans can be labeled as hypertensive and, of these, 11 million are not even aware that they suffer from the disease. Another factor that makes hypertension particularly dangerous is that it is an inocuous disease; there are no symptoms associated with the lower levels of the abnormal range, and as a result about two-thirds of those with hypertension are inadequately treated (National High Blood Pressure Education Program, 1973).

While hypertension is a symptom of an abnormal process, hypertension itself is not a killer. The causes of death associated with hypertension are congestive heart failure, stroke, renal failure, and coronary heart disease. Cardiovascular disease is the number one killer and because hypertension is directly related to the above-mentioned diseases, it can be seen that hypertension itself must be considered as a major etiological factor.

---

*Professor of Physiology and Biophysics, Director of Regional Primate Center, University of Washington School of Medicine, Seattle, Washington.

Variables Relating to High Blood Pressure

As indicated in Chapter 12, a great many factors have been correlated with the presence of hypertension. For instance, there is a direct relation with age in which diastolic blood pressure shows a steady increase from age 20 to age 60, then a decrease to age 80 (Paul, 1977). One obvious reason for the change in the direction of the curve between 60 and 80 is that severely hypertensive individuals are dying by age 60 and hypotensives or those with normal pressures are more likely to survive into their 80s. It has to be pointed out, however, that this correlation between age and blood pressure is not a universal phenomenon. There are certain cultures such as the Australian Aborigines and some African bushmen that do not show the relation (Paul, 1977). However, almost all Western industrialized countries reflect this relation.

A major factor in hypertension is genetics. Many twin studies have shown that there is a high correlation between siblings in blood pressures. This extends to identical twins that have been raised in different environments. The laboratory evidence for the genetic factor is reflected in that it has been possible to interbreed rats so that there are now several strains of spontaneously hypertensive rats. An interesting sidelight of this research is that one strain, the Okamoto strain, has a different physiological basis for hypertension than the Milan strain (Hallback et al. 1977). Therefore, although genetics is very important, hypertension is clearly not a monogenic disease but is definitely polygenic and multifactored.

Another important variable is race (National Center for Health Statistics, 1976). There is approximately twice the incidence of hypertension among black men than among white men. Black women are more prone to suffer from the disease and 50% of black women over the age of 60 have hypertension. This factor results in the statistic that between the ages of 25 and 44, a black person has 50 times the chance of dying of a complication of high blood pressure as a white person. Obviously, this is a situation where genetics could be playing an important role, but the possibilityof sociocultural factors being prominent is also high.

Obesity is another factor that is strongly correlated with hypertension (Paul, 1977). While the correlation is strong, the relation is small; that is, there is only about a 3-mmHg increase in blood presure for every 10 kg of excess weight. Since obesity is correlated with hypertension, it should follow that dieting will reduce pressure. During World War II a large set of experiments were carried out on the physiological aspects of starvation, and it was shown that mean blood pressure was reduced from 106 to 94 mmHg in those subjects undergoing starvation.

Finally, direct evidence of the role of sociocultural factors in hypertension can be provided by the findings that high blood pressure is inversely related to both income and level of education.

As can be seen, an array of variables appear to relate to hypertension. But while all of these variables are correlated with hypertension, we can draw no conclusions about cause or effect from these kinds of studies.

Etiologies of Hypertension

While there are multiple factors involved in producing high blood presure, it is possible to characterize some of the bases of hypertension into two major categories. Hypertension that is known to result from an obvious physiological malfunction is commonly known as "secondary." Preeminent in this category is renal hypertension, which comes about as a result of constriction of the renal artery or kidney disease. Clinically the role of the kidney can be easily demonstrated by those cases in which a person with hypertension has been found to have a constricted renal artery. After surgical correction of that situation, the hypertension often completely disappears. Experimental hypertension can be produced in the laboratory by decreasing the blood flow to the kidney by applying restricting clamps or otherwise reducing blood flow. Hypertension will develop over a period of time, but if the constriction is removed, then the hypertension will be reduced. However, as a complicating factor, if the hypertension is allowed to persist for several months, then removal of the clamps and reestablishment of normal blood flow into the kidney will not bring about a reduced blood pressure. These very dramatic demonstrations have focused attention on the kidney and its role in regulating blood pressure. It has been claimed that the kidney is responsible for all hypertension, but this is a hypothetical view that has yet to be proven.

Other pathophysiological mechanisms include tumors of the adrenal gland, which can increase the excretion of noradrenaline into the bloodstream. This in turn acts to constrict blood vessels. Tumors of the cortical portion of the adrenal gland may increase the output of aldosterone, with subsequent major alterations in the sodium–water balance in the body. Both of these forms of hypertension can be corrected by surgical techniques.

While important, secondary causes of hypertension are in fact a small percentage of the overall total. The much more important type of hypertension is "essential" hypertension, or "primary" hypertension. These terms seem to imply a knowledge of the causes of the disease, but in fact the basis for essential hypertension is not known, either because of the multiple factors (mosaic theory; Chapter 12) that may produce the disease or because the causative agent or mechanism has not been determined. However, the fact that we do not know the cause of the disease does not mean that nothing can be done about it. Treatment is available in a large number of forms, each of which requires continuous medication management for the rest of the individual's life. This added medication is accompanied by some very important side effects such as continued drowsiness, a light-headed feelng, and in many cases impotence. While only 30–35% of the people who have hypertension are currently being medicated, the importance of this medication cannot be denied. One recent study showed a 20% lower mortality for patients strongly encouraged to take medication (Kolota, 1979). Of course, one of the major problems is that medication noncompliance is very high. Patients frequently stop taking their medication when they begin to feel better and therefore the hypertension persists.

With regard to the etiology of the disease, there seems to be general agreement on one point: The psychological factor of "stress" appears to play an important role in the genesis of the pathology. We have already seen that in the clinical sense stress is never well defined and, therefore, the use of this term carries with it the inherent danger of its being applied as an explanatory concept. To have scientific meaning, an operational definition of stress must be established and the influence of stress-producing situations upon physiological mechanisms (which then disrupt normal regulation of blood pressure) determined. One of the major obstacles to scientific progress toward the understanding of this disease is the extremely broad range of situations encompassed by the term *stress*. The type of stress that is of concern here is psychological stress, as opposed to trauma or exercise, other disease, and so forth.

It is the purpose of this chapter to illustrate how this amorphous psychological phenomenon called stress could produce biological effects that might then lead to hypertension.

Physiological Characteristics of Essential Hypertension

Mean blood pressure is a function of the amount of blood being forced into the peripheral vasculature per unit time and the resistance to the flow of that blood within the vessels. This is indicated by the following formula:

$$\text{Mean blood pressure} = \text{cardiac output} \times \text{peripheral resistance}$$

This formula implies that if any one of these factors increases while the others are held constant, there will be an increased mean blood pressure. While there are several different forms of essential hypertension and several stages that the hypertension progresses through, it has been found that in the final form of fixed essential hypertension, the following physiological conditions exist:

1. Heart rate and stroke volume (the two components of cardiac output) are normal in people with essential hypertension; that is, cardiac output is normal.

2. Peripheral resistance is increased. While there are several factors that determine peripheral resistance, the major determinants are the viscosity of the blood and the lumen size of the blood vessels into which the blood is being forced. In essential hypertension viscosity is found to be normal; therefore the pathology must be in the vessel size, probably in the arterioles and in the form of a decreased lumen size of the vessels.
3. The increased peripheral resistance is distributed fairly evenly throughout the body. That is, the blood flow distribution in hypertensives is the same in the skin, the viscera, and the brain as it is in the normal person; it is increased somewhat in the muscles and decreased somewhat in the kidneys. In general, there are no major changes in the way blood is distributed between normal and hypertensive individuals.

The primary question to be examined in this chapter is what is the scientific evidence that links psychological stress to the physiological–anatomical process of permanently increased peripheral resistance, probably brought about by decreased arteriolar lumen size? Let us select four different hypotheses for the etiology of essential hypertension and indicate as precisely as possible how the stress factor interacts with the biological mechanisms responsible for reduction in the size of the lumen:

1. Frequently repeated episodes of increased blood pressure.
2. Disordered baroreceptor function.
3. Chronic low-level reductions in renal blood flow.
4. Excessive salt intake.

Each of these four hypotheses represents an illustration of how a single factor might influence blood vessel diameter. However, it must be made clear that there are many other factors hypothesized to bring about the same end result. Acknowledging the mosaic theory of hypertension, it could well be that all of these four factors are operating simultaneously or in any combination, or that many other factors could be operating as well. The object of focusing on four is to emphasize the fact that well-controlled laboratory experiments can provide evidence that demonstrates the potential for each one of these variables acting singly to produce enough of a physiological change to induce the pathological condition.

Experimental Situation

Relevant research findings have been obtained from animal experiments in which a 9- to 14-kg baboon has been adapted to chair restraint and trained daily to perform several tasks. In a special environmentally

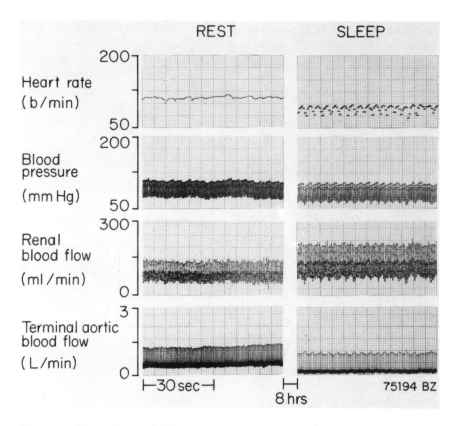

Figure 1. Comparison of CV responses associated with quiet rest and sleep. During sleep, heart rate is at a minimum and shows sinus arrhythmia, renal flow is at its maximum, and terminal aortic flow is at a minimum. These major differences in CV activity between awake resting and sleep occur in the presence of minimal differences in somatic activity. Reprinted from Smith et al. (1980b).

controlled chamber the animal is taught to rest quietly, press a lever for a food reward, turn an exercise wheel with his feet, and anticipate a very brief electric shock. After the animal has been well adapted and has learned these tasks, it is taken to surgery and under sterile conditions electromagnetic flow probes are placed on the renal and iliac arteries. A pressure cannula is placed in the axillary artery. After recovery from surgery the animal is returned to the training situation, and the cardiovascular changes that occur in conjunction with the various behaviors are recorded. The resultant cardiovascular (CV) changes accompanying each kind of behavior are demonstrated in Figs. 1–4.

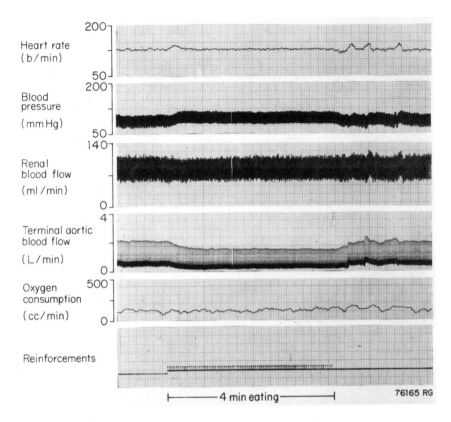

Figure 2. Cardiovascular response to ingesting periodically delivered applesauce (0.6 ml at a time). The CV response pattern associated with this behavior is a maintained 15–20 mmHg response in blood pressure and a maintained decrease in terminal aortic blood flow. There are no changes in heart rate or renal flow. Reprinted from Smith et al. (1980b).

While all of the responses are of interest and contribute to our knowledge about central neural control of the circulation, it is the response illustrated in Fig. 4 which represents the conditional emotional response (CER) that will be of direct concern. This CER response represents an objective definition of stress. There are, in fact, two independent measures of stress derivable from the same experimental condition. First, the behavioral definition of stress is found in the lever-pressing behavior. As a baseline response the baboon is trained to press a lever in order to receive an applesauce reward. After several minutes of lever pressing, an auditory signal is turned on that lasts for 1 minute. At the end of the minute a 1-

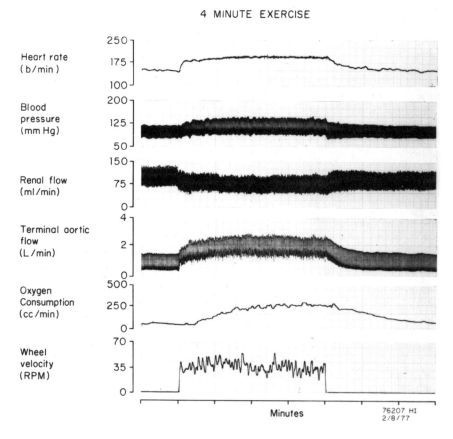

4 MINUTE EXERCISE

Heart rate (b/min)

Blood pressure (mm Hg)

Renal flow (ml/min)

Terminal aortic flow (L/min)

Oxygen Consumption (cc/min)

Wheel velocity (RPM)

Minutes

76207 HI
2/8/77

Figure 3. Cardiovascular responses to exercise. This pattern includes a rapid immediate increase followed by a slow increasing heart rate for the duration of the exercise. A similar sequence is seen in blood pressure. Renal flow shows an immediate maintained decrease and terminal aortic flow is immediately increased and remains so for the duration of the exercise. Steady, continually increasing oxygen consumption accompanies the CV pattern. Reprinted from Smith et al. (1980a,b).

second electric shock is applied. After seven or eight such presentations the animal shows the behavior illustrated in Fig. 4. When the auditory signal comes on, the animal stops pressing the lever, sits quietly for the 1-minute duration, and then, after the shock, proceeds to press the lever once again. This cessation or suppression of lever pressing provides us with a measurable objective definition of stress.

The second definition is a cardiovascular one. It can be seen that during the lever pressing all the variables of blood pressure, heart rate, and the blood flows are relatively constant. When the auditory signal occurs, there

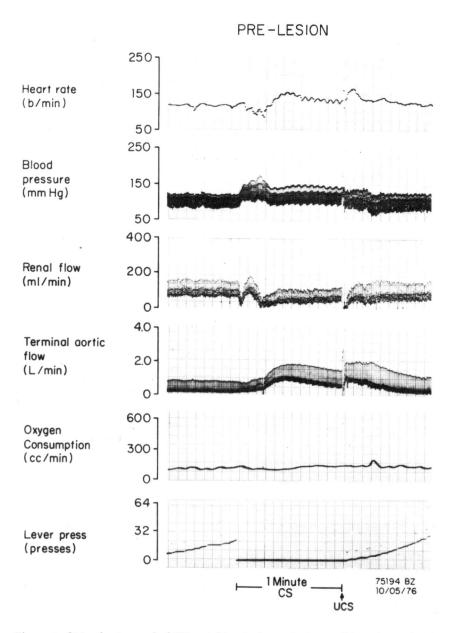

Figure 4. Strip-chart record of CV variables during a single conditioned emotional response trial. The bottom panel is the output of an incremental counter triggered each time the animal presses the lever. The counter was reset at conditioned stimulus (CS) onset. Reprinted from Smith et al. (1980a).

are both immediate and long-term changes that result in an increased heart rate, increased blood pressure, increased iliac blood flow, and a complex renal blood flow consisting of an immediate fast decrease followed by recovery to normal and then a subsequent slower delayed decrease in renal flow. This combination of cardiovascular responses then provides an additional definition of stress. With the experimental approach we are capable of examining the various hypotheses put forward. Figure 5 illustrates the cardiovascular responses to the CER situation in a series of six animals.

Hypothesis 1: Frequently Repeated Episodes of Increased Blood Pressure

It is evident from Fig. 5 that some animals respond to the stressful situation with very large increases in blood pressure and that some have relatively small increases. If an individual who showed a hyperreaction to a stressful situation in terms of increased blood pressure were exposed to many instances of stressful situations, then the arteriolar walls could be exposed to an exercise-like situation proposed in the first hypothesis. Other individuals who showed only small increases in blood pressure would not have their arterioles exposed to the large-magnitude changes in smooth muscle activity leading to constriction and relaxation of the arteries. It is a fact that smooth muscle continuously exposed to excessive loads will become hypertrophied, just like skeletal muscle contracting to lift heavy weights. However, when arteriolar smooth muscle hypertrophies, this results in a reduced lumen of the vessel as the developing media (middle layer of the arteriole) steadily encroaches upon it. This structural alteration could be the mechanism for the fixed, permanent hypertension (Folkow, 1977).

This illustration also points out how the genetic effect could become a predominant factor. If the inherent response to stress is to induce severe constrictions of the arteriolar musculature that subsequently produce the elevated blood pressure, then it would be exactly these individuals who hyperreact to emotional stimuli and happen to be exposed to many stressful situations who would eventually become afflicted with essential hypertension.

Hypothesis 2: Disordered Baroreceptor Function

Within the aortic arch and along the extent of the carotid artery, but particularly located in the bifurcation of this artery, are located sensory receptors that increase their firing rate when the artery walls are stretched. These receptor endings give rise to nerve fibers that run in the ninth and tenth cranial nerves and eventually enter the lower brainstem. In the stem,

273

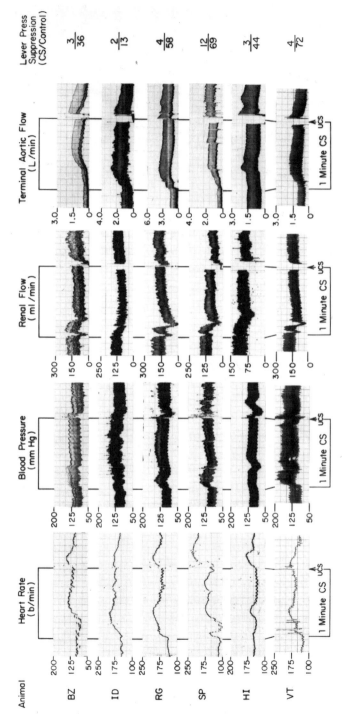

Figure 5. Single CER trials from six different animals. Data from animal VT (bottom row) were recorded at a slower chart speed. Lever press suppression refers to the number of lever presses performed during conditioned stimulus (CS) compared with the number of presses during the control minute immediately preceding CS onset. Reprinted from Smith et al. (1979).

they make a synaptic connection within the structure called the nucleus tractus solitarius, and the firing of the postsynaptic cells in this structure brings about activity in those nerve fibers proceeding from the central nervous system to the heart and the vasculature. These nerve fibers belong to the autonomic division of the nervous system and can produce either increases or decreases in heart rate and arteriolar diameter. This neuro-circuitry is an example of an autonomic reflex and the functional result of this reflex is the control of arterial blood pressure. Therefore these reflexes are known as baroreflexes. If something produces an increase in blood pressure, the pressure is reflected into the aortic arch and into the carotid arteries. The increased pressure stretches the walls of the arteries. This stretch changes the firing rate of the baroreceptors located in those walls, and the subsequent reflex is a slowing of heart rate and a dilation of the arterioles, leading to a return of blood pressure to more normal levels. The exact opposite situation holds if there is a drop in blood pressure and the change in the firing rate of the receptors is in the opposite direction. The subsequent effect is an increase in heart rate and a decrease in the diameter of the arterioles, both of which lead to an increase in pressure or what is in effect a return to normal pressure. Ordinarily these reflexes are extremely accurate, and blood pressure is kept in a very narrowly defined range. However, since these reflexes are part of central neural connections, it is clearly possible that the firing of the nerve cells in this reflex could be affected, particularly at the synapse at the nucleus tractus solitarius. It is possible that other neural activity could either facilitate or inhibit the firing of cells in this nucleus. If this reflex could be significantly modulated, then the ability of this reflex to return pressure to normal levels could be severely compromised and major alterations in mean blood pressure could ensue.

Evidence that these reflexes are indeed modifiable via other central neural activity and behavior itself is found in the following studies. If one measures heart rate, blood pressure, and other cardiovascular variables in an animal anesthetized with α-chloralose, one can introduce stimulating electrodes into various parts of the brain and elicit changes in the cardiovascular variables. While a large number of various patterns of cardiovascular responses can be found, the most dramatic are those in which stimulation simultaneously produces an increase in pressure with an increase in heart rate. This result can be achieved from several different locations within the brain. When one considers these changes, it is recognized that this sort of response should not occur if the baroreflexes are operating appropriately. In no case should an increase in pressure be accompanied by an increase in heart rate. A baroreflex should immediately decrease the heart rate and arterial constriction, which would result in pressure being returned to normal.

A number of years ago a series of studies were done in which the focus of attention was on the various neural structures that, when stimulated, produced simultaneous increased heart rate and blood pressures. These structures extended from locations in the posterior hypothalamus into the subthalamus and into the tectal region of the midbrain. The studies were carried out in cats, dogs, rats, and monkeys. These were anatomical studies based upon the ability to stain specifically those nerve fibers that, after having been physically separated from the cell bodies, proceeded to a degeneration phase. In this situation a particular silver stain can be utilized to stain only the degenerating fibers. In this fashion the nerve tracks associated with small lesions of various portions of the brain can be displayed. In these studies several routes of degenerating fibers were revealed that were expected; for example, the accumulation of fibers in the reticular formations of the brainstem. The reticular formation has been known for years to be a major route of autonomic fibers in the central nervous system. However, there appeared an unexpected projection from these higher regions into the lower brainstem to a nucleus called the inferior olive. This pattern of degeneration to the inferior olive was found in each case when the structure that was under investigation produced simultaneous increased heart rate and blood pressure. However, in subsequent studies in which fine electrodes were introduced into the inferior olive itself, no cardiovascular responses were generated. This dilemma was resolved only when the experiment illustrated in Fig. 6 was carried out. In this experiment the carotid sinus reflex was elicited by stretching the carotid arteries in a repeatable, systematic fashion. This stretching of the artery simulted a very large increase in blood pressure, and the immediate reflex response was the large decrease in heart rate and blood pressure shown in Fig. 6 which, under normal conditions, would have immediately returned an increased blood pressure to normal limits. This, in effect, was a maneuver to "fool" the system into believing that a high blood pressure was being produced within the arteries. It can also be seen in Fig. 6 that direct stimulation of the nucleus of the inferior olive produced no cardiovascular response whatsoever. However, the final panel illustrates that when stimulation of the inferior olive was carried out simultaneously with the elicitation of the baroreflex, the reflex (decreased heart rate and lowered pressure) was very greatly attenuated. This finding shows clearly that there are structures within the central nervous system that can severely modulate the baroreflex.

Knowing that there are neural structures that can produce modulation of the baroreflex, one would expect to observe these mechanisms in the normally behaving animal. As we look back at Fig. 5, we can see that in every case of the conditioned emotional response, there are simultaneous increases in heart rate and blood pressure that can be maintained. Thus in

276

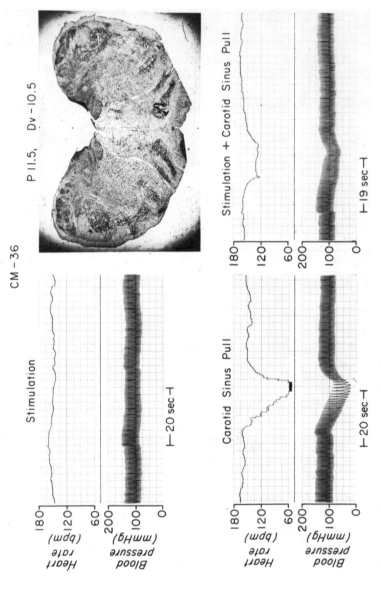

Figure 6. Control stimulation of the inferior olive and control carotid sinus reflex on the left. To the upper right the stimulation site in the inferior olive is indicated by an arrow. To the lower right is shown the inhibitory effect of inferior olive stimulation on the carotid sinus reflex. Reprinted from Smith and Nathan (1966). Copyright 1966 by the American Association for the Advancement of Science.

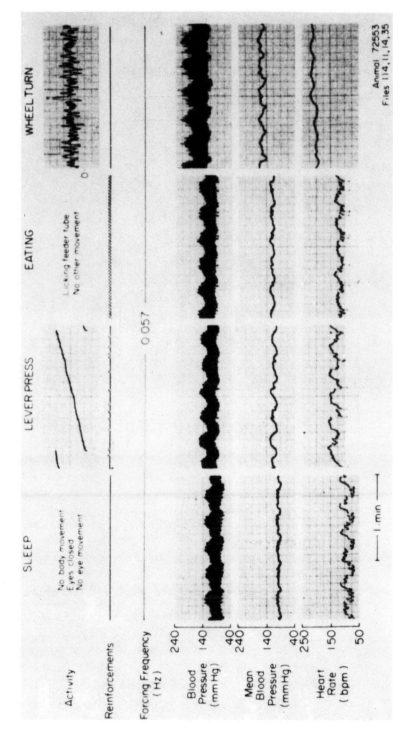

Figure 7. Records from driven trials (animal C). Sinusoidal alteration of blood pressure at 0.057 Hz. Reprinted from Stephenson et al. (1981).

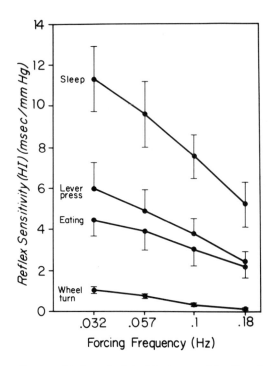

Figure 8. Baroreflex sensitivity calculated in terms of fractional changes in heart interval. Reprinted from Stephenson et al. (1981).

the normal situation there apparently is baroreflex modulation. This idea was put to a major test by Stephenson et al. (1981), who carried out a study using baboons instrumented as indicated previously and trained in a series of behavioral tests. In addition to the usual recording instruments, Stephenson placed an occlusion cuff around the descending aorta. By means of a precisely controlled system, he could increase and decrease the filling of this occlusion cuff in a cyclic fashion so that both the aortic arch and the carotid arteries would be exposed to cyclic variations in arterial pressure, depending upon the signals that were fed to the occlusion cuff. Using this sinusoidal variation in arteriole pressure, Stephenson then measured the changes in heart rate that accompanied these pressure changes. He could, in this fashion, derive an indication of the sensitivity of the reflex by comparing the change in the number of beats per minute as a function of the amplitude of the blood pressure change. The cyclic changes were then produced while the animal was in the process of carrying out several different behaviors. Figure 7 shows the cardiovascular responses to the cyclic changes while the animal was asleep, resting quietly, eating, or exercising vigorously to avoid shock. Figure 8 shows the analysis of the data and indicates clearly that the sensitivity of the baroreflex was altered dramatically by the kind of behavior in which the animal was engaged. It can be seen that during the wheel turning, to avoid shock the sensitivity was at a minimum. This would indicate that blood pressure and heart rate would then be allowed to go to a much higher level if the reflex sensitivity was measured during sleep; that is, the largest changes in heart rate to a given blood pressure change occurred while the animal was fast asleep.

This study provides definitive evidence in support of the idea that during stress the baroreflexes are inhibited, allowing blood pressure to increase. It is not too bold to assume that if the neural system involved in stress were chronically active, the baroreflex sensitivity would be continually turned down, higher levels of pressure would be allowed to occur, and this would be a potentially pathological situation that could lead to a condition of chronic hypertension. In this case a fixed hypertension might be brought about by the exaggeration of the "exercise" mechanism represented by the first hypothesis. However, it is also highly probable that the vascular diameter changes that are part of the baroreflex are affected by the behavior as well as the heart rate changes. Because of technical difficulties, it is not yet possible to determine directly the arterioral diameters in this unanesthetized preparation.

Hypothesis 3: Chronic, Low-Level Reductions in Renal Flow

The significance of this hypothesis is that when blood flow to the kidney is decreased, there is an immediate reaction on the part of the kidney to produce a substance called renin. Renin is a proteolytic enzyme produced by the kidney that splits an α-globulin in the blood to form a new chemical called angiotensin I. Angiotensin I is subsequently converted enzymatically within the lung to produce angiotensin II (AII). Angiotensin II is an active vasoconstrictor agent and a regulator of aldosterone. When the renin–angiotensin system was first discovered, it was felt that an explanation for all hypertension was at hand. Over the last 20 years it has been demonstrated conclusively that continued renin output is certainly not necessary for the establishment of all hypertension. However, a certain fraction of hypertension is indeed accompanied by increased elevated levels of renin. Thus it need only be shown that the renin is secreted aperiodically enough to produce the severe constriction that would then potentially lead to the fixed decreased lumen discussed under our first hypothesis. Therefore it is imperative to determine whether or not behavioral stress can alter the output of renin by the kidney. Blair (1976) carried out another study utilizing the baboon preparation, in which, in addition to several measuring devices, she implanted venous catheters

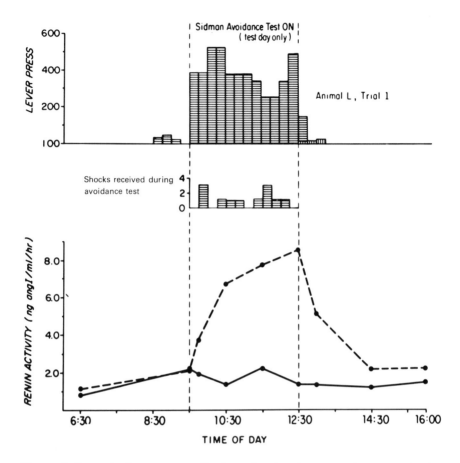

Figure 9. Example from one replication, showing lever-pressing rate, shocks received during avoidance test, and plasma renin activity. Control day values are denoted by the solid line and solid bars; avoidance test day values are denoted by the broken line and hatched bars. Note that plasma renin activity increased by 9:45 A.M. of the test day, before any shocks had been delivered. Reprinted from Blair et al. (1976).

from which blood samples could be taken remotely while the animal was carrying out various behavioral tasks. The stress task Blair used was called a Sidman avoidance task in which a signal is turned on and the animal must respond by pressing a lever at least once every 20 seconds or a brief shock is delivered. Shortly, the animals become so well trained that they press levers and are rarely exposed to the shock. However, this situation does produce elevated stress in the animal. Figure 9 shows the results of the study in which the renin activity levels were first determined over a control period before the signal for the avoidance condition was turned on. At 8:30 A.M. the avoidance condition was presented and the abrupt large-magnitude increases in renin that are associated with this period of stress are clearly evident. Again, it is obvious that if an individual's life were filled with many stressful events to which he or she happened to respond by increasing renin output, then the pathological conditions conducive to the establishment of essential hypertension would be imposed. Dengerink et al. (1983) have also shown that unpleasant environmental events such as noise will elevate AII in both rats and humans.

Hypothesis 4: Excessive Salt Intake

Over the years it has become apparent that the dietary intake of salt is a major factor in the production of hypertension. Just how this effect is produced is as yet unknown, but it is clear that almost any patient with essential hypertension who is put on a salt-restricted diet will show some amelioration of his hypertension. In addition to the increased fluid volume resulting from increased salt intake, there are several suggestions that salt plays a role in the hydration of the arteriolar walls, which could lead to increased thickening of the walls. There are other suggestions that the sodium content could play a role in the establishment of excitability levels of the smooth muscle cells within the arterioles; that is, an excess of sodium would interact with the calcium within the cell walls and the smooth muscle could become hyperresponsive, leading to a pathological constriction.

This is currently an active area of investigation and undoubtedly some answers will be forthcoming shortly. The following experiment demonstrates the relation between salt intake and stress in the production of hypertension. In this study Anderson (1982) utilized dogs that were trained to respond in an avoidance situation similar to that mentioned above. However, the dogs were also equipped with venous infusion cannulas so that additional salt loads could be introduced directly into the vascular system. The experiment was carried out with some animals simply receiving the salt load and others only being exposed to the avoidance situation. In each of these cases the dogs showed no systematic increases in arterial pressure over a period of weeks. However, when the salt load and the avoidance situation were combined, the animals showed dramatic increases in blood pressure such that in some instances the animals actually underwent a cerebral vascular accident; that is, a stroke was produced. This very dramatic experiment illustrates the importance of the stress factor in its interaction with physiological mechanisms, in this case, regulation of salt balance in the body and the subsequent development of chronic fulminating hypertension.

In each of the cases presented we have attempted to demonstrate the mechanisms by which a well-defined stress situation has interacted with physiological processes either to produce increased blood pressure itself or to alter major regulatory mechanisms such that a chronic essential hypertension condition could potentially be produced. Thus we see the complex relation that exists between biological and behavioral variables in the etiology of one of today's major health care problems.

References

Anderson, D. E. 1982. Behavioral hypertension mediated by salt intake. *In* O. A. Smith, R. A. Galosy, and S. M. Weiss, eds.: Circulation, Neurobiology and Behavior. New York: Elsevier Press; pp. 247–258.

Blair, M. L., E. O. Feigl, and O. A. Smith. 1976. Elevations of plasma serum activity during avoidance performance in baboons. American Journal of Physiology 231:772–726.

Dengerink, H. A., J. W. Wright, P. Thompson, and J. E. Dengerink. 1983. Changes in plasma angiotensin II with noise exposure and their relationship to TTS. Journal of the Acoustical Society of America (in press).

Folkow, B. 1977. Role of the vascular factor in hypertension. Contributions to Nephrology 8:81–94.

Hallback, M., J. V. Jones, G. Bianchi, and B. Folkow. 1977. Cardiovascular control in the Milan strain of spontaneously hypertensive rat (MHS) at "rest" and during acute mental "stress." Acta Physiologica Scandinavica 99:208–216.

Kolota, G. B. 1979. Treatment reduces deaths from hypertension. Science 206:1386–1387.

National Center for Health Statistics. 1976. Advance Data, Hypertension: United States. U.S. Department of Health, Education and Welfare, No. 2. Washington DC, U.S. Government Printing Office.

National High Blood Pressure Education Program. 1973. High Blood Pressure Information Center, Department of Health, Education, and Welfare Publication No. (HSM) 73-28. Washington DC, U.S. Government Printing Office.

Paul, O. 1977. Epidemiology of hypertension. *In* J. Gonest, E. Koiw and O. Kuchel (eds) Hypertension. New York: McGraw-Hill; pp. 613–630.

Smith, O.A., Jr., and Nathan, M. A. 1966. Inhibition of the carotid sinus reflex by stimulation of the inferior olive. Science 154: 674–675.

Smith, O. A., Hohimer, A. R., Astley, C. A., and Taylor, B. J. 1979. Renal and hindlimb vascular control during acute emotion in the baboon. American Journal of Physiology 236: R198–R205.

Smith, O. A., Astley, C. A., DeVito, J. L., Stein, J. M., and Walsh, K. E. 1980a. A functional analysis of hypothalemic control of the cardiovascular responses accompanying emotional behavior. Federation Proceedings 39: 2487–2494.

Smith, O.A., C. A. Astley, A . R.H ohimer, a nd R.B . Stephenson, 1980b. Behavioral and cerebral control of cardiovascular function. *In* M. J. Hughes and C. D.Barnes, eds.: Neural Control of Circulation. New York: Academic Press, pp. 1–21.

Stephenson, R. B., O. A. Smith, and A. M. Scher. 1981. Baroreceptor regulation of heart rate in baboons during different behavioral states. American Journal of Physiology 241:R277–R285.

14

Biofeedback and Psychophysiological Disorders

Jeffrey C. Steger, Ph.D.*

Introduction

It has been postulated that biofeedback techniques represent one of the most significant developments regarding psychophysiological research since the methodologies reported by Pavlov in the early twentieth century. Specifically, it has been noted that biofeedback experimentation often focuses upon the role of behavioral and environmental events as they interrelate with physiological processes (Shapiro and Surwit, 1976). According to Basmajian (1979, p. 1),

> Biofeedback may be defined as the technique of using equipment (usually electronic) to reveal to human beings some of their internal physiological events, normal and abnormal, in the form of visual and auditory signals in order to teach them to manipulate these otherwise involuntary or unfelt events by manipulating the displayed signals. This technique inserts the person's volition into the gap of an open feedback loop—hence the artificial name "biofeedback."

As applied to clinical problems, biofeedback is a generic term referring to the process of monitoring a physiological response system and providing specific information concerning this biological system. The information being monitored from this physiological system is presented in a simplified learning format so that the patient can acquire self-control or regulation of the biological function being monitored.

It is important to avoid the dichotomy between voluntary and involun-

*Assistant Professor, Department of Rehabilitation Medicine, University of Washington School of Medicine, Seattle, Washington. Present address: Department of Behavioral Science, Providence Hospital, Everett, Washington.

tary response systems postulated in many earlier studies concerning psychosomatic disorders. Specifically, biofeedback research has demonstrated that previously assumed "involuntary" biological systems, including heart rate, blood flow, and brain wave patterns, are all capable of being voluntarily regulated using appropriate feedback paradigms (Engel and Bleeker, 1974; Fahrion, 1977; Sterman, 1973). It may therefore be more useful to view physiological systems in terms of their accessibility or inaccessibility (regarding biofeedback monitoring) rather than in terms of voluntary or involuntary biological responses. In this way, the study of psychophysiological disorders is enhanced by biofeedback technology and the only limitations are those imposed by current methodology, rather than conceptual constraints.

Research Literature Considerations

Katkin and Murray (1968) have suggested that all rewards and punishments can significantly affect any learning paradigm, but that the biofeedback situation is primarily one in which information processing is the underlying mechanism determining the learning of a physiological response being monitored) and input (*to* the brain about the response) that is introduced into the feedback paradigm as a way to alter the physiological response of interest. Cybernetic and other synergistic control system formulations of biofeedback have been described by various authors (e. g., Mulholland, 1977; Anliker, 1977). While this model is enticing, it has not been applied extensively and the basic informational model of biofeedback is more parsimonious. The information model postulates simply that various methods of presenting information about physiological systems have differential effects on a person's ability to master the voluntary control of these systems.

A corollary to the informational model is the skills acquisition model as postulated by Lang (1974). In this model, it is stressed that the biofeedback paradigm is primarily a situation in which learned physiological control occurs in the form of complex human learning, such as the learning of a motor skill (Brener, 1974). In the skills acquisition paradigm, biofeedback is viewed as a function that guides the individual in his learning and which may serve to augment awareness of sensations and accompanying physiological responses that are more directly under his voluntary control as a means for mediating control over the desired biological system. In this particular view of biofeedback, the response-monitoring modality is viewed as an externalized sensory feedback mechanism that the individual uses as a calibrating mechanism for the less accessible internal system of feedback in his or her own visceral response, thereby allowing greater awareness of the response under study and generating greater control. This conceptualization has led researchers to investigate the differential effects of various types of instructions in the learned control of physiological systems and has looked at the individual's discrimination and awareness of internal changes during the biofeedback paradigm. One entire body of research literature focuses upon identifying which of these specific variables (learning, information processing, skills acquisition) is most salient in the biofeedback paradigm. As can be seen from this review, many biofeedback studies have focused upon issues only remotely related to clinical application, and the reader must carefully evaluate the extent to which such findings are pertinent to clinical populations.

Biofeedback Modalities

From a theoretical standpoint, there could be as many types of biofeedback equipment as there are specific biological responses in the human organism to be monitored. However, not all the physiological systems in the human body have been studied to the point where equipment exists that allows "real-time" measurement of the ongoing changes in these systems. The range of biofeedback equipment is currently restricted by the technological advancements to date. The major feedback modalities fall into the following categories:

1. Cardiovascular measurement systems (cardiac function and blood pressure monitoring).
2. Electromyographic measurements (EMG; muscle activity monitoring).
3. Peripheral vasomotor measurement (monitoring of the peripheral vascular system through thermistor or pulse volume assessment).
4. Electroencephalographic measurement (EEG; brain wave pattern monitoring).
5. Electrodermal measurement, or galvanic skin response (GSR; skin conductance or resistance monitoring).

As can be seen by this taxonomy, biofeedback technology is designed to monitor specific physiological response systems and each one of these systems has been investigated regarding its particular ability to treat various symptom problems and psychophysiological disorders. Also, each response system requires different electronic or mechanical tolerances and technical specifications for the feedback equipment. The implication of this fact is that different research designs and technical variations obfuscate comparisons across modalities. Furthermore, effective equipment is critical to clinical outcome and beginning practitioners would be well advised to become familiar with the technical requirements of various feedback modalities. The interested reader is referred to detailed discussions on this topic by Cohen (1979) and Peffer (1979).

While it has often been the custom to review biofeedback applications by each feedback modality (for example, Shapiro and Surwit, 1976; Blanchard and Young, 1974), the current chapter will keep the format of this book and focus upon different psychophysiological disorders. In many ways, a symptom-oriented format is more compatible with the review of biofeedback applications to clinical and medical problems, since one of the most significant features of biofeedback is its selective control of specific responses or patterns of response. This specificity of response monitoring is particularly relevant in managing psychophysiological and psychosomatic disorders, since the patient's physiological systems can be individually assessed. Thus the following review is organized according to some of the major psychophysiological disorders seen in medical practice and the ways in which biofeedback techniques have been applied in treating the various symptoms and problems.

Biofeedback Applications with Selected Symptoms

Pain

Pain is one of the most widespread and perplexing of the psycho-physiological disorders encountered in health care. As Fordyce and his colleagues have indicated, pain is most accurately viewed as a multifaceted phenomenon involving nociceptive stimulation and neurotransmission, sensation, pain behavior by the patient, responses to the behavior of the patient, and the suffering or emotional reaction of the patient to pain (Fordyce, 1976; Fordyce and Steger, 1979; Steger and Brockway, 1980; Steger, 1982). It is relevant to note that in using biofeedback with pain, it is assumed that components of the pain experience can be modified by learning to control physiological responses or emotions, and that in so doing the experience of pain can be lessened.

Pain is a complex problem and biofeedback applications to pain (particularly chronic pain) can be effective but must be carefully chosen and specifically applied in the context of a given symptom problem. The most common form of pain treatment to which biofeedback methodology has been applied involves the use of EMG feedback to reduce excessive muscle tension, which is hypothesized to be the major cause for or primary exacerbating variable in a person's painful experience. This particular application of feedback technology utilizes surface electrodes that monitor muscle tension and facilitates muscle contraction reduction. In turn, it is hypothesized that this type of relaxation will be related to symptom decreases for a variety of psychophysiological disorders related to tension and stress. The following review of specific pain-related symptoms is designed to demonstrate those psychophysiological problems that have been suggested to respond to biofeedback treatment of various modalities.

Headache

Tension or muscle contraction headache is probably the most common form of headache, typically characterized by a steady, dull ache or pain located somewhere in the occiput or posterior region of the head and often radiating around to the frontalis region. The frequency and duration of tension headache pain is often variable, may occur daily, and may last from a few minutes to several weeks. The modal pattern is headache pain of low to moderate intensity with moderate to high frequency. The common hypothesis regarding muscle tension headaches is that the pain results from sustained contractions of the skeletal muscles about the face, scalp, neck, and shoulders (Bakal, 1975; Martin, 1972). Sainsbury and Gibson (1954) and Haynes et al. (1975) have demonstrated that tension headache patients had significantly higher EMG levels during headache. Subsequent research has shown that tension headache treatment designed to decrease muscle tension often results in decreased emotional and physiological (i.e., pain sensations) symptoms and reduced medication usage related to headache pain (Budzynski et al., 1973; Hutchins and Reinking, 1976; Steger, 1978; Steger and Harper, 1980). Thus EMG feedback to the frontalis, cervical paraspinalis, and trapezius muscle groups has provided significant reduction of tension headache in several different studies involving numerous tension headache sufferers.

Another form of headache commonly assumed to fall in the category of psychophysiological disorder is the migraine headache. This syndrome is unlike the tension headache and is assumed to have a vascular etiology characterized by unilateral pain of a sharp, intense nature, typically occurring near the temples or behind the eyes. Migraine pain tends to be preceded by a predromal or aural phase consisting of photophobia, nausea, and mental confusion or "fuzziness." These pains are often accompanied by vomiting and are usually high-intensity, long-duration headache episodes that occur less frequently than tension headaches.

Another difference between tension and migraine headaches is that migraines tend to have a specific familial or hereditary component and are more consistently associated with a response to the cessation of prolonged stress (often characterized as a "rebound to stress" phenomenon) rather than an immediate response to stress as is observed in tension headaches (Budzynski, 1979). In an early application to migraine patients, Graham and Wolff (1938) demonstrated that scalp artery amplitude is increased with the severity of migraine headache. Sokolov (1963) demonstrated that varying intensities of averse stimuli generated different degrees of digital vasoconstriction in cephalic vasodilation. Other evidence exists demonstrating that migraine patients show an abnormal pattern of vascular blood flow (Lance, 1973) and that cranial artery variability is higher in migraine patients, indicating a general difficulty with stabilization of the autonomic nervous system mechanisms (Bakal, 1975). Sargent et al. (1972) reported that peripheral fingertip temperatures were significantly lower in patients suffering from migraines than in patients referred for tension headache.

These research findings suggest that alterations in peripheral blood flow patterns could be facilitated by thermal feedback technology and thereby generate improvement in migraine headache symptoms. Initial investigations in this area focused upon teaching individuals to either increase their peripheral fingertip temperatures or decrease their forehead temperatures (hypothesized to be incompatible with cephalic vasodilation) in an attempt to control migraine headache symptoms. This was shown to be effective in several studies using migraine patients, and thus the standard biofeedback treatment for migraine headaches has become the use of thermal feedback to provide peripheral vasomotor control via increasing temperature in the fingers (Sargent et al., 1973; Wickramasekera, 1973).

An additional form of biofeedback used in headache control is temporal artery pulse feedback. The relevance of extracranial pulse amplitude as an etiological mechanism in both tension and migraine headache has been suggested by several researchers. Specifically, Tunis and Wolff (1954) demonstrated that tension headache sufferers evidenced significant increases in average extracranial pulse amplitude during headache symptom conditions as compared to symptom-free conditions. In a similar conceptual application with migraine patients, Koppman et al. (1974) suggested that maladaptive vasodilation, as evidenced by dilated extracranial arteries (monitored through temporal artery pulse amplitude), could contribute to migraine headache symptoms. While both these studies suggest that responsivity to stress in the form of extracranial vasodilation is operative in tension and migraine headache symptoms, the only clinical research attempted to date involves migraine headache patients. In one study, it was demonstrated that by placing a sensor over the temporal artery on the side usually symptomatic during migraine episodes, seven of nine migraine patients showed significant decreases in extracranial pulse amplitude following 2–4 weeks of temporal artery feedback training using reflextive photoplethysmography (Koppman et al., 1974).

While it is clear that EMG and thermal feedback have consistently yielded positive treatment effects for both tension and migraine headache sufferers, it remains unclear as to which aspect of the biofeedback training procedure is the effective treatment ingredient. That is, to what extent is contingent EMG feedback versus generalized relaxation (often part of any effective therapeutic setting) contributing to tension headache reduction? One of the prototypical studies designed to answer this question was provided by Cox et al. (1975), who compared frontalis EMG feedback, simple relaxation, and a medication placebo group in the treatment of tension headache. It was found that the frontalis EMG feedback training group significantly decreased their headache symptoms and medication use more than the placebo capsule treatment group. However, the relaxation-alone group also demonstrated positive treatment effects and there was no statistically significant difference between the effects due to simple relaxation as compared to those resulting from EMG feedback. Similar results have been demonstrated by Haynes et al. (1975) and these raise the question as to the necessity for contingent EMG feedback in the treatment of tension headache. However, while decreases in EMG activity can be effectively demonstrated by relaxation-only groups (often as effective as the contingent EMG feedback groups), for the difficult clinical problem of chronic tension headaches, contingent feedback in combination with some stress management techniques is often required to effect significant long-term reduction in symptoms and medication use (e.g., Hutchins and Reinking, 1976; Steger and Harper, 1980).

Similar questions have been raised with regard to biofeedback applications with migraine headaches. While some researchers have demonstrated that thermal feedback results in significant improvement over other feedback or general relaxation strategies in the treatment of migraine headache (Sargent et al., 1973; Zamani, 1974), other clinical applications have not been as convincing. Kewman (1978) trained one group of migraine headache patients to raise their fingertip temperature using thermal feedback, a second group to lower fingertip temperature, and a third group received no biofeedback training but was instructed to monitor their headache incidence. All three treatment groups demonstrated significant decreases in migraine symptoms (the more significant reductions were reported by the two feedback groups as opposed to the self-monitored group). Thus contingent thermal feedback for teaching increased fingertip temperatures was not a necessary condition for migraine headache control. It has been noted that in almost all biofeedback treatment situations, several treatment components in addition to the specific contingent feedback are present, notably, general relaxation effects, home practice instructions, expectancy for treatment relief, some increase in sense of symptom and body control, and often specific cognitive and stress management techniques (e.g., Turk et al., 1979; Steger and Harper, 1980). Thus, in dealing with headache pain, it is important to remember that while several modalities of biofeedback have been effective, it is unclear what aspect of the feedback treatment procedure is providing the cure.

The detailed presentation of potentially confounding effects has been made for the psychophysiological symptom of headache, since this is one of the most common problems seen in health care. In addition, several researchers have indicated that less than 20% of the patients seen for headache complaints actually have significant muscle tension as the primary component of their symptoms and as many as 70% of these patients can have significant emotional and psychological problems (Harper and Steger, 1978). Thus careful consideration must occur in any psychophysiological workup for headache, and often a psychological evaluation as well as a biofeedback evaluation is needed.

General Musculoskeletal Pain

As with tension headache, musculoskeletal pain syndromes are usually assumed to be related to chronic and excessive contraction of the involved muscle groups. The application of biofeedback technology to musculo-skeletal pain problems other than headache typically involves a thorough neurological and physical examination by a physician trained in pain and neuromuscular disorders to rule out the extent to which respondent and ongoing organic pathology may be contributing to the experience of pain. Typically, however, most biofeedback referrals come much after the acute medical workup and are requested by the referring professional to help identify the extent to which muscle tension may be playing a role in the current symptom pattern. The following muscle tension- or muscle spasm-related symptoms have been effectively treated using electromyographic feedback: neck and shoulder pain, whiplash, spasmodic torticollis (Meares, 1973), upper back spasms, and various upper neck and shoulder pains related to muscle tension or spasm. Myofacial pain syndromes have also been effectively treated using EMG feedback technology (Clarke and Kardachi, 1977; Dohrmann and Laskin, 1978). It is typical for the patient referred for myofacial pain syndromes to have been evaluated by neurology and dental surgery professionals, so that any possible nerve damage is ruled out and the primary component to the current myofacial pain syndrome is assumed to be musculoskeletal in nature, involving chronic muscle contraction or muscle spasm. Other forms of myofacial pain that have been effectively treated using EMG feedback are temporal mendibular joint pain (Carlsson and Gale, 1977) and generalized myo-facial pain not related to the above-mentioned specific disorders that are assumed to be related to muscle tension.

Any pain syndrome can be exacerbated by stress, anxiety, and emotional tension and some patients respond to these stressful events by bruxating or tensing specific facial muscles that, when contracted over prolonged periods of time, generate the presenting symptom complaints. In these cases, biofeedback treatment often involves EMG monitoring of the specific muscle group combined with some general physiological monitoring for signs of stress reduction (e.g., decreases in heart rate and blood pressure or increased peripheral vascular functioning). In this way, the extent to which stress reduction and general relaxation occur in areas other than the specific symptom is assessed. The systematic interfacing of stress management and biofeedback techniques will be dealt with in more detail in the cardiovascular and stress reaction section of this chapter.

Chronic Pain

Applications of biofeedback technology have been used in attempting to deal with the more recalcitrant problem of chronic operative pain. Operant pain syndromes typically require a multidisciplinary team approach involving many aspects of progressive rehabilitation medicine, including physical therapy, occupational therapy, psychiatry, psychology, vocational counseling, biofeedback, and general stress management techniques. In the complex symptom of chronic pain, the application of a single modality must be carefully interfaced with a comprehensive treatment package. This is particularly true in the case of biofeedback, since a tendency exists for chronic pain patients and many other health care users to seek single-modality short-term interventions when a comprehensive, long-term program is needed. Thus it is often inappropriate for the biofeedback practitioner to attempt to treat a chronic pain problem when this treatment is isolated and not coordinated with a comprehensive program. However, when the biofeedback technology can be interfaced with an ongoing comprehensive program, this can be an appropriate and useful adjunct to therapy.

In the context of a chronic operant treatment program, biofeedback is often used as a method for teaching the patient to control muscle tension in the area of symptom involvement (when muscle tension is in fact contributing to the experience of pain). Also, biofeedback methods are used to teach general relaxation and stress-coping techniques, independent of muscle tension reduction related to the symptom, when general stress responsivity and hypersensitivity to tension are considered moderators of the patient's pain experience or when anxiety is felt to be a moderating variable in the experience of pain. In the latter situation, biofeedback methodologies using EMG feedback, thermal training, and skin conductance measures, as well as blood pressure or heart rate feedback, can be used as indicators to the patient of his or her ability to better cope with stress and tension by controlling the physiological concomitant of these emotional reactions. In addition, muscle atrophy or underuse of specific muscle groups has been identified as a component of some chronic pain patients' symptom complaints and in these cases EMG feedback designed to teach increased neuromuscular control and increased muscle activity can be a helpful adjunct to physical therapy and other aspects of the ongoing treatment program designed to yield increased muscle tone and endurance. As is obvious from this discussion, in the application with chronic pain patients, biofeedback is not so much a treatment modality by itself as it is a tool to be used in a highly individualized coordinated program designed for each patient's needs.

Low back pain is the most common form of chronic operant pain encountered by health care professionals. The general discussion of biofeedback applied to chronic operant pain also applies to those patients suffering from chronic low back pain, which has significant operant components requiring a comprehensive treatment program. There are some patients who experience low back pain (whether it be chronic or acute) who do not require a comprehensive pain treatment program, despite the fact that their pain symptoms are minimally related to ongoing organic pathology. In these patients, muscle spasms related to a specific precipitating event or chronic overuse of the involved muscles have generated the low back pain symptoms, but the patient has not fallen into a pattern of illness and pain behavior and is thus not yet an operant pain treatment candidate. In this situation, biofeedback has shown promise. In these cases, EMG feedback is used to identify specific muscle groups that contribute to the low back pain problem under varying conditions of movement activity and stress. This type of psychophysiological evaluation is often done in conjunction with a physical therapy assessment and is most effective when detailed observations of the covariation between muscle activity and varying degrees of physical activity and stress are obtained. The treatment then focuses upon reducing the EMG activity (via EMG feedback) in those muscles and under the condition determined (by the evaluation) to contribute to the back pain. This is the same model of biofeedback as applied to tension headaches.

A word of caution in the use of this model with chronic low back pain is in order. This "excessive tension" model has *not* been demonstrated to consistently yield effective low back pain treatment, except in those cases where back spasms are clearly present (by far the exception rather than the rule). However, a more recent conceptualization of the mechanism behind low back pain involves the concept of dysponesis. This model focuses upon the extent to which right- and left-side paraspinalis muscle groups are competing with each other (rather than coordinating their activity to enhance movement), thereby generating a disequilibrium in the skeletal muscle support system (Cram, 1981). Using this "disequilibrium" concept, EMG feedback methods monitoring right and left unilateral paraspinalis muscle activity have been designed to teach the patient how to equalize or equilibrate bilateral EMG activity in paraspinalis musculature during various back movement conditions where this type of cooperative effort is expected (e.g., sitting or standing in a normal, nonflexed position). This type of EMG treatment has been shown to be effective in decreasing reports of low back pain in several patients (Cram, 1981; Wolf, 1981). While these reports are preliminary, they point to the utility of biofeedback technology in serving as an assessment tool that can also serve as a treatment modality for psychophysiological disorders which have resisted more traditional approaches in the past.

The area of pain treatment remains a complex arena for the health care professional. Much experience in chronic and acute pain treatment, as well as biofeedback instrumentation and methodology, is required to apply feedback methods in pain management progress. The extent to which pain can be a function of factors other than psychophysiological variables like muscle tension and general sympathetic or autonomic nervous system activity makes this problem area more complex than most. The necessity of evaluating psychological, environmental, body mechanical, vocational, and chemical components in an individual's pain problem cannot be minimized. Thus, in applying biofeedback technology to any pain situation, many facets of treatment must be ruled out before biofeedback can be applied effectively.

Stress Reactions

Physiological reactions to stress that generate indentifiable and observable symptoms (for example hypertension, tachycardia, skin rash) are the types of disorders typically visualized when the terms *psychosomatic* or *psychophysiological* are encountered. In addition to these classic psychophysiological reactions, certain pain complaints can also be directly related to stress or emotional upset, but for the purpose of this section reference will be made only to specific psychophysiological reactions other than pain. Most of the disorders to be reviewed in this section can have definite and specific underlying organic etiologies and these must be ruled out before any biofeedback application is considered. This caution is obviously applicable to all aspects of biofeedback where organic tissue damage or disease processes can play a role in the symptom pattern reported by the patient.

Biofeedback technology is the most recent addition to an already existing set of therapeutic tools designed to treat psychophysiological reactions. Jacobsonian relaxation therapy (Jacobson, 1938), autogenic training (Luthe, 1969), and systemic desensitization (Wolpe, 1958) are all psychotherapeutic techniques designed to deactivate the patient's physiological reaction to stress and emotion and generate a relaxed and improved physical or emotional state. While these techniques have been proven to be effective in the treatment of many types of disorders (e.g., anxiety, phobias, insomnia), they all suffer from the same limitation; that is, none provides an inherent means to monitor the extent to which the patient actually becomes relaxed in response to the treatment. In these approaches, the therapist relies upon the patient's self-report of relaxation in assessing the extent of relaxation or reduced stress activity. Thus biofeedback methodology provides a needed increment in design technology for treating stress reactions by providing an objective measurement of various stress indicators as part of the treatment. Biofeedback systems provide diagnostic monitors of specific physiological responses that can be used at the same time as treatment modalities to generate decreases in reactivity to stress. In addition, these methods appear to have an additional advantage over the more traditional relaxation and stress reduction techniques, in that the latter rely upon generalized relaxation induction phrases and methodologies that may not work for all people in all situations, whereas biofeedback provides specific and individualized information about each person's physiological responses in any given situation. Thus it is reasonable to assume that learning occurs more consistently and more easily in these specific learing paradigms of the biofeedback model as opposed to the more general and less individualized situation of Jacobsonian relaxation, autogenic training, or systematic desensitization.

   Much of the work involving relaxation training using biofeedback has been done by researchers at the University of Colorado Medical School in Denver, Colorado, and a useful conceptualization of this biofeedback application comes from one of these researchers, Johann Stoyva. He suggested that the clinical use of biofeedback be divided into two primary approaches categorized as direct and indirect methods. As he perceived it (Stoyva, 1977), the direct application of biofeedback to psychophysiological disorders refers to identifying a specific physiological response assumed to be related to a specific stressful reaction (for example, increased heart rate in stress-induced tachycardia) and using the feedback paradigm as a method for reinforcing decreases in this particular response, thereby directly altering the person's reactivity to stress. In the indirect application of biofeedback to stress reactions, Stoyva postulated that an anxiety- or stress-related disorder be treated not by focusing upon a specific physiological concomitant or corrolary to the disorder but, rather, by using biofeedback as a method for generating generalized relaxation and reduced anxiety or stress. One example of this indirect method focuses upon muscle relaxation (through EMG feedback) as a means for generating generalized reduction to control a stress-related symptom like a skin rash. The assumption in this indirect biofeedback application is that other bodily physiological systems are altered as a result of training in general relaxation using EMG feedback. In either application, biofeedback methodology allows monitoring of various physiological response indicators, facilitating an objective assessment of the extent to which generalized relaxation effects and generalized decreased stress reactivity actually occur, whereas previous treatment interventions assuming generalized stress-coping training could only indirectly make these claims. With this set of considerations in mind, the following symptoms and disorders have been chosen to demonstrate typical biofeedback applications in stress disorders.

Cardiac Symptoms

While there is an extensive literature concerning the ability of normal subjects to alter cardiac functioning using various feedback methodologies, there has been relatively little clinical investigation regarding the use of biofeedback for medically and stress-related cardiac complications. The major areas of interest in cardiac symptom reduction involve arrhythmias and premature ventricular contractions (PVCs). For example, Engel and Bleecher (1974) found that paroxysmal atrial tachycardia could be brought under control using heart rate feedback. They also showed that heart rate feedback could be used in patients with ventricular arrhythmias secondary to coronary artery disease in order to decrease the frequency of arrhythmias resulting in a positive clinical outcome. In a similar application of heart rate feedback, Bleecher and Engel (1973a) and Miller (1975) demonstrated that patients with PVCs could demonstrate clinically significant (and often sustained) decreases in the frequency of arrhythmias. Finally, heart rate feedback was used by Bleecher and Engel (1973b) and Weiss and Engel (1975) to generate beneficial control in certain patients with coronary conduction defects. These studies combine to suggest that significant reductions in heart rate can result from feedback paradigms in highly stressed individuals showing abnormally high heart rate and arrhythmia problems. However, these findings are in direct contradiction to the results of studies in normals, where it was very difficult to demonstrate significant reductions in heart rate using feedback methods. This suggests that the clinical utility of biofeedback with cardiac problems only reveals itself under situations where reactions to tension- and stress-coping mechanisms are salient.

Biofeedback treatment methods have been developed that effectively treat the following disorders: cardiovascular and heart rate feedback paradigms, sinus tachycardia (Scott et al., 1973; Vaitl, 1975), atrial fibrillations (Bleecher and Engel, 1973b), Woff–Parkinson–White (WPW) syndrome (Bleecher and Engel, 1973a), and ventricular ectopic rhythms (Weiss and Engel, 1971; Pickering and Miller, 1977). As can be seen from this brief review, the application of biofeedback to psychophysiological reactions involving cardiac symptoms appears promising. The specificity and individualization of training responses in difficult cases where other methods have been ineffective is perhaps one of biofeedback's most useful characteristics.

Hypertension

Two types of blood pressure monitoring systems have been developed and historically used biofeedback evaluation and treatment of essential hypertension. One of these is a miniaturized cannule transducer implanted in one of the major arteries that provides a continuous measurement of blood pressure and blood flow volume (Fey and Lindholm, 1978). This technique minimizes artifacts resulting from measurement variance, since it does not require an uncomfortable technique and repeated administration (for example, use of a sphygomanometer). The most prevalent method, however, for monitoring blood pressure makes use of the common occluding cuff and stethoscope for determining systolic and diastolic pressure by monitoring Korotkoff sounds (Tursky et al., 1972; Engel et al., 1981). This system is often referred to as the "constant cuff" system, since the occluding cuff remains on the arm constantly throughout the monitoring of blood pressure, although it is periodically deflated to avoid negative side effects from continual occlusion of the arteries. In this way, continuous (through the use of implanted cannulae) or intermittent (occluding cuff) information regarding diastolic and systolic blood pressure can be used in evaluating the effects of various relaxation techniques. Using one of these blood pressure monitoring systems, the patient is trained to alter his or her diastolic or systolic blood pressure and the feedback device provides information and reinforcement regarding the learning occurring during the feedback session.

The significant clinical reduction of blood pressure has been demonstrated in several studies involving patients suffering from mild and moderate hypertension. Benson et al. (1971) used the cuff system to teach patients to significantly lower their systolic blood pressure. These patients showed significant decreases in blood pressure after the feedback training, which had not been demonstrated during 16 pretreatment monitoring sessions. Similar results have been demonstrated in several studies and it is generally concluded that constant cuff or cannula implant feedback technology is effective in teaching hypertensive patients to lower their blood pressure (Fey and Lindholm, 1978; Tursky et al., 1972; Engel et al., 1981; Krist and Engel, 1975).

Despite consistent clinical findings, the role of contingent blood pressure feedback in controlling hypertensive responses is not at all clear; nor has the value of such procedures for long-term change been established. Surwit et al. (1978) compared the results of three treatment groups in differentially affecting blood pressure in borderline hypertensives. One treatment group received specific binary feedback for reductions in blood pressure and heart rate (the constant cuff method of Schwartz et al., 1972). The second group received analog feedback for forearm and frontalis EMG relaxation, and a third treatment group underwent a meditation–relaxation procedure (Benson, 1975). The results of this study demonstrated that all three treatment groups showed significant reductions in blood pressure following treatment, with no significant clinical differences observed between these treatment groups. Thus, while the blood pressure feedback group was effective in generating clincally relevant and significant decreases in blood pressure for hypertensives, so were the EMG feedback and general meditation (relaxation) treatment procedures used in the other two groups. As in the case of pain control, it can be seen that several mechanisms may be operating in the biofeedback control of blood pressure in hypertensives. In a recent review of biofeedback and other hypertensive treatments, Reeves and Shapiro (1978) concluded that "since biofeedback and relaxation techniques have resulted in equivalent blood pressure reductions, it would seem the less costly and simpler relaxation procedures would be the treatment of choice. However, the combination of biofeedback and relaxation has produced the most substantial (*blood*) pressure reductions." Unfortunately, the differential or additive effects of each of these treatment components in hypertensive intervention is yet to be investigated. Also, while EMG feedback (Patel and North, 1975) and blood pressure feedback (Schwartz et al., 1972; Fey and Lindholm, 1978) continue to appear as the primary biofeedback methods used for controlling hypertension, it appears that a combination of these two feedback modalities in addition to stress reduction techniques and cognitive therapy might be the most effective treatment.

Anxiety

Anxiety and general tension are two common psychosomatic disorders. Recent clinical studies involving the application of biofeedback to chronic anxiety have generated compatible results suggesting that muscle relaxation can have a beneficial effect on anxiety and the physiological systems controlling it. In this application of feedback technology to a psychophysiological disorder, it is assumed that excess muscle tension contributes to overall physiological activity and bodily responses and can be interpreted by the brain as a component of increased arousal or anxiety. Thus the focus of treatment is to decrease EMG activity and hopefully generate a decrease in anxiety symptoms. Using frontalis EMG feedback, Raskin et al. (1973) were successful in showing some improvement in anxiety symptoms for four out of ten chronic anxiety patients. A more convincing intervention was demonstrated by Townsend et al. (1975) when they compared EMG feedback training to group psychotherapy in the treatment of chronic anxiety. In this paradigm, decreases in EMG were the focus of the biofeedback treatment and this treatment group generated significantly more improvement in measures of mood disturbance, trait anxiety, and state anxiety than did the psychotherapy group.

Other more specific applications to the problem of anxiety involve the treatment of specific phobias where a specific physiological response is monitored (e.g., muscle tension) that is assumed to contribute to the patient's perception of arousal and fear in the specific phobic situation. Using this paradigm, Reeves and Mealiea (1975) effectively treated two cases of driving and flying phobia using EMG feedback. While these applications to anxiety and phobic situations are preliminary, they again demonstrate a possible advantage of biofeedback methodology in treating psychosomatic disorders. Specifically, feedback technology allows the therapist to monitor the target physiological index primarily related to the psychosomatic disorder being treated and can provide individualized training based on the specific physiological reaction of the individual patient in each fearful or stressful situation.

Insomnia

Insomnia is another psychosomatic illness that has been associated with overreactivity to stress and an inability to consistently relax and control the autonomic nervous system. Using frontalis EMG, positive treatment effects have been demonstrated for insomnia in several studies (Hauri et al., 1976; Freedman and Pabsdorf, 1976; Corsi et al., 1976; and Borkavec, 1976). While these studies involved multiple case investigators, Haynes et al. (1979) contrasted general relaxation instructions with specific frontalis EMG feedback in a controlled clinical outcome study. They demonstrated that the biofeedback treatment group was significantly more effective in generating decreases in sleep disturbance when compared to the relaxation group in a set of insomniacs. This set of results is preliminary in nature, since some of these studies used electroencephalographic monitoring of sleep latency brain wave patterns to verify the subjective report of sleep disturbance, while others did not, thus obfuscating direct comparisons of results.

Another form of feedback intervention that has been proposed but not tested in a controlled clinical setting involves electroencephalographic (EEG) feedback. In this application, patients with insomnia are trained to generate brain wave patterns compatible with sleep [for example, teaching the patient to increase the predominance of theta waves (3–7 Hz), assumed to be associated with sleep]. While these preliminary findings are interesting, the differential effectiveness of relaxation versus EMG feedback versus EEG feedback has yet to be demonstated in the treatment of sleep onset insomnia. However, it does appear that some form of autonomic nervous system deactivation occurs as a result of relaxation (EMG feedback) and brain wave patern alteration (EEG feedback) and may be useful in facilitating sleep and controlling sleep disturbance disorders.

Miscellaneous Stress-Related Disorders

There have been periodic case reports in the literature involving various psychophysiological disorders that have been effectively treated with biofeedback. While none of the following symptoms have been studied in a controlled manner involving the application of feedback technology, the systematic application of biofeedback in an attempt to control the physiological response associated with each of these symptoms has been consistent with the methodology applied in the more common and better controlled psychophysiological disorders like tension headaches and hypertension. The following is a list of psychosomatic disorders that are typically assumed to be stress related and which have positively benefited from some form of biofeedback intervention:

1. Asthma—monitoring of respiratory resistance (Khan, 1977), of EMG (Kotses et al., 1976, 1978).
2. Ulcerative colitis—abdominal EMG relaxation (Steger, 1976).
3. Tinnitus—monitoring EMG (House, 1978; House et al., 1979).

In addition to the above case examples of biofeedback intervention with stress-related physical reactions, there have been anecdotal findings suggesting that skin rash reactions can be effectively improved through direct biofeedback methods (thermal feedback to decrease the blood flow to the involved area assumed to be the direct source of the symptom), as well as by indirect techniques (electrodermal and GSR feedback to decrease skin conductance measures as a way to indirectly reduce the rash by generalized anxiety reduction). All of these reports remain preliminary but once again indicate that the application of biofeedback methodology to psychophysiological disorders is primarily limited by the creativity of the therapist and the technical monitoring capabilities of the feedback equipment.

Peripheral Vascular Symptoms

Control of digital skin temperature through biofeedback instrumentation and learning paradigms has been cited previously in the control of migraine headaches (Sargent et al., 1973). In addition to the application to headache problems, other peripheral vascular symptoms have been effectively treated using thermal feedback technology. The major disorder related to peripheral vasomotor dysfunction is Raynaud's phenomenon, characterized by a significant decrease in blood flow to the periphery, resulting in extreme cases in gangrene and amputation of the digits. In

addition, pain and decreased fine motor coordination are often concomitants of the Raynaud's disease process and generate significant
impairment and discomfort for patients with this disorder. This particular
set of symptoms has not necessarily been connected with stress, although,
as reviewed earlier in this chapter, it has been demonstrated that, in
general, peripheral vasomotor activity appears to covary with levels of
stress. As in the application to migraine headache, the common concept-
ulatization of thermal feedback is utilized in the treatment of Raynaud's
phenomenon, since Raynaud's patients have significantly lower than
average peripheral fingertip temperatures.

In the standard thermal feedback paradigm a thermistor ($0.1-0.01°$ F
sensitivity) is taped to the involved peripheral digit to monitor peripheral
fingertip temperature. With this technique thermal information from the
thermistor is translated into an audio or visual signal where increases or
decreases in skin temperature are indicated by corresponding increases or
decreases in the signal. Using this paradigm, ideopathic Raynaud's
phenomenon was shown to be significantly clinically improved by Taub
(1977) and Surwit et al. (1978). In a similar application, Greenspan et al.
(1980) demonstrated that thermal feedback was significantly more
effective in decreasing symptoms related to peripheral vascular disease
than was general relaxation therapy.

Other vascular symptoms have also been treated using biofeedback
technology. In the area of sexual dysfunction, both erectile failure and
orgasmic dysfunction have been reported to relate significantly to blood
flow patterns in the male and female, respectively (Barbach, 1975).
Erectile failure (where organic pathology like diabetes is not present)
is primarily related to decreased blood flow into the penile vasculature,
resulting in decreased erection strength. Erection has been monitored
using biofeedback technology through both penile temperature and
the circumference of the penis via penile plethysmograph (Barlow
et al., 1976). In using biofeedback to monitor erectile difficulties, it can be
seen that the feedback modality might also serve as an effective treatment
technique providing specific information to the patient regarding his
ability to increase either his penile temperature (theoretically only
possible by increasing the blood flow into the penis and therefore the
strength of the erection) or his penile circumference (a more direct
measure of erection). This hypothesis was effectively tested when it was
demonstrated that men suffering from erectile failure could learn to
significantly increase their erectile capabilities using feedback from a
penile plethysmograph (Csillar, 1976).

In an application of orgasmic dysfunction in women, EMG monitoring
of vaginal muscle activity was used as an indication of the strength of
orgasmic response. In this application, women were taught to increase
their EMG activity during masturbation as a way to train orgasmic

response initially in masturbatory activity and then to generalize this to intercourse. This was found to be successful in one case of female orgasmic dysfunction using EMG feedback (Perry and Whipple, 1981). It has been hypothesized that monitoring vaginal or labial temperatures is another way to increase female orgasmic response, since increased vascularity is assumed to result from increased blood flow to the vaginal area. However, this form of thermal feedback has not been applied in a controlled manner to women with orgasmic dysfunction, nor have the other applications of biofeedback for sexual dysfunction (erectile failure) been tested regarding the most critical issue in this area: the extent to which these improved sexual responses generalize to the partner situation.

Gastrointestinal Disorders

Gastrointestinal (GI) disorders have previously been mentioned as psychophysiological symptoms related to stress. Specifically, reference was made to EMG feedback in the treatment of ulcerative colitis, and this is one of the major applications of biofeedback methodology for GI disorders. In this method, feedback technology is used to decrease stress responsivity and yield clinical improvement in any GI disorder exacerbated or caused by stress and tension. However, there are some GI disorders that are not necessarily a direct reaction to stress but which are symptoms resulting from specific dysfunctional physical systems in the gastrointestinal tract. This is not to imply that stress or muscle tension cannot play a role in any functional GI disorder (including these listed in this section). These particular GI disorders are separated and placed under this heading, however, since the biofeedback methodology focuses on the specific physiological response system that has been diagnosed as dysfunctional and is the major cause of the symptom pattern. The following is a list of such GI disorders that have positively benefited from the use of feedback technology:

1. Functional diarrhea—monitoring of Borgorygmi (Furman, 1973).
2. Functional encopresis—monitoring of anal sphincter pressure (Kohlenberg, 1973).
3. Fecal incontinence—monitoring and feedback from anal sphincter EMG activity (Schuster, 1977).
4. Urinary retention and incontinence—monitoring of urinary sphincter EMG (Pearne et al., 1977).

In all the cases listed, patient control of the dysfunctional response had been unsuccessful with a variety of other techniques, including generalized relaxation and nonspecific tension reduction of the involved muscle groups. Once again, the specific nature of biofeedback intervention allowed the patient to gain control of the dysfunctional physiological response by being provided accurate and immediate information from this system.

Speech Disorders

As in the case of gastrointestinal disorders, speech disorders have responded well to preliminary applications of biofeedback technology. Again, it is not assumed that speech disorders are necessarily related to stress or anxiety. Instead, a specific physiological system is usually involved that can be brought under voluntary control through biofeedback applications. As in the case with gastrointestinal disorders, speech disorders involving different physical systems have been identified and in each case a monitoring system specifically designed for the involved physical response was built and used to provide feedback to the patient in an effort to gain control over the previously dysfunctional system. The following is a list of speech disorders that have been effectively treated using biofeedback technology:

1. Stuttering—EMG monitoring of the muscles involved specifically in speech (Hanna et al., 1975; Lanyon, 1977).
2. Subvocalization—EMG monitoring of external sternocleidomastoid and related area activity (Hardyck and Petrinovich, 1969).
3. Voice quality deficits—EMG monitoring of the muscles involved in speech (Daly and Johnson, 1974).

While promising, these applications must be considered preliminary, since they primarily involve case studies of the application of specific feedback modalites in single cases.

Seizure Disorders

One of the most widely discussed and renowned areas in biofeedback is the area of electroencephalographic (EEG) feedback. This type of feedback has been used in monitoring seizure activity as well as attempting to control it through providing feedback to the individual regarding brain wave activity. Initial interest in brain wave pattern monitoring using biofeedback technology did not stem from seizure patients but, rather, from the observation that yogi meditators exhibiting significant pain control produced significant increases in the percentage of alpha brain wave activity (Kamiya, 1969). This observation, once verified and replicated, led to a series of investigations that demonstrated that subjects could learn to alter their brain wave activity when provided specific and contingent feedback using electroencephalographic monitoring equipment (Kamiya, 1969; Beatty and Legewie, 1977). In an application of the implications of these findings, Sterman and his colleagues attempted to apply EEG methodology to the evaluation and treatment of seizures. Specifically, he argued that if normal subjects could be shown to generate learned brain wave pattern conditioning, it might be possible to teach epileptics to alter their brain wave patterns to become more "normalized," in this way decreasing or preventing seizure activity. He chose standard EEG feedback techniques that monitor brain activity (EEG) across several frequency ranges: theta (3–7 Hz), alpha (8–12 Hz), and beta (13–30 Hz). His "target" EEG frequency was the 12–14 Hz sensory motor rhythm (SMR) occurring over the Rolandic fissure of the sensory motor cortex to monitor psychomotor activity in patients suffering from psychomotor epilepsy. In this paradigm, a light would go on or off whenever the patient demonstrated normalized versus epileptiform brain wave patterns and in this way a conditioning and learning situation was established. Using this technique, it was demonstrated that epileptic patients could significantly decrease their epileptiform brain wave activity by increasing SMR predominance, resulting in decreased seizure frequency and seizure medication intake (Sterman et al., 1974). Although this biofeedback is promising, the clinical application is typically complex and requires expensive and sophisticated computer technology and personnel.

Nevertheless the area of brain wave control in humans perhaps best illustrates how the technology developed for biofeedback applications has facilitated research results that have moved us beyond the antiquated notion of voluntary versus involuntary systems to the level of synergistic feedback mechanisms in human physiological conceptualization.

Conclusion

Biofeedback methodology has advanced significantly in recent years, yet many clinical applications remain on an experimental level. It has been demonstrated that biofeedback technology can generate positive clinical effects in various psychophysiological disorders, particularly those symptoms related to muscle tension and stress. In general, the more specific the symptom and the more closely it is related to a given physiological response, the more likely it is that some biofeedback system exists to yield clinical effective treatment.

In dealing with psychophysiological symptoms, it is important to remember that despite the focus upon specific physiological responses in biofeedback paradigms, most psychosomatic disorders are multifaceted and seldom related only to physical factors. Thus multimodal evaluation and treatment where several health care specialities are required are a common and often necessary part of any health care strategy for psychophysiological symptoms.

This chapter has presented various intervention strategies involving biofeedback technology and it should be apparent that much research remains to be completed before many of those strategies can be indicated as clear "treatments of choice" for a given symptom. Controlled studies that account for such nonspecific variables as placebo and expectancy effects are present in only a few feedback treatment areas and much more research is needed to separate the effective from the irrelevant treatment components. In particular, it is important to remember that inexpensive intervention strategies like simple relaxation have been shown to provide powerful results with many psychophysiological disorders. Thus, in evaluating cost-effectiveness considerations, biofeedback intervention should be compared to less costly yet effective strategies shown to benefit psychosomatic symptoms. In this way, a stepwise treatment strategy might evolve where treatment initially utilizes readily available, inexpensive, self-monitoring techniques (e.g., home relaxation tapes, home exercise, and deep-breathing activities) and progresses to more specific and costly intervention (e.g., cardiac feedback, EMG monitoring) when the first level of intervention proves ineffective.

References

Anliker, J. 1977. Biofeedback from the perspectives of cybernetics and systems science. In J. Beatty and H. Legewie, eds.: Biofeedback and Behavior. New York: Plenum Press; pp. 132–145.

Bakal D. H. 1975. Headache: A biophysical perspective. Psychological Bulletin 82:369–382.

Barbach, L. 1975. For Yourself: The Fulfillment of Female Sexuality. Garden City, New York: Doubleday.

Barlow, D. H., W. S. Agras, G. G. Abel, E. B. Blanchard, and L. D. Young. 1976. Biofeedback and reinforcement to increase heterosexual arousal in homosexuals. Behavior Research and Therapy 13:45–50.

Basmajian, J. (ed.). 1979. Biofeedback—Principles and Practice for Clinicians. Baltimore, Maryland: Williams and Wilkins; p. 1.

Beatty, J., and H. Legewie. (eds.). 1977. Biofeedback and Behavior. New York: Plenum Press.

Benson, H. 1975. The Relaxation Response. New York: William Morrow.

Benson, H., D. Shapiro, B. Tursky, and G. E. Schwartz. 1971. Decreased systolic blood pressure through operant conditioning techniques in patients with essential hypertension. Science 173:740–742.

Blanchard, E. B., and L. D. Young. 1974. Clinical applications of biofeedback training: A review of evidence. Archives of General Psychiatry 30:573–589.

Bleecher, E. R., and B. T. Engel. 1973a. Learned control of cardiac rate and cardiac conduction in a patient with Wolff–Parkinson–White syndrome. New England Journal of Medicine 288:560–562.

Bleecher, E. R., and B. T. Engel. 1973b. Learned control of ventricular rate in patients with atrial fibrillation. Psychosomatic Medicine 35:161–170.

Borkavec, T. T. 1976. Physiological and cognitive processes in the regulation of anxiety. In Schwartz, G. and Shapiro, D., eds.: Consciousness and Self-Regulation: Advances in Research. New York: Plenum Press.

Brener, J. 1974. A general model of voluntary control applied to the phenomena of learned cardiovascular change. In P. A. Obrist, A. H. Black, J. Brener, and L. V. DiCara, eds.: Cardiovasculary Psychophysiology. Chicago, Illinois: Aldine; pp. 15–38.

Budzynski, T. H. 1979. Biofeedback strategies in headache treatment. In Basmajian, J., ed.: Biofeedback: Principles and Practice for Clinicians. Baltimore, Maryland: Williams and Wilkins; pp. 132–152.

Budzynski, T. H., J. M. Stoyva, C. S. Adler, and D. J. Mullaney. 1973. EMG biofeedback and tension headache: A controlled outcome study. Psychosomatic Medicine 35:484–496.

Carlsson, S. G., and E. N. Gale. 1977. Biofeedback in the treatment of long-term temporomandibular joint pain: An outcome study. Biofeedback Self-Regulation 2:161–171.

Clarke, N. G., and B. J. Kardachi. 1977. Treatment of myofascial pain-dysfunction syndrome using biofeedback principle. Journal of Periodontology 46:643–645.

Cohen, B. 1979. Basic biofeedback electronics for the clinician. In Basmajian, J., ed.: Biofeedback: Principles and Practice for Clinicians. Baltimore, Maryland: Williams and Wilkins; pp. 257–268.

Corsi, R., B. Frankel, and K. Gardner. 1976. EMG biofeedback and autogenic training as relaxation techniques for chronic sleep-onset insomnia. Proceedings of the Biofeedback Research Society Seventh Annual Meeting, p. 8.

Cox, D. J., A. Freundlich, and R. G. Meyer. 1975. Differential effectiveness of electromyographic feedback, verbal relaxation instructions and medication placebo. Journal of Consulting and Clinical Psychology 43:892–898.

Cram, J. 1981. Dual channel EMG feedback in treating chronic low back pain. Poster presented at the Annual Midwinter Conference of the Biofeedback Society of America, Vail, Colorado.

Csillar, E. R. 1976. Modification of penile erectile response. Journal of Behavior Therapy and Experimental Psychiatry 7:27–29.

Daly, D., and H. P. Johnson. 1974. Instrumental modification of hypernasal voice quality in retarded children: Case reports. Journal of Speech and Hearing Disorders 39:500–607.

Dohrmann, R. J., and D. M. Laskin. 1978. An evaluation of electromyographic biofeedback in the treatment of myofascial pain-dysfunction syndrome. Journal of American Dental Association 96:656–662.

Engel, B., and E. Bleecker. 1974. Application of operant conditioning techniques to the control of cardiac arrythmias. In J. Obrist, J. Black, J. Brener, and J. DiCara, eds.: Cardiovascular Psychophysiology. Chicago, Illinois: Aldine; pp. 52–59.

Engel, B. T., K. R. Gaarder, and M. S. Glasgow. 1981. Behavioral treatment of high blood pressure: I. Analysis of intra- and inter-daily variations of blood pressure during a one month baseline period. Psychosomatic Medicine 43:255–270.

Fahrion, S. 1977. Autogenic biofeedback treatment for migraine. Mayo Clinic Proceedings 52:776–784.

Fey, S., and E. Lindholm. 1978. Biofeedback and progressive relaxation: Effects on systolic and diastolic blood pressure and heart rate. Psychophysiology 15:239–247.

Fordyce, W. 1976. Behavioral Methods for Chronic Pain and Illness. St. Louis, Missouri: C. V. Mosby.

Fordyce, W. E., and J. C. Steger. 1979. Behavioral management of chronic pain. In

J. Brady and O. Pomerleau, eds.: Behavioral Medicine: Theory and Practice. New York: Williams and Wilkins; pp. 125–153.

Freedman, R., and J. D. Papsdorf. 1976. Biofeedback and progressive relaxation treatment of sleep onset insomnia. Biofeedback Self-Regulation 1:253–271.

Furman, S. 1973. Intestinal biofeedback in functional diarrhea: A preliminary report. Journal of Behavior Therapy and Experimental Psychiatry 4:317–321.

Graham, J. R., and H. G. Wolff. 1938. Mechanism of migraine headache and action of ergotamine tartrated. Archives of Neurology and Psychiatry 39:737–763.

Greenspan, K., P. F. Lawrence, D. B. Esposito, and A. B. Voorhees. 1980. The role of biofeedback and relaxation therapy in arterial occlusive disease. Journal of Surgical Research 29:387–394.

Hanna, R., F. Wilfling, and B. McNeil. 1975. A biofeedback treatment for stuttering. Journal of Speech and Hearing Disorders 40:270–273.

Hardyck, C. D., and L. F. Petrinovich. 1969. Treatment of subvocal speech during reading. Journal of Reading 1:3–11.

Harper, R., and J. Steger, 1978. Psychological correlates of frontalis EMG and pain in tension headache. Headache 18:215–218.

Hauri, P., P. J. Phelps, and F. B. Jordan. 1976. Biofeedback as a treatment for insomnia. Proceedings of the Biofeedback Research Society Seventh Annual Meeting, p. 34.

Haynes, S. N., D. Moseley, and W. T. McGowan. 1975. Relaxation training and biofeedback in the reduction of frontalis muscle tension. Psychophysiology 12:547–552.

Haynes, S., H. Sides and G. Lockwood, 1979. Relaxation instructions and frontalis electromyographic feedback interventions with sleep-onset insomnia. Biofeedback and Self-Control 1977–1983; pp. 113–121.

House, J. W. 1978. Treatment of severe tinnitus with biofeedback training. Laryngoscope 88:406–412.

House, J. W., L. Miller, and P. R. House. 1979. Severe tinnitus: Treatment with biofeedback training—Results in forty-one cases. Transactions of the American Academy of Ophthalmology and Otolaryngology 84:697–703.

Hutchins, D., and R. Reinking. 1976. Tension headaches: What form of therapy is most effective? Biofeedback and Self-Regulation 1:183–190.

Jacobson, E. 1938. Progressive Relaxation, 2nd ed. Chicago, Illinois: University of Chicago Press.

Kamiya, J. 1969. Operant control of the EEG alpha rhythm and some of its reported effects on consciousness. In C. T. Tart, ed.: Altered States of Consciousness. New York: Wiley.

Katkin, E. S., and E. N. Murray. 1968. Instrumental conditioning of autonomically mediated behavior: Theoretical and methodological issues. Psychological Bulletin 70:52–68.

Kewman, D. C. 1978. Voluntary control of digital skin temperatures for treatment of migraine headaches (doctoral dissertation, University of Texas at Austin, 1977). Dissertation Abstracts International 38:3400B.

Khan, A. U. 1977. Effectiveness of biofeedback and counter-conditioning in the treatment of bronchial asthma. Journal of Psychosomatic Research 21:97–104.

Kohlenberg, R. J. 1973. Operant conditioning of human anal sphincter pressure. Journal of Applied Behavior Analysis 3:201–208.

Koppman, J. W., R. O. McDonald, and M. G. Kunzel. 1974. Voluntary regulation of temporal artery diameter by migraine patients. Headache 14:133–138.

Kotses, H., K. D. Glaus, P. L. Crawford, J. Edwards, and M. Scherr. 1976. Operant reduction of frontalis EMG activity in the treatment of asthma in children. Journal of Psychosomatic Research 20:453–459.

Kotses, H., K. D. Glaus, S. K. Bricel, J. Edwards, and P. L. Crawford. 1978. Operant muscular relaxation and peak expiratory flow rate in asthmatic children. Journal of Psychosomatic Research 22:17–23.

Krist, D. A., and B. T. Engel. 1975. Learned control of blood pressure in patients with high blood pressure. Circulation 51:370–378.

Lance, J. W. 1973. Mechanism and Management of Headache, 2nd ed. London, England: Butterworths.

Lang, P. J. 1974. Learned control of human heart rate in a computer directed environment. In P. A. Obrist, A. H. Black, J. Brener, and L. V. DiCara, eds.: Cardiovascular Psychophysiology. Chicago, Illinois: Aldine; pp. 392–405.

Lanyon, R. I. 1977. Effect of biofeedback-based relaxation on stuttering during reading and spontaneous speech. Journal of Consulting and Clinical Psychology 45:860–866.

Luthe, W. (ed.). 1969. Autogenic Therapy, Vols. I–VI. New York: Grune and Stratton.

Martin, M. J. 1972. Muscle-contraction headache. Psychosomatics 13:16–19.

Miller, N. E. 1975. Applications of learning and biofeedback to psychiatry and medicine. In A. M. Freedman, H. I. Kaplan, and B. J. Sadock, eds.: Comprehensive Textbook of Psychiatry—II. Baltimore, Maryland: Williams and Wilkins; pp. 28–41.

Mulholland, T. B. 1977. Biofeedback method for locating the most controlled responses of EEG alpha to visual stimulation. In J. Beatty and H. Legewie, eds.: Biofeedback and Behavior. New York: Plenum Press; pp. 115–121.

Patel, C. H., and W. R. S. North. 1975. Randomized controlled trial of yoga and biofeedback in management of hypertension. Lancet pp. 93–95.

Pearne, D. H., S. D. Zigelbaum, and W. P. Peyser. 1977. Biofeedback-assisted EMG relaxation for urinary retention and incontinence: A case report. Biofeedback and Self-Regulation 2:213–217.

Peffer, K. 1979. Equipment needs for the psychotherapist. In J. Basmajian, eds.: Biofeedback: Principles and Practice for Clinicians. Baltimore, Maryland: Williams and Wilkins; pp. 257–268.

Perry, J., and B. Whipple. 1981. Pelvic muscle strength of female ejaculators: Evidence in support of a new theory of orgasm. Journal of Sex Research 17:22–39.

Pickering, T. G., and N. E. Miller. 1977. Learned voluntary control of heart rate and rhythm in two subjects with premature ventricular contractions. British Heart Journal 39:152–159.

Raskin, M., G. Johnson, and T. J. W. Rondestved. 1973. Chronic anxiety treated by feedback-induced muscle relaxation. Archives of General Psychiatry 28:263–267.

Reeves, J. L., and W. Mealiea. 1975. Biofeedback assisted cue-controlled relaxation for the treatment of flight phobias. Journal of Behavior Therapy and Experimental Psychiatry 6:105–109.

Reeves, J. L., and D. Shapiro. 1978. Biofeedback and relaxation in essential hypertension. International Review of Applied Psychology.

Sainsbury, P., and J. F. Gibson. 1954. Symptoms of anxiety and tension and accompanying physiological changes in the muscular system. Journal of Neurology, Neurosurgery, and Psychiatry 17:216–224.

Sargent, J. D., E. E. Green, and E. D. Walters. 1972. The use of autogenic feedback training in a pilot study of migraine and tension headaches. Headache 12:120–125.

Sargent, J. D., E. D. Walters, and E. E. Green. 1973. Psychosomatic self-regulation of migraine and tension headaches. Seminars in Psychiatry 5:415–428.

Schuster, M. M. 1977. Biofeedback treatment of gastrointestinal dysfunction. Medical Clinics of North America 61:907–912.

Schwartz, G. E., D. Shapiro, and B. Tursky. 1972. Self control of patterns of human diastolic blood pressure and heart rate through feedback and reward. Psychophysiology 9:270 (abstract).

Scott, R. W., E. B. Blanchard, E. D. Edmundson, and L. D. Young. 1973. A shaping procedure for heart-rate control in chronic tacydardia. Perceptual and Motor Skills 37:327–338.

Shapiro, D., and R. W. Surwit. 1976. Learned control of physiological function and disease. In H. Leitenberg, ed.: Handbook of Behavior Modification and Behavior therapy. Englewood Cliffs, New Jersey: Prentice-Hall.

Sokolov, N. E. 1963. Perception and the Conditioned Reflex. New York: Pergamon Press.

Steger, J. 1976. Abdominal EMG Biofeedback Treatment of Ulcerative Colitis. Paper presented at the annual meeting of the Western Psychological Association, Seattle, April 1976.

Steger, J. 1978. Personality and pain ratings in biofeedback treatment. Archives of Physical Medicine and Rehabilitation 59:551.

Steger, J. C. 1982. Chronic pain management in the rehabilitation setting. In R. Berni, ed.: Rehabilitation Nursing and Patient Teaching. New York: Wiley.

Steger, J. C., and J. A. Brockway. 1980. Treatment of chronic pain in the disabled. In D. Bishop, ed.: The Management of Behavioral Problems in the Disabled. Baltimore, Maryland: Williams and Wilkins, pp. 272–301.

Steger, J., and R. Harper. 1980. comprehensive biofeedback versus self-monitored relaxation in the treatment of tension headache. Headache 20:137–142.

Sterman, M. 1973. Neurophysiologic and clinical studies of sensorimotor EEG biofeedback training: Some effects on epilepsy. Seminars in Psychiatry 5:507–525.

Sterman, M. B., L. R. Macdonald, and R. K. Stone. 1974. Biofeedback training of the sensorimotor electroencephalogram rhythm in man: Effects on epilepsy. Epilepsia 15:395–416.

Stoyva, J. M. 1977. Why should muscle relaxation be clinically useful? Some data and 2½ models. In J. Beatty and H. Legewie, eds.: Biofeedback and Behavior NATO Conference Series. New York: Plenum Press; pp. 85–94.

Surwit, R., R. Pilon, and C. Fenton. 1978. Behavioral treatment of Raynaud's disease. Journal of Behavioral Medicine 1:323–335.

Taub, E. 1977. Self-regulation of human tissue temperature. In G. Schwartz and J. Beatty, eds.: Biofeedback: Therapy and Research. New York: Academic Press; pp. 147–168.

Townsend, R. E., J. F. House, and D. Addario. 1975. A comparison of biofeedback mediated relaxation and group therapy in the treatment of chronic anxiety. American Journal of Psychiatry 32:598–601.

Tunis, M. M., and H. G. Wolff. 1954. Studies on headache: Cranial artery vasoconstriction and muscle contraction headache. Archives of General Psychology 71:425–434.

Turk, D. C., D. H. Meichenbaum, and W. H. Berman. 1979. Application of biofeedback for the regulation of pain: A critical review. Psychological Bulletin 86:1322–1338.

Tursky, B., D. Shapiro, and G. E. Schwartz. 1972. Automated constant cuff-pressure system to measure average systolic and diastolic blood pressure in man. IEEE Transactions on Biomedical Engineering 19:271–276.

Vaitl, D. 1975. Biofeedback—Einsatz in her Behandlung einer Patienten mit Sinustachykardie. In Legewie and Nusselt, eds.: Biofeedback Therapie. München, Germany: Urban and Schwarzenberg; pp. 21–25.

Weiss, T., and B. T. Engel. 1971. Operant conditioning of heart rate in patients with premature ventricular contractions. Psychosomatic medicine 33:301–321.

Weiss, T., and B. T. Engel. 1975. Evaluation of an intra-cardiac limit of learned heart rate control. Psychophysiology 12:310–312.

Wickramasekera, I. 1973. Temperature feedback for the control of migraine. Journal of Behavior Therapy and Experimental Psychiatry 4:343–345.

Wolf, S. 1981. Biofeedback Applications to Chronic Low Back Pain Patients During Dynamic Movement. Paper presented at the annual meeting of the Biofeedback Society of America, Louisville, Kentucky.

Wolpe, J. 1958. Psychotherapy by Reciprocal Inhibition. Stanford, California: Stanford University Press.

Zamani, R. 1974. Treatment of Migraine Headache: Biofeedback versus Deep Muscle Relaxation. Paper presented at the Fifth Annual Meeting of the Biofeedback Research Society, Colorado Springs, Colorado.

15

Behavioral Problems
in Pediatric Practice

Eric Trupin, Ph.D.,* Robin Beck, M.D.,† and
Peter Fehrenbach, Ph.D.‡

It comes as no surprise to primary care physicians that a recent survey of
pediatricians (American Academy of Pediatrics, 1978) indicated that the
greatest area of change in clinical practice over the past ten years was the
amount of time spent counseling patients and families. This finding is
consistent with the growing evidence that there is a dramatic increase in
the prevalence of children manifesting "clinically significant psychiatric
disorders" (Goldberg et al., 1979). Even the most rigorous epidemiological
studies that have utilized stringent diagnostic criteria have arrived at
incidence rates for serious childhood behavior disorders to be no lower
than 11.8% in the United States (Gould et al., 1981). This percentage does
not include severely disturbed or psychotic children.

The enormity of this public health problem is dramatized when one
relates those statistics to actual numbers of children. Six million children
between 5 and 19 require some form of treatment for their behavior
disorders (Goldberg et al., 1979). These children rarely receive treatment
during the early stage of difficulty. When they do, it is often at a time when
their behaviors have already seriously impacted on the systems outside
the framework of their families, thus setting in motion a complex
psychosocial dynamic that impedes the likelihood of a rapid decrease in
symptomatology and subsequent positive outcome.

*Associate Professor, Department of Psychiatry and Behavioral Sciences, University of
Washington School of Medicine, Seattle, Washington.
† Clinical Assistant Professor, Department of Family Medicine, University of Washington
School of Medicine, Seattle, Washington.
‡ Post Doctoral Fellow, Department of Psychiatry and Behavioral Sciences, University of
Washington School of Medicine, Seattle, Washington.

It has become increasingly clear that biological factors and the rate of maturation, both cognitively and physically, as well as social factors play an important role in the adaptive responses of children. For example, male children manifest a much higher incidence of behavioral problems and specific learning disorders than females. This finding is probably influenced to a major extent by differing rates of development of functions associated with cerebral lateralization as well as social factors (Townes et al., 1980). In addition, boys show much higher rates of aggression than girls in early childhood (Maccoby and Jacklin, 1974). Early problems with aggression for boys are known to be predictive of later serious psychiatric disorders and tend to be persistent personality characteristics for boys, but not for girls (Kagan and Moss, 1962). Thus social experience may reinforce or exaggerate constitutionally rooted differences.

In addition to the above-mentioned prevalence data, we can now predict that 20% of all children with a chronic medical illness will experience the persistent sequelae of behavior and learning difficulties. If we broaden our definition of psychosomatic illness to include all behavioral consequences of physical illness, the array and frequency of behavior disorders that children display in medical settings is extraordinary (Showalter, 1979). A recently published encyclopedia of pediatric psychology (Wright et al., 1979) decribes 114 medical/psychological problems that often present themselves in a primary health care setting. The problems range from asthma and arthritis to phobias and tracheotomy addiction, to name just a few.

What role does the primary care physician play in this public health crisis? The role that is essential and associated with positive treatment outcome is no different than that of providing any other form of health care—essentially, to attempt treatment strategies that are coherent, logical, efficient and which have proven to be effective and economical for patients. These interventions are predominantly derived from behavioral and social learning theories. When these strategies fail, one assumes the problem to be deeply embedded and complex and then it is time to acquire consultation (psychiatrist or psychologist) or make a referral to a mental health specialist.

The primary care physician functions as the individual who promotes mental health in order to avoid the onset of emotional disturbances by developing the capacity of children and families to deal with crises and problems prior to their onset or in their earliest and for that matter most rectifiable stage. Education, in order to enhance "wellness," is the primary principle in treating behavior disorders in children.

Numerous studies have demonstrated that differing parental styles influence a child's psychosocial adjustment. Parents who are both *permissive* and *rejecting* frequently raise aggressive children (Feshbach, 1970). *Restrictive* and *rejecting* parents tend to produce children who engage in self-aggressive behaviors and who are vulnerable to depression. Parents who set up rules and contingencies in a consistent fashion but who also display warm nurturing behavior tend to produce children with the highest rates of psychological adjustment (Baumrind, 1971). These parents are seen as *restrictive* and *warm*. This chapter will attempt to help primary care physicians to teach and promote this style in families.

Now that the enormity of the problem has been conveyed, let us define the key treatment principles and suggest some strategies we have found effective for children in primary care settings. Let us keep in mind at the outset that there is no disagreement with the notion that human behavior is the result of many complex internal and external ecologies. But there are empirically derived behavioral principles that have been demonstrated to rapidly induce a reduction in maladaptive behavior. It is necessary, however, to abide by a principle of therapeutic parsimony (Graziano, 1975). This principle basically requires that when a child presents a behavior problem, the physician attempts the simplest explanation and, further, prescribes strategies that are easily employed, monitored, and evaluated. However, it is incumbent upon the practitioner to understand and be aware of the fluid and progressive nature of child development, both physically and cognitively. Knowledge of the child's developmental tasks always allows for more precise prescriptions and enhances one's skill in primary prevention with families.

The information to follow should allow the reader to do the following:

1. Understand basic behavioral principles as they apply to children in a primary care setting.
2. Develop an appropriate treatment strategy for a variety of common pediatric problems and be able to evaluate its effectiveness.

Behavior Change Strategies

The Experimental Analysis of Behavior

For the busy practicing primary care physician to adopt an intervention for behavioral problems, the intervention must be efficiently prescribed and must provide the best chance for successful outcome. The approach to behavioral problems described below meets both of these requirements.

The tenets of this approach are derived from the following behavioral rules:

1. All behavior has consequences.
2. All high-rate behavior is frequently reinforced.

Certainly these rules are simplifications, but they are easily remembered and lead to the formulation of potentially useful interventions, no matter what the characterizations of a specific behavior problem.

This treatment approach to behavioral problems is empirical—something must be measured, usually the behavior to be changed. This is so fundamental that it deserves elaboration. The application of behavioral tactics in any setting is an experiment, just as arriving at a medical diagnosis is a form of hypothesis testing. The relations or principles are well defined. However, in applying these principles in the clinical setting, the practitioner will be working with a unique individual in a unique environment and discovering which of many possible consequences result in desired behavioral change. Generalizing successful applications from one setting to another is appropriate for the practitioner as well as the patient. If previously successful strategies do not work, the experiment has revealed something unique about the subject or the environment. These are the most challenging situations that may tax the imagination of the practitioner, parent, or child. Understanding behavioral principles and applying them in practice is not likely to be static or dull.

Measuring behavior in a quantitative way is basic to successful intervention for the behavioral scientist and the practitioner. The easiest thing to measure about a behavior is how frequently it occurs. There are many variations of this fundamental measurement. However, one very important point should be made: The majority of all behaviors that present in the physician's office labeled as problems by a parent or teacher are problems of behavioral frequency. In fact, the frequency of the behavior, rather than the behavior itself, is often the clinical problem. This resolves many issues for the parent and physician, who does not have to label behavior as "good" or "bad." In other words, it is all right to have a temper tantrum, but one five times daily may result in consternation for an otherwise sympathetic parent. An experimental analysis of behavior only gives us the tactics to apply in an attempt to change the frequency of a behavior.

Basic Tactics to Change Behavior

Up to this point, behavior has been discussed from an experimental approach. Problem or deviant behavior is behavior that is occurring at an unacceptably high frequency and determined by its consequences. In this section, behavioral tactics basic to intervention in any environment will be introduced. There are two general classes of tactics applied in the clinical setting: tactics to increase the frequency of desired behaviors and tactics to decrease the frequency of unacceptable behavior.

Discriminated Attention to Behavior. Attention to behavior may take many forms, from smiling and words of approval to anger and disapproval in both expression and tone of voice. Both may be consequences that increase the behavior they follow (we would like to think that children and other adults want approval; unfortunately, this is not always so). The important point about attending is which behavior to attend to. This leads to the tactic that is discriminated attention to "good" behavior. The word *good* has been added here to emphasize the fact that while children (and adults) display lots of behaviors, some of these behaviors can be lived with (e.g., quiet independent play, reading, helping with chores, etc.) and some of them cannot be lived with (e.g., tantrums, fighting, physical abusiveness toward parent or peer, etc.). Most parents would like to increase the frequency of the former and reduce the latter; thus *good* is defined. Since children generally will work for parental attention, behaviors followed by parental attention will increase in frequency. Discriminated attention to "good" behavior is the most powerful way to change behavior in a desired way. It forms the basis of successful intervention for behavioral problems, no matter what other behavioral tactics are applied.

Discriminated attention is also an important developmental tactic. Parental attention to the newborn infant can be characterized as nondiscriminatory and given on a continuous schedule. These parental behaviors may be inappropriate for the infant during the second 6 months of life(see Case 1). While the definition of discriminated attention may seem obvious, it is best to demonstrate or model attending behavior for a parent, for example, a smile, a nod, positive physical contact such as touches or hugs, words of approval or praise for the work or activity of another, and so on.

Contingencies, Reinforcers, or Bribery. The most common form statements take when contingencies are applied is the "if ... then" statement. For example, a parent may say to a child at bedtime, "If you brush your teeth and get your pajamas on, I will read to you for half an hour." This statement is quite clear in specifying what is desired of the child and what the consequences will be. Noncompliance by the child means going immediately to bed. Often contingencies of the following type are heard: "If you don't sit still, I will spank you." Subsequent observation reveals that the child does not still and may or may not be spanked. This parent might complain that the child "doesn't listen," for most parents do not follow through with these contingencies or threats and are poor punishers. For words to have meaning, they must relate in a direct way to what happens in the environment. "Listening" by the child is merely having the relation between behavior and consequences clearly specified and consequences that are effective in producing the desired behavior.

Parents may object to using contingencies or bribery. This is usually expressed as a wish for some internal state within the child that results in "good" behavior. Usually it is expressed as a question: "Why isn't this child 'motivated' or 'responsible'?" These parents are using contingencies. They just have not overtly specified them for the child or have made the consequences too obscure or too remote in time to directly affect behavior. In responding to these objections, it is helpful to point out contingencies that all societies apply to their members, for example, "If you break the law, you will go to jail." Every day individuals operate under many different and sometimes conflicting contingencies. They generally fall into two classes, those that promise positive consequences and those that threaten negative or aversive consequences. As a general rule, those that are more positive, that is, promise a reward (something worth working for), are more successful in maintaining changeworthy behavior.

TACTICS USED TO DECREASE THE FREQUENCY OF BEHAVIOR

The following sections deal with tactics that help reduce the frequency of behaviors. They are forms of punishment. Many parents equate punishment with physically negative consequences, for example, slapping or spanking. These consequences can change behavior, but to be effective, they must immediately relate to a specific behavior and they must be unusual, unique, or painful. In other words, physical negatives, to be effective for the child, must stand in sharp contrast to the usual interaction with the parent. Is there a place for physically negative or painful consequences in raising children? When a parent is truly frightened for the well-being of a child, they may use physical punishment effectively. An example might be when a toddler walks over to the wall socket with a screwdriver or runs into a busy street. While both situations might have been prevented, if they occur, they are life-threatening. Physical punishment administered in this situation can certainly stop the behavior if it is in sharp contrast to the parent attending to other more acceptable behavior at a high rate. However, if parental attention only occurs when the toddler approaches the wall socket or runs into the street, punished or not, these behaviors may remain at an unacceptably high rate, with tragic consequences. Alternatives to physical punishment that have proven more effective in reducing the frequency of behavior are as follows.

Not Attending or Ignoring Behavior. Since children will, as a rule, work for parental or other adult attention, not attending to specific behaviors should result in a decrease in their frequency. The application of this tactic occurs frequently on a daily basis as the complement of discriminated attention to "good" behavior. Problem behaviors, by definition, occur at an unacceptably high rate; that is, they have already been reinforced. Depending on the setting—home, nursery, or classroom—it may or may not be possible to apply this tactic, particularly if there are others, such as peers, who are attending to the problem behavior as well. The tactic of not attending or ignoring behavior has very limited applications as an intervention for deviant behavior. During the preschool years, it has been useful in managing high-rate crying or persistent nighttime awakening during the second 6 months of life, and crying or whining in the younger preschooler if these behaviors are labeled as problems by parents.

Timeout. Timeout is the physical removal of a child from the setting in which reinforcers are available. It is a form of punishment. Like all punishment, by itself, timeout only results in a decrease in deviant behaviors for which it is the consequence. In combination with an environment rich in discriminated attention to other behavior, timeout is a very powerful and effective intervention. This combination of interventions in the home or school is so commonly applied that in the remainder of this chapter discriminated attention/timeout will be abbreviated DA/TO. Placing the emphasis on discriminated attention to good behavior emphasizes the most important variable for successful application of these tactics. Since the advent of an experimental analysis of behavior, timeout has been studied extensively and applied in many settings (Patterson, 1971). The following are the criteria that need to be met for its successful application:

1. The behaviors leading to placement in TO need to be clearly identified by parent and child.
2. The consequences need to be clearly stated for the child and carried out by the parent.
3. The parent utilizes TO in an unemotional, nonpunitive manner.
4. Time spent in TO is less important than setting a criterion to end TO.
5. TO is controlled by the parent, not the child.
6. TO works best in environments where discriminated attention to "good" behavior is occurring at a high rate.

The room chosen for timeout and its stimulus properties have not been critical to successful application of this tactic in the home. The child's room works well as a TO room, provided that the door can be closed and locked if necessary. The behaviors that will result in TO are identified, for example, peer aggression, tantrums, etc. When they occur, the parent may say, "I have asked you not to do that. You are going to your room until you have been quiet for five minutes." The child is accompanied to the room by the parent, the door closed and controlled or locked with a slide bolt if necessary. No matter what the child does in the room, the door is not opened until the 5-minute criterion is met.

In the above example, the statement governing the application of TO is quite clear. The behavioral consequences, once applied, will be effective even if the child does not understand the words, as will be seen in the case studies described below.

Applying behavioral tactics in the home with parents as the agents of intervention and the data collectors has been well described and widely practiced (Graziano, 1975). Often home-based intervention replicates an experimental design where behavioral frequency is measured during a baseline period, during an intervention phase, followed by multiple replications of these two conditions, that is, ABAB . . . . This design has the attributes of using the individual child as his or her own control and allowing repeated evaluation of the intervention. This study design is important for the experimenter studying the effect of specific interventions on target behavior tactics; it may or may not be appropriate in day to day practice. The practitioner is less concerned about convincing an independent and skeptical audience than about the effectiveness of a specific tactic. However, he or she is just as concerned as the experimenter about measuring the outcome of intervention, so that in practice an AB design is frequently used, that is, where no reversal occurs or, as in some instances described below, only the intervention phase is employed.

Two cases are presented in which similar behavioral problems were managed in 4-year-old boys. The first case models the best of the applied behavior studies reported in the literature (Zeilberger et al., 1968). In the second case, intervention occurred in a busy medical practice with fewer resources.

CASE 1

A 4-year-old boy was enrolled in a study to help modify screaming, fighting, disobeying, and bossing behaviors occurring at home. During observation in the home, the mother's behavior was noted to be inconsistent when the problem behaviors occurred, and often she reinforced these behaviors with excessive attention. Experimental sessions were held for 1 hour daily. One or more observers independently kept data on three behavior categories for the child—physical aggression, yelling, and bossing—and any intervention given to the child by his mother at 20-second intervals. The mother's behavior was recorded with regard to verbal and physical contact with her son at 20-second intervals. A   baseline period extended for ten sessions, followed by an experimental period, a return to base line, and a final experimental period. In the experimental periods, the mother was given the following instructions:

1. After your son acts aggressively or disobediently, take him to the TO room (a bedroom with no toys or other items to interest children).
2. As he is taken to the TO room say, "You cannot stay here if you fight," or "You cannot stay here if you do not do what you are told." Make no other comments.

3. Place him in the TO room quickly with no conversation. Shut and hook the door.
4. He must be quiet for 2 minutes before he can come out of TO.
5. When it is time to come out, take him back to his regular activities without comment.
6. No long explanations are to be given about the TO program. A short explanation may be given later, if you desire to do so, at a time when the undesirable behaviors have not occurred.
7. Ignore undesirable behavior not specified for TO. Do not attend to them by looking suddenly or making comments.
8. Ignore undesirable behavior that you learn about in retrospect.
9. Reinforce desirable cooperative play frequently without interrupting it.
10. Always reward cooperation.
11. Treats may be given for a period of desirable behavior.
12. Continue the program outside of observation sessions.

The results of the intervention for each problem behavior observed during the different conditions were recorded by the observers. The data on aggressive behavior are shown in Fig. 1. The percentage of intervals was calculated by dividing the number of 20-second intervals scored for aggressive behavior by the total number of 20-second intervals of observation. This data is plotted through baseline and subsequent conditions. These data are typical of the ABAB design, using the individual child as the control and from which the experimenter and independent reader can make judgments as to the effectiveness of the intervention. In the case of aggressive behavior, both experimenter and parent agreed that the reductions produced during the experimental conditions when DA/TO was in force were significant and desirable.

CASE 2

A mother and her 4-year-old son were referred to the clinic by Children's Protective Services (CPS) workers after the father had beaten his son severely for the second time. The father had admitted himself to the psychiatric ward of a local hospital. In the examining room, the child had torn the instruments off the wall, emptied drawers, flooded the sink, bitten his mother, thrown an object at his mother, and broken her glasses. She asked, "What can I do?"

Further history revealed that the mother was a retired airline attendant and the father a musician. The marriage was precipitated by her pregnancy and had been stressful to both parents financially and emotionally. They lived in a small studio apartment. No relatives lived nearby. They had one neighbor couple with whom they were close and who had a son the same age. The mother spent all day with her son. Because of physical aggressiveness by her son, the neighbors no longer let the boys play together. The mother could not go to the store or to restaurants because of his behavior.

When asked what behaviors she liked in her son, she was unable to specify any. When asked what she did not like, she immediately listed tantrums,

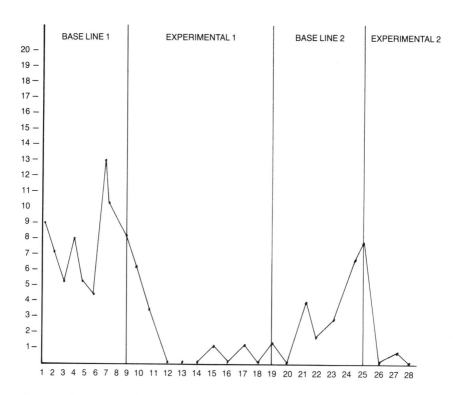

Figure 1. Percentage of intervals scored for aggressive behavior.

hitting and biting her and the neighbor's child, and not listening or doing as told. Also, she added that it took her 2 hours to get him to bed at night. When asked to describe what she did when the above problem behaviors occur, she described her usual response as sitting down with her son to explain why such behavior is bad. When very angry, she spanked him. She readily agreed to cooperate with the following program.

1. The importance of her attention in maintaining behavior was explained. She was told about the importance of attending to "good" behavior. Words, phrases, and physically positive gestures (touches, hugs) were modeled in the examination room. Over the next week she was asked to observe her son and record the behaviors she liked and can attend to.
2. TO was described and to be implemented for tantrums, hitting and biting, and disobeying. TO was to occur swiftly and on every incidence of the above behaviors. After the behavior occurred, she was to say, "I am sorry; I asked you not to do that. You are going to your room until you have been quiet for 5 minutes." Similarly, for disobeying, "I asked

you to _____; because you disobeyed you are going to your room . . . ."
She was to get a slide bolt for the door so it could be controlled. When
TO was over, the door was to be opened and she and her son return to
activities in progress. She was told to increase the activities he enjoyed
doing with her so that there is sharp contrast between being in TO and
being out. She was asked to record the total time in TO for each day.
3. Contingencies were described and the verbal behavior modeled. A
   bedtime contingency was described: "It is time for bed. If you brush
   your teeth and get your pajamas on, I will read to you for half an hour."
   Also, "It is bedtime now, you may get up once to use the bathroom. If
   you get up again, I will close the door." Other contingencies and how
   they are used were described and modeled. Emphasis was placed on
   keeping her son successful in meeting the contingencies and on trying
   to use contingencies that provide reinforcers rather than avoid
   punishment.

The above interactions were written specifically for the mother and her son.
Explanation of the tactics and how they are implemented and modeling the
verbal behavior were provided with both parent and child present. The
written instructions were sent home with the parent, with an example of how
to record the total time in TO each day. Any questions that arose at home
were answered by phone follow-ups daily. The mother was to return to the
clinic in 1 week.

The data collected by this parent are presented in Fig. 2. The mother
reported that after the third day none of the target negative behaviors
occurred. She spoke in an animated fashion about many of her son's
acceptable behaviors. The neighbor's son was now coming over frequently to
play with her son. She never missed reading to him at bedtime. Observations
in the exam room were useful. At the first visit, physical contact between
mother and son was limited to physically negative interactions and no social
positives. On follow-up, there were frequent touches, smiles, nods, and verbal
positives. Over the subsequent 2 months, TO was used on one occasion for 15
minutes following a tantrum. Following the father's discharge from the

Figure 2. Total timeout recorded in Case 2.

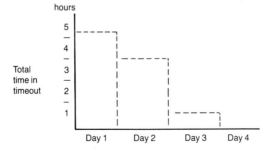

hospital, both parents returned to the clinic and were pleased with their son's behavior. The tactics were being applied when necessary and the parents had independently managed a new problem behavior successfully. The mother and son were seen subsequent to the parents' divorce, which occurred within a year of the initial visit. Although separation was a stressful event, neither parent identified specific behavioral problems in their son as related to the separation. Further follow-up of mother and son was lost when she moved closer to her parents and other relatives.

These two examples of the use of DA/TO (plus contingencies in the latter case) demonstrate many important differences in an applied behavioral study and the clinical practice of medicine. The former is characterized by much more comprehension and reliable data collection, a large time investment on the part of the experimenter, and, while intensive, a brief involvement with the family over a period of weeks. This contact is initiated by and limited to the resolution of the behavioral problems.

In the clinical practice of medicine, the implementation of DA/TO involved minimal physician (experimenter) time, less than 1 hour for the initial visit. The data collected were less comprehensive but allowed the physician and parent to document success or failure of the intervention. Baseline information must often be reconstructed from verbal reports from the parent: for example, "What behaviors do you like?" "What behaviors don't you like?" To understand what consequences are maintaining the problem behavior, the physician must ask, "What do you do when your child has a tantrum?" These questions have been extremely useful in reconstructing the "baseline" data. Observation of the effectiveness of the parents' verbal commands in the examining room is also useful. In Case 2 above, the mother's "words" had no effect on the child's behavior; the implication being that, at least in the recent reinforcement history of this child, the mother's words were not related in a meaningful way to what happened to the child. Other baseline information is available to the careful observer. Perhaps the most powerful learning tactic applied by any organism is imitation. Often the child who emits physically aggressive behavior, for example, hitting and slapping, is imitating parental behavior. One can ask, "If physical punishment is used in the home, what kind is it and how often does it occur?"

Verbal behavior also gives information about past learning experiences. There is nothing intrinsically troublesome or negativistic about the 2-year-old, for example. However, when the 2-year-old in the exam room says, "No!" "Don't!" or "Stop that!" at every opportunity, one can guess that the freedom provided by competent ambulation is providing an environment rich in those verbalizations from parents or older siblings.

Finally, the physician's contact with families is periodic over many years and based on providing medical care for health maintenance and acute illnesses, as well as for behavioral problems. As a resource to a family, the physician's role is not only to intervene when possible but, if intervention fails, to find an appropriate referral resource for the family. Identification of the family who will require referral for behavioral problems is a problem in practice. The case managed in practice and described above is an example of successful intervention; that is, total time in TO fell rapidly and TO was not applied after 3 days. This pattern is so typical of the successful application of DA/TO that the need for reassessment and/or referral can be easily identified:

1. Total time in TO remaining at a high level beyond 3 days.
2. Failure to record data.

Both of these criteria can be easily documented and lead to appropriate referral or altered intervention. Experience teaches that in the above situation, for whatever reasons, parents are not providing discriminated attention to acceptable behavior; that is, the rapid falloff in total time in TO is probably less a measurement of the "success" of TO than one of the effectiveness of DA to acceptable behavior.

Discriminated attention can be applied at any age and in any setting; TO is limited mostly to the preschool years and only rarely applied in the form described above beyond that time. How early can TO be used in conjunction with DA? To answer this question another case will be presented from practice.

CASE 3

A young scientist brought her daughter, now 12 months old, into the office with the complaint that she had starting having tantrums. At the slightest frustration, she would throw herself to the floor (she had begun walking at 8 months of age), arch her back, scream, kick, and become inconsolable. This began to occur approximately 3 weeks prior to the office visit and was then occurring two or three times daily during the few hours the mother and daughter spent with each other.

Both parents worked; a live-in housekeeper cared for this child and their 4-year-old son during the day. The mother was very attentive to her daughter. Many social and physical positives occurred in the exam room. She was concerned that her attempts to console or ignore her daughter during tantrums had no effect. She specified many of her daughter's behaviors that she liked. She was distraught that the limited time they spent together was always disrupted by tantrums.

The mother was experienced in managing behavioral problems and data collection with her 4-year-old. Briefly DA/TO was reviewed with her, modeled, and written instructions were given.

The following data were reported by phone in 3 days following the office visit. The data were gathered over 3 hours on each of the 3 successive days (see Fig. 3). No tantrums occurred on day 3. This is the youngest child in which a combination of DA and TO has been applied in our practice.

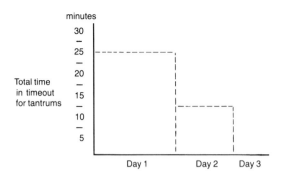

Figure 3. Total timeout recorded in Case 3.

The following case represents an example of intervention by a practitioner who utilized all of the tactics introduced above and a special variation on the use of discriminated attention.

CASE 4

A mother and her 2½-year-old daughter came to the clinic with the complaint that the daughter awakened from sleep and cried until she was given a glass of water. This occurred every night and often twice nightly between 2:00 and 4:00 A.M. The father is a painter who contracted to paint television transmitter towers and other hazardous jobs in various cities throughout the United States. The family spent approximately 6 months each year living in motel or hotel rooms. The mother stayed with her daughter all day. The nighttime awakening was disturbing her husband's rest and had become a major problem.

On questioning, the mother stated that when her daughter awakened at night and cried, she got up immediately, held her, and gave her a glass of water. Further questioning revealed that the daughter had two to three tantrums daily and bedtime was a protracted process in the evening that was usually disruptive for both parents. When asked what her daughter did that she liked, the mother listed many things, including playing quietly, drawing or coloring, helping with daily activities, and so on. The mother added spontaneously that her problem with these activities was that while the daughter would color or draw for a few minutes, she would then start throwing crayons or toys. The mother's response was to go over, pick the objects up, and help her daughter begin a new task. This occurred so frequently that the mother had almost no free time during the day to get anything else done. Intervention prescribed in this case included the following:

1. Tantrums. DA/TO as described in the previous cases. The total time in TO each day was to be recorded.
2. Nighttime awakening and crying. The mother was to enlist the support

of her husband for the following week. When her daughter awakened and cried, they were not to enter her room. Alternatively, they were to record the total crying time each night and report the results by phone at the end of the week.
3. Task change. The mother was to observe her daughter's play during the day. For 1 hour she was to record the total play time on each task before her daughter threw objects, had a tantrum, or merely changed activities. Tantrums were to result in TO. From this information she was to decide how long to let her daughter remain on a task before joining her in the activity *before* she emited the objectionable behavior. While playing with her daughter, she was to use verbal praises and introduce a new task or activity and then withdraw. Over the week she was permitted to increase the intervals of independent play before intervention but was to avoid extending them to the point where objectionable behaviors recur.

The total crying time at night dropped from 30 to 10 minutes and did not occur after the second night. The mother's verbalization of this experience was that it seemed that her daughter was "relieved" not to have to awaken and cry at night. Tantrums were no longer occurring at the former high rate, and the total time in TO data was similar to that reported in Case 3. Before ending the phone conversation, the mother also reported that she had kept data on the total time that she spent either interacting with her daughter or cleaning up from previous activities before and subsequent to the intervention prescribed as in item (3) above. She reported that she kept this data throughout the week, recording the total time spent directly with her daughter or on related tasks (cleaning up) for the same 1-hour period each day. Her total time spent dropped from 50 minutes per hour before intervention to less than 10 minutes per hour at the end of the week, and objectionable behaviors such as breaking crayons or throwing objects were no longer occurring.

No longer attending to nighttime crying resulted in a rather dramatic and rapid decrease in the frequency of the behavior. When nighttime crying is operant (high rate and determined by its consequences), the termination of attention will almost always result in the disappearance of the behavior in two nights. It is usually safe to assume that nighttime crying is operant during the second 6 months of life. It is during this time that parents need to think about attention and its consequences on behavior. Persistence of operant nighttime crying beyond the first year of life is not an uncommon problem with the first child or in special situations such as the family described above, where the mother maintained the behavior inadvertently while attempting to avoid disturbance of her husband's sleep.

The variation of discriminated attention introduced in this case in item (3) above is a well-described tactic. The objectives were clearly to intervene before the objectionable behavior occurred and to increase independent playtime or "attention span" by slowly increasing the interval before the mother intervened with social positives and task change. While the physician could not think of an easy way to document the consequences of this intervention, the mother did! The mother in this case had not only intervened successfully and kept data using DA/TO, but had generalized those skills to another problem in which she had been given only basic directions on the use of a "differential schedule of reinforcement."

Adolescents

Just as with younger children, a number of behavioral techniques are available to the physician for use with older children and adolescents. In this section, the behavioral management of pediatric problems with older children will be illustrated with case examples. These cases have been selected to illustrate variations on already described techniques. While in each case the procedures used were effective with the particular problem, the case studies have been chosen because they demonstrate behavioral intervention strategies that are potentially useful with a variety of problems.

The basic principle of behavior change with adolescents remains that behaviors are believed to be developed and maintained by their consequences. Behaviors tend to occur with more frequency when followed by a reward or reinforcer. In evaluating a behavioral problem in pediatric practice with adolescents, it is often helpful to first determine what possible reinforcers are being obtained or given as a consequence of engaging in the problem behavior. In a number of cases, the simple elimination of the reinforcement may result in a decrease in the problem behavior. Extinction, when used in conjunction with positive reinforcement of other more acceptable behaviors, has been shown to be an effective aid to the pediatrician dealing with behavioral problems. A simple case example of the use of extinction of inappropriate behavior and positive reinforcement of more desirable behavior is illustrated in the following case example.

CASE 5

Brian was a 15-year-old boy with a history of mild asthma. His asthma seemed to have a relatively high allergic component and he never had required treatment with steroids. However, one day while playing softball, he had an asthmatic attack that was more serious than average. He was able to control the attack with the usual methods, including the use of a bronchodilator. In the weeks following this particular attack, Brian began to focus more on his own breathing, complaining of shortages of breath. A pulmonary function examination by his physician revealed no physiological basis for the complaints. Further interviews with Brian and his parents revealed that Brian was receiving considerable attention and sympathy whenever he made a complaint about his diminished breathing ability. Furthermore, Brian's asthma and current complaints had become the focus of a great deal of the regular family conversation and the basis for much of the parents' interactions with him, to the exclusion of other more appropriate topics and issues. It was therefore recommended that the parents begin to ignore Brian's complaints, except when it was clear that he was in real respiratory distress. In addition, the parents were encouraged to give considerable attention to, and to show more interest in, other things that Brian might talk about (e.g., school activities, sports). While Brian's initial reaction to the parents' change in behavior was to escalate his complaints, within a few days the frequency of complaints of shortages of breath diminished and more acceptable verbal behavior increased.

Children are known to experience a variety of fears, most of which are transient and resolve spontaneously. However, a significant number of children develop fears that can persist even into adulthood. The physician is likely to encounter significant instances of fear in the course of clinical practice that can have a direct impact on the efficiency and utilization of medical procedure themselves, for example, extreme fear of injections, blood drawings, and so on. The pediatrician is also likely to be asked for help in dealing with the fears of children and adolescents that are causing considerable disruption in the lives of the patient and his or her family. The following case study is an example of how the pediatrician can advise and work with the parents in the process of reducing a significant fear in an adolescent boy. The procedures are based on self-control procedures described by Graziano (1975).

CASE 6

John was a 12-year-old boy with normal intellectual development who had for at least 3 years experienced nighttime fears. The problem had begun around the time of the parents' divorce, at which time John became increasingly reluctant to go to bed, expressed a fear of the dark, and insisted that lights and a radio be left on, and repeatedly awakened the mother and two older teenage siblings during the night. Initially, the problem was dealt with by the mother's reassuring the child that there was nothing to fear and generally attempting to comfort him when upset. However, after some time her patience became severely strained and her approach to the problem was to be more punitive, but with no decrease in frequency of attention. The older siblings also became critical of the "babyishness" of their younger brother. Yet the problem persisted with varying degrees of severity for several years, causing significant family distress until a new approach was taken.

The intervention selected was based on the rationale that fear behaviors are learned and can be maintained by reinforcing social consequences, and that nighttime fears escalate from the initial cue of being told to go to bed through a series of self-stimulating cognitions that tend to increase the child's arousal. For example, children will self-stimulate by evading vivid frightening images and misconceptions and by repeating a variety of fear-related statements to themselves. The attention the child receives during the night inadvertently reinforces these cognitive and associated fear behaviors. The plan of the intervention was to interrupt this escalating pattern early in the sequence and to reinforce more adaptive coping behaviors on the part of John.

With the exception of the first session, the treatment was carried out in the home by the mother. The first sessions involved the pediatrician instructing John in three ways he could make himself not be afraid of the dark. These included relaxation (lying down and relaxing), pleasant visual imagery (selecting and imaging some pleasant activity or event), and self-talk that emphasized being brave (saying things like, "I am brave. I can handle being in the dark."). John was told that these exercises, which were to be practiced with his mother, were to help him overcome the teasing of his older siblings. The mother was instructed to lead John in these exercises every night at a specified time just before bedtime. She was also given instructions in how to implement a reward system for both successful practice and the successful completion of five consecutive nights without disruption or resistance to going to bed with the lights out. The rewards were in the form of points, with the accumulation of a specified number of points resulting in a highly desirable activity—being allowed to ask and take a friend to a professional baseball game.

With the aid of the intervention, rapid improvements in the fear behavior was reported by the mother. John was able to have five consecutive fearless nights within the first week of the onset of the program. Follow-up evaluation suggested that the previously highly disruptive and frustrating problem had been greatly reduced.

Despite tremendous advances in our knowledge of a variety of diseases and technical advances in their treatment, patient compliance with prescribed treatment regimes remains a major problem. Noncompliance can be especially problematic in teenagers with insulin-dependent diabetes mellitus, both because a great deal of the treatment ignores self-management and because good compliance is necessary for reasonable disease control. The following case illustrates how behavioral methods can be used to increase patient compliance.

CASE 7

Jennifer was a 13-year-old girl who was first hospitalized and diagnosed as having juvenile onset diabetes mellitus when she was 10 years old. Immediately after the original diagnosis was made, she was reported to have engaged in a variety of "acting out" behaviors on the hospital ward. However, within a brief period of time, she came to accept the diagnosis and soon took over the major responsibilities of the self-management, including urine and blood testing, injections of insulin, and adherence to the recommended diet. She reportedly did reasonably well until age 13, when she was hospitalized for acute ketoacidosis. While in the hospital, she admitted to her family and pediatrician that she had not taken her insulin for 2 days prior to the admission. Her only explanation at the time was that she was "tired of taking the shots." Subsequent assessment revealed that both Jennifer and her parents had an excellent understanding of the disease process and the rationale for the particular treatment regimen she was supposed to follow.

However, Jennifer acknowledged considerable feelings of anger toward her father, although she denied that these feelings were in any way related to her parents' current separation and divorce plans, or to the noncompliance. Jennifer was discharged from the hospital with a referral to a child psychiatrist, but the family did not follow up on this recommendation.

Three months later, Jennifer was readmitted to hospital by her pediatrician for acute diabetes ketoacidosis. During the admission it again became clear that Jennifer had not been consistently following her diet, had lied about test results, and had on occasion not taken her insulin injections. After she was medically stabilized, a meeting was held with Jennifer, her mother (with whom she was living), her pediatrician, and a consulting psychologist. All parties present agreed, including Jennifer, that her noncompliance was a serious problem and that a referral for family counseling would definitely need to be followed this time. However, until such time that Jennifer could be trusted to reassume primary responsibility for her own tests and injections, a mechanism for ensuring compliance on an outpatient basis would be necessary. A behavioral contract was negotiated between Jennifer and her parents and witnessed by her pediatrician. A behavioral contract stipulates those behaviors required of both parties and specifies the consequence for successfully completing or failing to complete the required behavior. Jennifer and her mother agreed to follow the contract. Jennifer was to show each of her morning Chemstrip results to her mother for inspection. If the results of the test were below specified limits, both injections that day were to be given in the mother's presence. If after 2 months there were no further hospitalizations, the contract was to be renegotiated and possibly eliminated.

This contract had built into it a powerful reinforcer for this 13-year-old girl—the privilege of giving herself her own injections privately rather than in what she considered the embarrassing position of being visually monitored by her mother. On the other hand, it ensured that if an injection was skipped, it would most likely be picked up on the blood glucose test and appropriate action could be taken to bring her back under control.

The contract appeared to be successful in its goal of keeping Jennifer in compliance and was dropped after 2 months of good control. After 6 months, Jennifer had not been rehospitalized and had regained 15 pounds lost in the previous 6 months. Brief family therapy had been completed, and the crisis surrounding the parents' divorce had been for the most part resolved. In addition, a number of issues typical of early adolescence were dealt with and were seen as contributing to the noncompliance (e.g., anger with parents, rebelliousness, increased sensitivity about body image and being different). The behavioral contract allowed these issues to be worked on in counseling, while giving the pediatrician the assurance that her insulin injections would continue to be given.

It is our hope that the procedures described in these case studies will provide the practitioner with the impetus to attempt similar interventions with patients and generalize these approaches with a wide range of childhood behavior problems.

References

American Academy of Pediatrics. 1978. Pediatric practice patterns. Pediatrics 62:627–665.

Baumrind, A. 1971. Current patterns of parental authority. Developmental Psychology Monographs 1:1–103.

Feshback, S. 1970. Aggression. In P. H. Mussen, ed.: Carmichael's Manual of Child Psychology, Vol. 2. New York: Wiley.

Goldberg, I. D., D. A. Regier, T. K. McInerny, I. B. Pless, and K. J. Roghmann. 1979. The role of the pediatrician in the delivery of mental health services to children. Pediatrics 63:898–909.

Gould-Schwartz, M., R. Hitzig-Wunsch, and B. Dohrenwend. 1981. Estimating the prevalence of childhood psychopathology. Journal of Child Psychiatry 20:462–476.

Graziano, A. M. 1975. Behavior Therapy with Children II. Chicago, Illinois: Aldine.

Kagan, J., and H. A. Moss. 1962. Birth to Maturity. New York: Wiley.

Maccoby, E. E., and C. N. Jacklin. 1974. The Psychology of Sex Differences. Stanford, California: Stanford University Press.

Patterson, G. R. 1971. Families: Applications of Social Learning Theory to Family Life. Champaign, Illinois: Research Press.

Schowalter, J. F. 1979. The chronically ill child. In J. D. Noshpitz, ed.: Basic Handbook of Child Psychiatry, Vol. 1. New York: Basic Books; pp. 432–436.

Townes, B., E. Trupin, D. C. Martin, and D. Goldstein. 1980. Neuropsychological correlates of academic success among elementary school children. Journal of Consulting and Clinical Psychology 48:675–684.

Wright, L., A. Schaefer, and G. Solomons. 1979. Encyclopedia of Pediatric Psychology. Baltimore, Maryland: University Park Press.

Zeilberger, J., S. E. Samsen, and H. N. Sloane. 1968. Modification of a child's problem behaviors in the home with the mother as therapist. Journal of Applied Behavioral Analysis 1:47.

16

Chronic Pain

John D. Loeser, M.D.* and Wilbert E. Fordyce, Ph.D.†

The management of patients with chronic disease is becoming an increasing part of the physician's task; a major portion of these patients suffer from chronic pain. The cost to society, in medical bills, compensation payments, and loss of productivity, is staggering. The numbers seem to grow each year. Indeed, we may be living in an epidemic of chronic pain. Pain clinics are springing up throughout the industrialized Western nations, whereas there were only a dozen of them a decade ago. A brief review of American health care in the 1980s leads one to the conclusion that physicians do a good job alleviating acute pain but often utilize therapeutic strategies that perpetuate chronic pain. One may reason that persistence of pain into chronicity is a rough index of limitations in the health care system and its attendant concepts and methods. The prevalence of chronic pain suggests that acute and chronic pain may have very different anatomical, physiological, and psychological substrates. However, most American patients and their physicians labor under the delusion that all pains are due to some form of tissue pathology and that therapeutic success will occur only if the source of the pain is identified and excised.

This model for pain is derived from the concepts of René Descartes, who was the foremost philosopher of the French Enlightenment. Descartes divided human existence into "mind" and "body." For him, pain was a reflex response to a physical stimulus, predictable and explicable if the stimulus was known. For us, it is apparent that the physical characteristics

---

*Professor, Department of Neurological Surgery, University of Washington School of Medicine, Seattle, Washington.

† Professor, Department of Rehabilitation Medicine, University of Washington School of Medicine, Seattle, Washington.

of the pain stimulus are often indeterminate. Just what is the etiology of chronic low back pain? Is there any noxious stimulus? Even when the stimulus is more apparent, as in acute pain, the stimulus alone does not reliably predict the individual's response. If you do not consider the model one has for an illness important, consider how you would treat a patient using St. Augustine's concept: "All diseases of Christians are due to demons."

The Cartesian model makes pain the response to a physical stimulus. This concept ignores the range of responses to a stimulus and cannot even begin to explain those pains not related to tissue damage.

A more serviceable model can be built around four concepts: nociception, pain, suffering, and pain behavior (Fig. 1).

Nociception is defined as the detection of potentially tissue-damaging thermal or mechanical energy by specialized nerve endings connected to Aδ and C fiber afferents. A wide variety of anatomical and physiological studies have conclusively shown that nociception is a specific peripheral sensory system. It is not due to excessive or abnormal patterned activation of larger afferent fibers involved in light touch or proprioception.

In the intact animal, nociception usually leads to *pain*, which is defined as a perceived noxious input to the nervous system. The linkage between nociception and pain can be interrupted by surgical, pharmacological, or psychological means, emphasizing that nociception is a peripheral event; pain is a feature of the spinal cord and brain. Not only is there nociception in the absence of pain, but there is clearly pain without nociception.

Figure 1. Pain model. From J.D. Loeser *in* M. Stanton-Hicks and R.A. Boas, editors: Low Back Pain. New York: Raven Press. Copyright 1980.

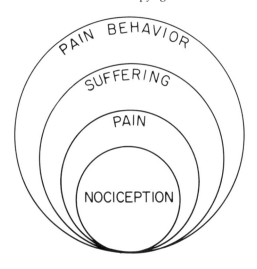

Consider the long list of pain states associated with injuries to the central or peripheral nervous system, often called "central pain states" (Table 1).

Every one of these diseases is characterized by chronic pain in the absence of any evidence for ongoing nociceptive activity. Indeed, in phantom limb pain not only is there no evidence for tissue damage where the pain is perceived, but the painful body part is itself absent. A meaningful concept of pain must include an explanation for those types of pain unrelated to noxious stimulation. The absence of such a concept leads to absurd surgical and pharmacological therapies, based more upon social convention than scientific realities. For example, if you have the pain of tic douloureux in your nose, no one advocates surgical excision of that part of your physiognomy. In contrast, myriads of patients with tic douloureux perceived in their teeth have those cosmetically and functionally important structures avulsed, even though there is not a shred of evidence that dental extractions eliminate the pain of tic douloureux. A similar error is made by prescribing narcotics for chronic usage to patients with tic douloureux: These drugs are antinociceptive and do not alleviate central pain states unless soporific levels are attained.

We do not understand the neural mechanisms of central pain states: They can be conceived as "errors in information processing" or "short circuits." It is essential when evaluating studies of pain to discriminate pain due to nociception from pain due to something wrong within the nervous system. Both are equally real but have widely disparate anatomical and physiological substrates. Experimental pain studies, with a few recent exceptions, have focused upon nociception, but the findings are often extrapolated to the clinical setting, where the presence of nociception is dubious. Cognitive factors can be shown to modify the response to an experimenter-controlled noxious stimulus, but they may not act in a similar fashion in clinical pain states. It is not at all clear that classic laboratory sensory physiology studies have any relevance to chronic pain.

Pain usually leads to *suffering*, which is defined as a negative affective

Table 1. Central Pain States

Thalamic syndrome	Phantom limb pain
Tic douloureux	Arachnoiditis
Postherpetic neuralgia	Atypical facial pain
Post-thoracotomy pain	Causalgia
Nerve root avulsion pain	Neuralgias
Post-thoracotomy syndrome	

response engendered by pain and by such diverse phenomena as depression, isolation, anxiety, and fear. People may suffer for a variety of reasons. English speakers tend, however, to use the language of pain to describe all the phenomena of suffering. A book entitled *Worlds of Pain* (Rubin, 1976) is, in fact, about the suffering of a poor, immigrant population in the Chicago stockyards at the turn of the century. *A Just Measure of Pain* (Ignatieff, 1978) describes penitentiary life in the early industrial age. Neither volume discusses pain; both are concerned with suffering. Consider this quotation:

> Art is pain. It must be. And the rubbish that passes for art today—the lazy, effortless, casual, thrown-together, doodled rubbish—is the result of the modern world's fear of pain and demand for an anesthetic.
>
> B. Levin, *Horizon Magazine*

Finally, we have all probably used the phrase, "So-and-so is a pain in the neck" (or elsewhere). We do not mean that our neck hurts, nor that so-and-so resides in our neck; we mean that so-and-so is causing us to suffer. Similar linguistic examples abound. The way we utilize language clearly constrains the way we (both patients and physicians) think. Our health care delivery systems reinforce this error: Patients who complain of pain are presumed to have a noxious etiology and the potential role of affective factors is ignored. Illich (1976) stated eloquently, "Medical civilization, however tends to turn pain in to a technical matter and thereby deprives suffering of its inherent personal meaning."

It is important to recognize that nociception, pain, and suffering are private, internal events that cannot be quantified or proven to exist. *Suffering* usually leads to *pain behavior*, which is the interaction between the individual and the surrounding world. Pain behavior is defined as any and all outputs of the individual that a reasonable observer would characterize as suggesting pain, such as (but not limited to) posture, facial expression, verbalizing, lying down, taking medicines, seeking medical assistance, and receiving compensation. Like any other form of behavior, pain behaviors are measurable. Indeed, it is the patient's pain behaviors that the physician evaluates in the establishment of diagnosis and treatment outcome. All behaviors are influenced by their consequences, especially if they have been present over time. Environmental contingencies will alter the likelihood of the elaboration of a specific behavior. Neurosurgeons and orthopedists have long claimed that back surgery was more successful on private paying patients than those covered by workmen's compensation. Such a recognition of behavioral or environmental contingency factors in no way excludes psychodynamic explanations of human behavior, for it is obvious that both past affective experiences and present contingencies will influence behavior. The important point is to acknowledge that events outside of the patient often play a major role in the genesis of pain behavior.

The task of the clinician is to determine which of the four factors, nociception, pain, suffering, and pain behavior, are playing significant roles in the genesis of the patient's problem, and then to direct therapies at the appropriate etiological factors. The obligation of the basic scientist is to recognize that experiments involving portions of the neural or psychological substrates of acute pain do not encompass the universe of phenomena related to a patient's pain. It is for these reasons that we must recognize the differences between acute, chronic, and experimental pains. What they have in common is very limited. Experimental and acute pains almost exclusively involve nociception. Chronic pain often has little evidence for any nociceptive activity and is more often related to pain in the absence of nociception or to affective and environmental factors. This is reflected in the frequent meaninglessness of data derived from experimental pain studies when applied to patients with chronic pain. Indeed, close scrutiny has led many to the viewpoint that chronic pain and acute pain have nothing in common save for the four-letter word *pain*. Therapies, whether pharmacological, physical, or surgical, that are highly successful in controlling acute pain are not only ineffective in the patient with chronic pain, but often add to the patient's pain behavior. We have seen a significant number of chronic pain patients who are surgical veterans, professional doctor shoppers, and massive overutilizers of drugs. They reach our pain clinic carrying shopping bags full of medications; their physicians have become a way-station in the patient–prescription relationship. Their pain behavior is florid. Doing nothing other than helping them to cease their medications and increase their activity levels has, for many of these unfortunates, eliminated their pain behavior. Narcotics and sedative–hypnotic drugs (diazepam is the worse offender) are among the causes of chronic pain. They are significant contributors to depression. Patients frequently cannot discriminate between nociception and falling blood levels of these drugs. Similarly, inactivity and immobilization, which effectively palliate acute pain, only add to chronic pain behavior. The significant factor again appears to be the prominent role of nociception in acute pain and its absence in chronic pain, and the importance of affective and behavioral factors in chronic pain.

It is important to discriminate between chronic pain due to cancer and that due to a benign disease process. The pain associated with uncontrolled cancer is due to continuous and often increasing tissue damage; hence it is best described as long-standing acute pain and should be treated with therapies aimed at reducing nociception. Benign diseases causing chronic pain are rarely associated with nociception and are rarely ameliorated by antinociceptive measures.

No single methodological approach is likely to explain all of the known phenomena of pain. It is obvious, we hope, that the brain is the organ of the mind and the source of all complex behaviors. Although we may not understand the electrochemical processes by which the brain works, we do know which organ to study.

This book focuses upon human behavior and its role in the genesis of illness. Patients with chronic pain manifest many phenomena that suggest that the interaction between the patient and his or her environment is a major cause of illness. Pain behavior frequently can be traced to either a payoff (something desirable happens if the patient manifests pain behavior, such as attention from the spouse or financial compensation) or avoidance of something undesirable (such as getting out of a stressful job or avoiding personal contact with a threatening individual or situation). In addition, there are some patients who continue to seek medical attention solely for the opportunity to have some form of personal interaction (social reinforcement) with another human being. Yet others appear to emit pain behaviors and limit activity in the incorrect assumption that continuing an activity that produces a modicum of distress will lead to an increase in suffering. Such may have been true during the healing time of an injury but may no longer be valid. In all four instances, it is not nociception that generates the patient's pain behavior. The physician must look outside the patient to find the cause of the patient's chronic illness.

To understand the behavioral perspective of chronic pain, we must first consider the characteristics of a behavioral approach.

The Cartesian model is both a "mind–body dualism" and a stimulus–response model. In the context of pain, the assumption is made that the "response of pain" (really pain behavior) is to the stimulus of nociception. Therefore the symptoms of pain—the pain behaviors—are but extensions or reflections of the underlying tissue damage and associated nociception. The implication of this concept is that one must understand and modify the alleged underlying tissue damage and nociception if pain relief is to occur.

A behavioral perspective departs from that kind of biomedical model by focusing on the behavior itself, in this case, the pain behaviors. Behavior—actions of the organism—is not to be understood solely as extensions or reflections of underlying processes within the person, but has significance in its own right. It follows from such a view that we must look at the factors that influence behavior. Many of those factors are to be found in the interaction between the person and both the immediate and anticipated environments.

A second characteristic of the behavioral perspective is that the criterion of change is change in the patient's behavior. If one's intervention has not resulted in a behavioral change, nothing of confirmable merit has been accomplished. The evaluation of the pain problem and its treatment both must focus on the pain behaviors, that is, what the patient does. What may have originated as symptoms of underlying tissue damage at the time of onset due to nociception may at some later point in chronicity have become the problem itself. The linkage between nociception and pain behavior, perhaps close at the onset, may in chronicity be loose or nonexistent. The problem now is pain behavior. This is what must be changed.

A third proposition characterizing the behavioral approach is awareness of the necessity of operationalizing procedures and the assessment of their effects in behavioral terms. The units of change are units of behavior. These must be measured as precisely as possible in order to assess effects.

There is a spectrum of ways in which the functioning of humans may be viewed. At one extreme is what might be termed a "structuralist" view. The person develops a "personality structure" or configuration of attitudes or motivations and these guide or direct ensuing behavior, with only modest attention to the "here-and-now" environment. At the opposite extreme is an "environmentalist" perspective, in which an individual's behavior is seen as under the control of environmental stimuli or perceived environmental consequences, with only limited attention to effects of prior experience. Both extremes obviously oversimplify. Here we take an "interactionist" view. Prior experiences leading to selective stimulus perception and selective anticipation of consequences will exert influence on the person's functioning, though that influence will become operative only in response to environmental events. Environmental stimuli and contingent environmental consequences will also exert significant influence. It has been said that environmental consequences mold behavior but that stimulus control maintains it. Within the context of an interactionist perspective, the following concepts are fundamental to understanding the role of learning/conditioning (i.e., behavioral) factors on chronic pain:

1. Behavior is changeable. The processes that define change are largely understood as learning processes.
2. Behavior tends to increase in rate if followed promptly and systematically by positive (as defined by the individual) consequences, that is, positive reinforcement.
3. Behavior tends to diminish in frequency and ultimately disappear under either of two conditions:
   a. Previously sustaining positive reinforcement is withdrawn (extinction).
   b. A behavior incompatible with the behavior to be diminished is effectively positively reinforced and thereby becomes established.

4. The definition of "reinforcer" is both circular and idiosyncratic. If a consequence, when presented, increases behavior, it is a positive reinforcer. Or, if a consequence, previously occurring in a contingent manner, when withdrawn results in a decrease of a behavior, it, too, is for that person a positive reinforcer.

Reinforcers gain their influence on our behavior from past experience and therefore depend for their effectiveness on the individual's particular learning experiences. There is a whole technology having to do with the scheduling and delivery of reinforcement to which the interested reader is referred (Reese, 1966; Berni and Fordyce, 1977; Marr and Means, 1981).

There appear to be two general ways in which conditioning factors may come to exert influence and, in some cases, virtually totally control pain behaviors.

One course of conditioning is direct positive reinforcement of pain behaviors, paraphrased as, "When I hurt (emit pain behaviors) 'good' things happen that otherwise would not." Stated more formally, the emission of pain behaviors is followed contingently by positive reinforcement. The principle obvious clinical examples of this are PRN medication regimens, attention from physicians, spouses,and important others occurring on a pain behavior contingent basis, and rest, whether prescribed or self-selected, as a treatment modality.

The example of PRN medication as a source of conditioning effects should be evident. A PRN regimen requires that one must emit some form of pain behavior in order to receive or have sanctioned consumption of the analgesic. If sedation or relaxation, for example, are pleasant to the individual, a positive reinforcer has been made contingent upon pain behavior and a conditioning paradigm has been set up. Of course, if sedation is aversive, no such effect can be expected.

The attention factor should also be evident. Spouses and others often extend special amounts or forms of attention to one who is suffering.

One of the clearest examples of the potential impact of conditioning effects in general and selective attention or social responsiveness in particular on pain behaviors is illustrated in a study by Block et al. (1980). Chronic pain patients in evaluation had characterized their respective spouse's typical responses to indications of patient suffering (i.e., pain behaviors). From those data, patients were divided into those reporting more and those reporting less support by their spouses. They were then interviewed in a room with a one-way mirror. For half of each interview, they were informed correctly that their spouses were observing; for the other half of the session instructions were that a "neutral" health care professional was observing, which was also true. Appropriate controls for sequence effects were imposed. During each half of the interview patients were asked at one point how much pain they were experiencing at the

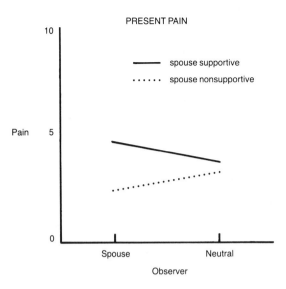

Figure 2. Results of interview experiment. From Block et al. (1980).

moment. Figure 2 shows the results and indicates that reported subjective distress, a form of pain behavior, varied systematically as a function of the subject's believing that it was the spouse or a neutral person who was observing. In conditioning terms, spouses presence had, for the supportive spouse subgroup, become a conditioned discriminated stimulus, which in turn evoked increments in pain behavior. Conversely, where the spouse had come to be discriminated as nonsupportive, decrements in suffering were reported.

Rest has special significance. First, it is typically and wisely prescribed as an important element of treatment for acute pain. Second, many people find it reinforcing to "take it easy." Third, sanctioned or prescribed rest also has the effect of precluding the person from doing something that may be aversive, not only "pain," but other activities (e.g., going to a job). Therefore rest should be seen as a potential reinforcer. It may be prescribed and maintained on a pain behavior contingent basis. To do that sets up a potentially influential conditioning paradigm.

There is a second and perhaps more important way in which learning or conditioning factors may play a role in the maintenance of a pain problem. Avoidance learning is a well-established and well-documented pheno-menon. It is manifested in either escape or avoidance behavior. *Escape* behavior is defined as behavior that effectively terminates an aversive stimulus, for example, removing one's hand from a hot stove, thereby terminating the aversive pain of the heat. *Avoidance* behavior is behavior that postpones an aversive stimulus, for example, avoiding placing one's hand on the hot stove to postpone—presumably indefinitely—the aversive stimulus.

Avoidance learning might also be termed indirect positive reinforcement, because the behavior leads indirectly to reinforcement. The aversive stimulus is avoided or terminated, a positive consequence. Whatever the terminology, there appear to be two important ways in which avoidance learning may play a role in chronic pain. One is that pain behaviors may lead to "time out"* from aversive events. A housewife who dislikes vacuuming rugs or scrubbing walls may find prescribed rest for back pain very reinforcing, for it not only postpones the aversive stimulus of pain or suffering she expects to arise from moving the involved body parts but also avoids the aversive stimulus of the disliked housework. Similarly, the impotent male is likely to find prescribed rest and avoidance of sexual activity reinforcing because it avoids both anticipated pain from movement of the involved low back and the psychological suffering from exposure to defective ability to achieve an erection. Potential examples are legion.

A number of well-established facts about avoidance learning are important to remember. Once established, it takes relatively little continuing reinforcement to maintain an avoidance response (Reese, 1966). In addition, there is always the risk that each time the person engages in the avoidance behavior in order to postpone (i.e., avoid) pain/suffering, that same avoidance response is also reinforced in yet another way; another activity that is also aversive may be avoided.

It is common to see patients with chronic pain long after a relatively minor injury. There is no reason to expect the healing process to require more than a few weeks, yet pain behaviors persist indefinitely. These patients frequently have problems coping with the stresses of everyday life. Avoidance learning or indirect positive reinforcement seems to play a major role in their pain behavior.

There is a second way in which avoidance learning seems often to play a role in the maintenance of a pain problem beyond healing time. This derives from the concept of *conditioned aversive stimuli*. It has long been observed that stimuli occurring contiguously to aversive stimuli tend, over many repetitions, to take on aversive properties themselves. A simple illustration of this phenomenon could be found in an unwise mother who speaks only to her children to criticize them. Initially the criticism is

---

*Traditional behavioral science use of the term *time out* has been as in time out from positive reinforcement, as when a child is sent to his or her room as punishment. The choice here is to use it in a more socially conventional sense, akin to a hiker taking time out to rest when tired.

aversive; ultimately the mere sight of that mother, or the sound of her voice, could become aversive to those children.

The relevance of conditioned aversive stimuli as an aspect of avoidance learning to chronic pain is that stimuli contiguous to nociception and ensuing pain behaviors may themselves take on the aversive properties. To illustrate, consider back sprain and the ensuing guarding behavior as in moving gingerly. Were one to guard long enough through excessive reclining and restricted movement, aspects of the multitude of proprioceptive and kinesthetic cues that always occur when one is moving could themselves take on aversive properties. Suppose, for example, that a person learned early in life of a back pain problem where walking more then 100 feet produces a sharp increase in pain/suffering. Were that pattern to persist for a significant number of "trials," observation by the person that the 100 foot mark was being approached well could take on aversive properties. The result could be that mere perception of approach of 100 feet could lead to experiencing the aversive stimulus' avoidance behavior (stopping to recline) and could be expected to follow.

This type of conditioning effect can be perceived as superstitious overguarding behavior. The person makes the mistake of thinking that since it was the case that certain amounts of movement led to pain and suffering, movement will, long after healing time, continue to have similar effects. As a consequence, the person continues to engage in guarding behavior that, in the sense of tissue damage, is quite unnecessary. There is the incorrect (i.e., "superstitious") anticipation of nociception and it is followed by overguarding.

The importance of anticipated aversive consequences and associated guarding behavior to an understanding of chronic pain could easily be underestimated. The phenomenon of avoidance learning usually is not considered by physicians or by patients in regard to pain problems. Typically, pain is understood as a warning signal cuing the person that to continue with a pain-producing activity will both increase pain and threaten further body harm. That view may also be stated as implying a positive correlation between exercise/activity and pain/suffering (as in pain complaints). That is, "the more I do the more I will hurt and the less I do the less I will hurt." This axiom is illustrated by a physician's prescription to work to tolerance, for example, "Let pain be your guide," an all-to-often prescribed dictum to pain patients. The axiom is also apparent when family members caution the pain patient to stop an activity when pain arises. That in turn promotes avoidance learning. But is the axiom true in chronic pain?

One study by Fordyce et al. (1981) challenges the validity of this axiom. The authors observed 25 chronic pain patients who were performing perscribed exercises "to tolerance," defined as, "do (the exercise) until

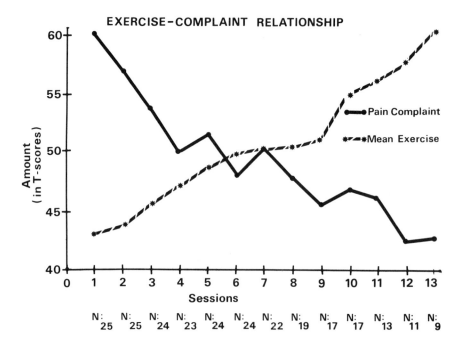

Figure 3. Exercise–complaint relationship in experiment.

pain, weakness, or fatigue cause you to want to stop. You decide when to stop." All sessions were observed and both the amounts of exercise performed and the number of visible or audible indicators of pain/ suffering (i.e., pain behaviors) were recorded. Therapist–observers maintained a neutral, nonprotective, nonencouraging posture during the sessions. Results as shown in Fig. 3 fail to show the expected positive correlation between exercise and pain complaints. To the contrary, the results were consistently and overwhelmingly negative. The more exercise performed, the fewer were the pain complaints.

Outside the context of the management of chronic pain, it does not surprise us that the more one does, the better one feels, at least up to some point. But in the context of chronic pain the situation is readily observed to be very different. People are laboring under the conviction that pain is a warning signal and that when pain/suffering occurs, one should take precautionary action. Treatment decisions, prescription of rest, and so forth, continue to be made almost universally under this misconception.

A behavioral approach to the evaluation and management of the patient

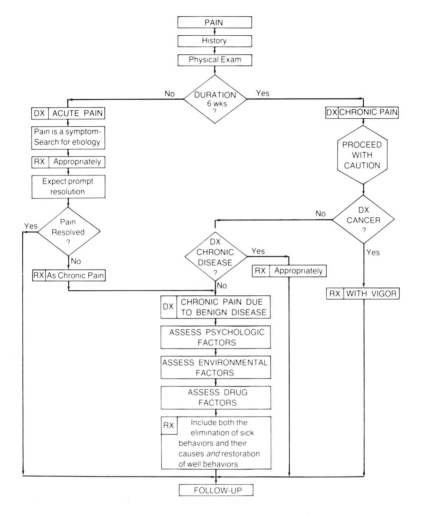

Figure 4. An algorithm for evaluation and management of pain.

with chronic pain is illustrated in Fig. 4 and can be summarized by the following points:

1. In trauma-induced pain persisting beyond expected healing time, the possibility of little or no linkage between pain behaviors and alleged or inferred nociception should be considered. There may now be a problem relating to learning or conditioning.
2. So-called "psychogenic" or "conversion reaction" concepts, for example, are by no means the only logical alternative to pain

behaviors not supported by physical findings. Moreover, such concepts are burdened by allegiance to a disease model concept of behavior that is at variance with voluminous contradicting empirical data. It is not necessary to postulate, and frequently it would be quite incorrect to infer, that the existence of a now learned/conditioned pain problem (we suggest the term *operant pain*) relates to some personality or motivational problem.

3. In chronic pain, evaluation should examine as much as possible what the person does—his or her actions. One should not rely solely either on physical findings data past their healing time or on simple verbal report or body language data from the patient. Such information as diary records show time distribution among sitting, standing/ walking, and reclining, and frequency counts as to activities engaged in derived from checklists and the like, can provide much useful additional information from which to assess the problem.

4. Since both family members' responses to pain behaviors and their observations of the patient provide critical information, patient evaluation should always include an interview of the spouse or other significant individuals.

5. Analgesics or medications such as muscle relaxants or sedative– hypnotics as well as pain-contingent rest should be understood as having potentially powerful consequences. If they are prescribed on a *pain behavior* contingent basis, there is major risk of extending the duration and severity of the pain problem. If used at all, they should be on a time-contingent regimen, that is, with fixed time intervals between doses.

6. Social feedback can, if improperly programmed, worsen the problem. Family members should be helped to recognize this and to respond so as to not reinforce pain behaviors.

7. Activation of the chronic pain patient who has a reduced activity level is essential. It usually can be readily accomplished by prescription of an incremental working-to-quota regimen of exercise.

A final, very important point needs to be considered. In acute illness, reduction or elimination of symptoms usually leads to a resumption of effective "well" behavior. In chronic illness, reduction of symptoms or impairment is by no means automatically followed by resumption of effective well behavior. Many factors play a role in this observation. Inactivity leads to poor muscle and joint tone and easy fatiguability. Nociceptive stimuli may thus temporarily follow even minimal exercise. Disuse leads to skill reduction. Some people are more likely to get sick or to remain so because they have defects in their ability to cope with the demands of life. For others, long periods of being grounded by, for example, chronic pain will have led to the loss of access to opportunities for jobs. For these reasons and others, it is essential in the management of chronic pain that the treatment program consider the use of what the person will do when the pain subsides, and maximize the likelihood of achieving those goals, for example, through vocational guidance and placement, family planning with regard to recreational patterns, and developing more gratifying life-styles.

References

Berni, R., and Fordyce, W. E. 1977. Behavior Modification and the Nursing Process, 2nd ed. St. Louis, Missouri: C. V. Mosby.

Block, A. R., E. F. Kramer, and M. Gaylor. 1980. Behavioral treatment of chronic pain: The spouse as a discriminative cue for pain behavior. Pain 9:243–252.

Fordyce, W. E., R. McMahon, G. Rainwater, S. Jackins, K. Questad, T. Murphy, and B. de Lateur. 1981. Pain complaint–exercise performance relationship in chronic pain. Pain 10:311–321.

Illich, I. 1976. Medical Nemesis. New York: Pantheon Books.

Ignatieff, M. 1978. A just measure of pain: the peniteniary in the industrial revolution, 1750–1850. New York: Pantheon Books.

Loeser, J. D. 1980. Perspectives on Pain. Proceedings of First World Conference on Clinical Pharmacology and Therapeutics. London: MacMillan Publishers Limited; pp. 313–316.

Marr, J., and B. Means. 1981. Behavior Management Manual: Procedures for Psychsocial Problems in Rehabilitation. Hot Springs, Arkansas: Arkansas Rehabilitation, Research and Training Center.

Reese, E. P. 1966. The Analysis of Human Operant Behavior. Dubuque, Iowa: William. C. Brown.

Redd, W., and A. Vazquez. Conditioned version in cancer patients. Behavior Therapist, April 1981 (invited discussion).

Rubin, L. B. 1976. Worlds of pain: Life in the working class family. New York: Basic Books.

17

Depressive Illness
and Medical Practice

John A. Chiles, M.D.,* Nicholas G. Ward, M.D.,† and
Joseph Becker, Ph.D.‡

Depression is one of the most common major illnesses in the United States. Several million persons a year require treatment for depression, their numbers far exceeding the treatment resources available from psychiatric specialists. Hence many depressed patients first seek medical assistance from their family physician or internist. The lifetime risk of this disease is 8–12% for men and 20–26% for women, and while the morbidity and mortality of depression cannot be accurately assessed, they are a major public health concern (Weissman et al., 1981), with the loss of work hours and productivity and the adverse interpersonal effects of depression on family and friends representing a significant social cost. In addition, suicidal ideation, suicide attempts, and suicide are distressingly common with this group. People with depressive illness kill themselves at approximately ten times the frequency of patients with other psychiatric diagnoses.

Some patients who suffer from depression experience it as primarily an emotional and psychological problem, and talk about it in those terms. However, the family doctor will see, in the course of his or her career, many people with depression who present with a physical complaint. Often these patients will have symptoms of undetermined cause and will seem to amplify these symptoms. The family practice physician needs to know appropriate precedures for diagnosing depression so that these

*Associate Professor, Department of Psychiatry and Behavioral Sciences, University of Washington School of Medicine, Seattle, Washington.
†Associate Professor, Department of Psychiatry and Behavioral Sciences, University of Washington School of Medicine, Seattle, Washington.
‡Professor, Department of Psychiatry and Behavioral Sciences, University of Washington School of Medicine, Seattle, Washington.

patients may be started on the most effective treatment course. Our purpose in this chapter is to provide a framework for such a diagnostic interview, review the more important differential points, look at the developing biological correlates of depression, and review the currently available treatment methods, with a brief discussion as to what the future might hold.

Diagnosis of Depression

"A man must swallow a toad in the morning if he is to assure himself that nothing worse will happen to him that day." This bit of seventeenth century graffito reflects the state of mind dysphoria, which, when persistent, is a primary ingredient of depression. It is a prolonged and pervasive emotional state for which patients use a number of words to describe: depressed, sad, blue, hopeless, bored, gloomy, dejected. Some depressed patients will deny that they are depressed but, instead, will acknowledge anhedonia, the loss of ability to experience pleasure. The patient often has negative thoughts about himself, the world, and the future, and is often in a state of giving up, feeling that nothing he or she does seems to make any difference anyway. Dysphoria is a prominent disturbance of emotion in depression. Anxiety is another important emotional ingredient (or contaminant) of depression, present in up to 50% of depressed patients. Anger may be present, especially in patients with long-standing depression and more severe interpersonal difficulties.

While the emotional aspects are important, it is necessary for the clinician to realize that depressive illness is more than just an emotional state. To diagnose every patient who is sad and woebegone as depressed, especially when somatic therapies are being considered, is a mistake. Such emotional reactions are often appropriate temporary responses to stressful life events.

There are a number of nonspecific and specific psychological and psychiatric reasons to be excessively worried. Nonspecifically, there is a virtual army of the "worried well," of which we have all been members at one time or another. This "temporary hypochondriasis" is not a psychiatric disorder or a personality problem, but seems to occur in the context of the widely researched notion that increased stress leads to increased visits to the doctor. For a thorough discussion of hypochondriasis, see Altman (1975). A visit to the doctor can represent a need for *education* (a second-year medical student worried about having cancer), *support* (a patient who develops chest pain in a recurrent grief reaction on the anniversary of his father's death by heart attack), *ventilation* (a patient who is for some reason blocked from expressing a powerful emotion), or *advice* (how to deal with a family parent, how to apply for unemployment insurance). A well-organized physician's office should have a file on the area's various support services to which the patient can be referred (Barsky, 1975).

Depressive illness, by contrast, is a more complex syndrome. In addition to emotional disturbances, depressed patients have cognitive, behavioral, physiological, and sometimes perceptual troubles. The diagnosis requires an evaluation of each of these areas.

Cognition

Cognition, or how we think about things, is awry in the depressive. Depressed patients describe recurrent themes in their thinking, for example, hopelessness, blameworthiness, pessimism, somatic complaints, and lack of energy. Suicidal ideation is frequently found in depressive cognition. An important part of the psychotherapy of depression has to do with making the patient aware of this repetitious and unproductive thinking in such a way that it can be changed. Psychotic depressives suffer the same style of cognition, carrying it further to delusions of blame, worthlessness, poverty, and body dysfunction. The blame is perversely expansive; patients take "credit" for negative events far beyond their control. As they talk of their imagined poverty and disintegrating bodies, their affect is congruent with the despair they express, an important differential point between the delusions of psychotic depression and those of schizophrenia.

Perceptual disturbances occur in several forms in depression, including illusions, depersonalization, and, the most dramatic, hallucinations, found in approximately 25% of psychotically depressed patients. The hallucinations follow the theme of the depression and are almost always congruent with the patient's affect. Auditory hallucinations are condemnatory and derogatory; visual hallucinations are of frightening, sometimes horrible scenes; olfactory hallucinations are foul and putrid odors.

A last cluster of cognitive disturbances in depression is indecisiveness, poor memory, and disrupted concentration. The worse the depression, the more frequent are the complaints of these problems. The memory deficits are certainly related to inattention and decreased concentration, but how much they might relate to other aspects of memory is unknown.

Behavior

Depressive behaviors fall into two groups: those observable in any given interview and those that occur over time. The more severe the depression, the more pervasive the behavior. A decrease in activity, psychomotor retardation, is the most common interview behavior. Answers are quite brief and a long time in coming. There is no spontaneity, and at his most severe, the patient is unresponsive, a dejected and passive individual.

Not infrequently one may observe what seems to be the opposite behavior, psychomotor agitation. Patients appear in great distress, wringing their hands, pulling their hair, pacing, and moaning. Again, this behavior is increasingly evident with more serious depression. Occasionally, some patients combine elements of both retardation and agitation, with latency of speech and hand wringing occurring simultaneously.

Over time, depression results in a decrease in productive physical activity and social withdrawal. Performance at work and home deteriorates, and social contact diminishes. Those who maintain frequent contact with the depressive, such as family members, often describe a painful overinvolvement with the patient, especially if the patient begins to talk about suicide. As one spouse put it, "I am constantly fighting against being sucked into this giant vacuum cleaner." And even the depressed Antonio observed, in Shakespeare's *Merchant of Venice*, "In sooth, I know not why I am so sad. It wearies me. You say it wearies you."

Physiology

The more severe the depression, the more severe the physiological disturbances. The vegetative functions such as appetite, sleep, energy level, libido, and bowel functions are impaired, resulting in insomnia, anergy, and constipation. However, some depressed patients have an increase in sleep and appetite—hypersomnic, hyperphagic depressions. Unfortunately, these specific increases are not predictive for one kind of therapy over another.

Depression in its severe form is hard to miss. In its many variations, however, it provides more than its share of diagnostic problems. The American Psychiatric Association (1980), in its *Diagnostic and Statistical Manual of Mental Disorders*, stated a rational and uniform way of diagnosing major depressive illness. Inclusion and exclusion criteria are utilized. In this system, a patient has a major depressive episode when he has a prominent and relatively persistent dysphoric mood and has at least four of the following eight symptoms, each being present for at least 2 weeks:

1. Poor appetite and significant weight loss *or* increased appetite and significant weight gain.
2. Insomnia or hypersomnia.
3. Psychomotor agitation or retardation.
4. Anhedonia or pervasive decrease in sexual drive.
5. Anergy or fatigue.

6. Feelings of worthlessness, self-reproach, or excessive or inappropriate guilt.
7. Complaints or evidence of decreased ability to think or concentrate, or indecisiveness not associated with marked loosening of associations or incoherence.
8. Recurrent thoughts of death, suicidal ideation, or suicide attempt.

Exclusion criteria include schizophrenia, a schizophreniform disorder, a paranoid disorder, organic mental disorder, or uncomplicated bereavement.

Severity

Several able reviews of methods for assessing the severity and/or subtype of depression are available (Hammen, 1981). Some widely used clinical scales can be quickly and easily administered by office staff or self-administered by the patient. The Beck depression inventory and the Zung self-rating depression scale (Zung, 1965) are among the most commonly used of these measures. Such self-report measures have limitations but if used prudently, they can be helpful in checking on clinical impressions. The Beck depression inventory is somewhat more heavily weighted toward psychological depressive symptoms, and the Zung inventory toward somatic depressive symptoms. Therefore the Beck inventory is probably more useful for detecting milder depressives. The number of false negative scorers can be reduced by astute clinical observation and by using data from collateral informants. Scales such as those of Beck and Zung provide a basis for estimating *severity of depression*, but not for establishing a *diagnosis of depression*. Some clinicians and investigators regard the Hamilton rating scale for depression (Hamilton, 1960) as the most valid measure of severity of depression. However, administration of this instrument requires an interview.

Differential Diagnosis

As we have seen, depression has a number of components, and each of these components can be a problem in its own right, without being part of a syndrome of depression. Insomnia, fatigue, pain, anxiety, and sexual dysfunction are problems that can be included in the syndrome of depression, but they may also have some other etiology. Thus the diagnosis of depression must be made on the basis of positive findings, and not on exclusion.

Differentiating between grief and depression may be difficult, since many of the symptoms of depression are present in grief and may persist for several months. Grief usually differs from depression in that self-esteem tends to be preserved and anhedonia tends not to be fixed. The loss of a loved one commonly provokes feelings of guilt that one did not do enough for the deceased, but these feelings do not translate into a sense of worthlessness. A depressed person often experiences a pervasive loss of interest in life activities, while the person in grief will find that he or she may at times still enjoy some activities. About 10% of people who are experiencing grief will go on to develop a clinical depression. These people tend to be isolated, either by "preference" or by the realistic lack of a social support system, and should be treated.

Depression in Medical Settings

While it was once believed that many depressions in adolescent, geriatric, and pain patients were "masked" and not readily evident, further research has not supported this. Depression in children, adolescents, and older adults can be diagnosed by using criteria very similar to those used with younger adults. In geriatric psychiatry, the term *pseudodementia* has been applied to patients thought to be demented but who lost their "dementia" when treated with antidepressants. While some patients have all of the somatic, cognitive, and perhaps perceptual disturbances of depression but deny dysphoria, careful interviewing will usually reveal anhedonia and anxiety. Patients with chronic pain complaints frequently present with this pattern of symptoms. They have the depressive syndrome but deny the depressive mood.

It is now clear that in much of the work on masked depression, it was the examiner who was masked, not the patient. The most obvious symptoms of the patient were taken as the entire problem, and more subtle psychological and emotional difficulties, for example, anhedonia, were not correctly evaluated. The concept of masked depression remains pertinent in individuals who have depression and some other psychiatric disorder; for example, depression and alcoholism, or depression and delinquency. Each problem may require a separate treatment strategy, and it is unclear how the successful treatment of one problem will affect the other. The causal versus coincidental relations in these combination disorders is also unclear.

Depression occurring in a medical setting presents a number of diagnostic and treatment problems. A patient may develop a depression as a consequence of a serious medical illness. Another patient may have a depression, a primary affective disorder, and also a medical illness, with the two more or less coincidental. Yet another patient may have depressive symptoms that are an integral part of the illness itself. Differentiating these possibilities is a sometimes impossible job. Some medical illnesses, and some medications, appear to cause depression, and the depressive symptoms may be the first, or the most prominent, or occasionally the only manifestation of the illness or drug problem. An adequate medical history and physical workup is an essential part of the initial evaluation of depression.

Occasionally, the specific nature of a symptom may help in differentiating a depression from a medical condition. A man who develops impotence but who still has nocturnal penile erections does not have diabetic impotence and may well have depression. A woman who complains of dysphoria and fatigue being worse in the morning is less likely to have a medically based cause for her symptoms. Most people with chronic medical illnesses tend to feel fatigued and dysphoric as the day progresses. People who complain of feeling fatigued and yet have insomnia are not likely to be in a hypometabolic state, where hypersomnia would be expected with the fatigue, but they might be depressed.

A complete list of medical conditions that can be associated with depression would probably include all medical conditions. Those conditions traditionally associated with a high risk for depression include malignancies (e.g., cancer of the pancreas), chronic infectious illness (e.g., mononucleosis, hepatitis), endocrinopathies (e.g., thyroid disease), vitamin deficiencies (e.g., B_6, B_{12}), and neurological illness (e.g., multiple sclerosis). Depressions secondary to medical illnesses respond to treatment of the underlying disorder. Unless it is treated, the patient will continue to be at risk for depression even though there may be some response to antidepressant therapy. A final notion to keep in mind is that many a doctor has made the mistake of using an initial negative evaluation in a depressed patient as the basis for attributing later findings to "functional" causes. Very difficult decisions are sometimes required in, on the one hand, avoiding repetitive and costly medical evaluations and, on the other, being alert for emerging medical difficulties.

Drug Misuse and Depression

Depressions can be both drug induced and occur with drug withdrawal. Increasing age and prior depressions make drug-induced depressions more likely. The Physician's Desk Reference (PDR) lists many drugs that "might" cause depression. Drugs that commonly produce this risk include alcohol, antihypertensives, antipsychotics, and barbiturates. Oral contraceptives have been implicated, with some evidence that they interface with pyridoxin absorption as a way of producing depression. Women with estrogen-induced depression may be more likely to have hypersomnia, fatigue, and hyperphagia. Treatment with 25–50 mg of pyridoxin twice a day has been reported to highly effective. If a medication is suspected, a drug holiday should be considered, and, if done, usually proves to be informative. Rapid withdrawal can lead to depressive symptoms. Benzodiazapines are an example of such a drug. Orderly and gradual withdrawal is the solution. Some drugs produce sedation and psychomotor slowing (e.g., barbiturates) or akinesia (e.g, antipsychotics). These symptoms should not be mistaken for depression.

Somatization

In practice, the most common differential problem for the family physician is distinguishing depressions from the troublesome, more general category of patients who seem to be excessively worried: the problem of patients who amplify their bodily symptoms. Depression is the most common reason for this amplification, occurring in up to 50% of medical patients with symptoms of undetermined cause. The physical complaint is usually a minor one; that is, the loss of function is much less than the patient's complaint about it, or the complaint is about loss of a vegetative function—sleep, appetite, sex. Often these patients will minimize or deny their depression, but an interview for depression is necessary. Look especially for hopelessness ("I know I won't get better"), worthlessness ("I'm not worth treating"), blameworthiness ('I deserve to be sick"), and an episodic history of the same troubles in the past (Dubovsky and Weissberg, 1978; Lipowski, 1979; Nemiah, 1975).

Biological Correlates of Depression

Several biological ideas concerning depression have evolved from research in the past 20 years. Four avenues of biological etiology are currently being explored. The first involves a suspected deficiency in neurotransmitters associated with depression. The central catacholamine, norepinephrine, and the indolamine serotonin have been thought to be, separately or together, deficient in depressed individuals. Drugs that increase the amount of these neurotransmitters or enhance their availability have been found to be efficacious in depression. These drugs include monoamine oxidase inhibitors, tricyclics, amphetamines, and the serotonin precursor L-tryptophan. Some patients with depression have lower levels of metabolites of these two neurotransmitters. Specifically, levels of 5-hydroxyindolacetic acid (5-HIAA), a metabolite of serotonin, are lower in the cerebrospinal fluid of depressives, and levels of 3-methoxy-4-hydroxy-phenylglycol (MHPG), a metabolite of central norepinephrine, are lower in the urine of some depressives.

   A second biological abnormality noted in depression is insensitivity in the hypothalamopituitary axis. A majority of depressives have a high steroid output, with a possible failure of the brain's normal inhibitory influence on the release of adrenocorticotropic hormone and cortisol. Some depressives have been noted to have increased cortisol secretion, abnormal nocturnal release of cortisol, and inadequate suppression of cortisol by dexamethasone. Many depressives have diminished levels of thyroid-stimulating hormone and decreased response to injections of thyroid-releasing hormone.

A third hypothesis holds that the cholinergic–adrenergic neurotransmitter balance is important in that an imbalance leads to depression or mania. The fourth hypothesis states that there is an electrolyte membrane potential disturbance and that depression may be associated with an accumulation of intracellular sodium, with a lowering of the resting membrane potential. To date, there are no specific laboratory tests for the diagnosis of depression, nor have any laboratory tests been shown to specifically indicate one antidepressant treatment over another.

Biological Treatment of Depression

Two recently described methods that fall mostly in the somatic treatment method should be briefly mentioned. The first is sleep deprivation, or, more accurately, rapid eye movement (REM) deprivation. Some significantly depressed individuals report improvement in their depressed state after one or two nights of either total or REM sleep deprivation, but the stability of this improvement has not yet been established. Swedish studies indicate that if this sleep deprivation is continued twice a week for 2–3 weeks, more permanent improvement ensues. Running on a regular basis has recently been touted as a treatment for depression, but the claim is still under investigation and has not yet been fully substantiated.

Tricyclic Antidepressants

By far the most common drug treatment for depression in the United States is the use of tricyclic antidepressants. Until recently, there were six tricyclic antidepressants available in the United States. These were two dibenzazepines, imipramine and desipramine; three dibenzocycloheptenes, amitriptyline, nortriptyline, and protrityline; and the dibenzoxepin doxepin. At the time of this writing, a number of drugs, the so-called second generation of antidepressants, are being scheduled for release on the U.S. market. Some of these will be mentioned in our section on what the future holds for the treatment of depression.

The tricyclic antidepressants are most useful in what has been called the acute, primary, unipolar, severe, autonomous depressive syndrome. These patients have the following characteristics: recurrent depressive episodes, psychomotor retardation, no clear precipitant, an autonomous quality to the depression, a family history of similar illness, and an age over 40. In addition, males tend to respond somewhat better to tricyclic antidepressants than females. The presence of clear physiological disturbances, such as middle and late insomnia and anorexia with weight loss, may be predictive of improved response. As depressed patients move farther from this set of depressive characteristics, their response to tricyclics tends to lessen. In addition to the use of tricyclics with the above-mentioned depressive syndrome, there are reports and studies in the psychiatric literature of the efficacy of tricyclics in some conditions of anxiety, adult minimal brain dysfunction, and obsessive–compulsive disorders. These drugs should not be tried in any of these conditions by anyone not thoroughly familiar with this literature.

There is variability in the absorption, metabolism, and excretion of tricyclic antidepressants; thus dosages and blood levels will vary widely among individuals. Blood levels of these drugs are now available through many hospital and commercial laboratories and appear to be related to therapeutic response. While there may be some variability from lab to lab and appropriate ranges for each lab should be known, the generally accepted therapeutic plasma levels for selected tricyclics are as follows: amitriptyline, 125–250 ng/ml; nortriptylone 50–140 ng/ml; imipramine 150–300 ng/ml; and doxepin 75–200 ng/ml. Doses of 100 mg a day (75 mg for nortriptyline) or over are often needed to attain these plasma levels. The half-lives of these drugs are usually over 20 hours, so that once-a-day dosing is often sufficient.

The tricyclic antidepressants are drugs with multiple chemical actions that affect a variety of organ systems. Full knowledge of the drug's side effects and patient susceptibility is essential. The major side effects and complications of tricyclics involves their anticholinergic properties, autonomic effects, cardiotoxicity, and interactions with other drugs. The anticholinergic effects produce, perhaps, the most common complaints, since these frequently occur within the therapeutic range of the tricyclics. The complaints include dry mouth, blurred vision, constipation, and urinary retention. Tolerance usually develops to these side effects. Autonomic effects include drowsiness, ataxia, orthostatic hypotension, fine tremor, and partial impotence and retarded ejaculation in the male. Orthostatic hypotension is far more common in geriatric patients and may occur at very low doses. Cardiac effects include the quinidinelike action of slowed conduction and repolarization and the possible induction of arrhythmias. Recent studies indicate that new arrhythmias are quite uncommon at normal therapeutic plasma levels. Idiosyncratic sensitivity reactions can occur with the tricyclics, as with all other drugs, and the tricyclics have occasionally been noted to activate manic psychosis or schizophrenia in a predisposed patient. The tricyclic antidepressants will potentiate other drugs. They increase the effect of alcohol by about one-third on a drink-by-drink basis. Most troublesome is the interaction they have with other anticholinergic compounds to produce an atropinelike toxic delirium.

Monoamine Oxidase Inhibitors

Monoamine oxidase inhibitors (MAOIs) are effective with the same group of depressions as the tricyclics. In addition to treatment response, they are similar to the tricyclics in many ways in terms of their physiological properties, side effects, and complications. However, the MAOIs have almost nonexistent anticholinergic properties and are not associated with nearly as many withdrawal symptoms as the tricyclics. Also, the MAOIs may be specially effective in patients with "atypical" depressions in which anxiety, panic attacks, multiple phobias, and/or hypochondriasis predominate. Unfortunately, these advantages are usually more than outweighed by the synergistic action of MAOIs with other sympathomimethic compounds. These drugs can interact with tyramine, a pressor substance found in a wide variety of foods, precipitating severe and possible fatal hypertensive crises. Any patient placed on these drugs should be given a list of foods and substances to be avoided. For this reason, and because of the lack of evidence that MAOIs are more efficacious than tricyclics, tricyclics may be preferred as the initial drug of treatment for severe depression. Tricyclics and MAOIs can be combined if this is done in an inpatient setting where diet can be controlled and the two drugs are started simultaneously and at about one-half their normal dose. In changing from a MAOI to a tricyclic, a drug-free hiatus of 7 days is recommended. If a patient is on a tricyclic and this has proved ineffective, small doses of a MAOI may be added.

Electroconvulsive Therapy

The electrical induction of six to ten modified grand mal seizures is effective short-term treatment for severe, psychotic, endogenous, refractory depressions. It may be the initial treatment of choice in acutely suicidal and depressed patients and pregnant women. Recent advances in electroconvulsive therapy (ECT) include the delivery of a unilateral electrical charge and much better control of the amount and duration of the electrical current. The disadvantages of ECT include a variable period of confusion following the treatment, the risks of general anesthesia, and the fact that the relapse rate from this treatment is greater than with treatment by antidepressants. In addition, this treatment has a negative image for much of the general public and is frightening to many patients. When possible, a patient should be given an adequate trial of antidepressant medication before ECT is undertaken.

While the antipsychotic medications have questionable or no intrinsic antidepressant properties, they are useful in the management of some patients with psychotic depressions. If the delusional or hallucinatory components of the depression are clear-cut, particularly if the delusions are of a hypochondrical nature, an antipsychotic agent used in the first several weeks of treatment will help to contain the psychotic component. When there is a diagnostic question between schizoaffective illness and depression, a combination of a tricyclic and neuroleptic may be indicated, particularly until the syndrome can be clarified. These agents are synergistic, and when one is discontinued, the dose of remaining medication usually needs to be raised.

Advances in the Biological Treatment of Depression

The 1980s should see the introduction of a number of antidepressant compounds, some of which are in general use in other parts of the world. These have been grouped together and labeled the "second generation" of antidepressant drugs. These drugs will include additional tricyclics such as trimipramine, clomipramine, and amoxapin; tetracyclics including maprotiline and mianserin; bicyclics including viloxazine and zimelidine; and, lastly, some drugs that bear very little structural similarity to medications currently on the market. Trazadone is an example of this diverse group. Each of these medications should be reviewed as the literature becomes available. They will all have claims of offering some advantages over current tricyclics, especially in the areas of side effects and rapidity of action. The literature, particularly as it compares these new drugs with established methods of treatment, should be critically reviewed. These medications have definite pharmacological implications for further research into the biochemistry of depression. The farther these drugs move from the current pharmacological profile of antidepressants, the more they will offer possibilities for reevaluating the various theories on the biological correlates of depression.

References

Altman, N. 1975. Hypochondriasis. *In* J. J. Strain and S. Grossman, eds.: Psychological Care of the Medically Ill. New York: Appleton-Century-Crofts.

American Psychiatric Association. 1980. Diagnostic and Statistical Manual of Mental Disorders, 3rd ed. (DSM III). Washington, DC: American Psychiatric Association.

Barsky, A. J. 1979. Patients who amplify bodily sensations. Annals of Internal Medicine 91:63–70.

Dubovsky, S. L., and M. P. Weissberg. 1978. Clinical Psychiatry in Primary Care. Baltimore, Maryland: Williams and Wilkins; pp. 1–20.

Hamilton, M. 1960. A rating scale for depression. Journal of Neurology, Neurosurgery, and Psychiatry 23:56–62.

Hammen, C. L. 1981. Assessment: A Clinical and Cognitive Emphasis. *In* L. P. Rehm, ed.: Behavior Therapy for Depression: Present Status and Future Directions. New York: Academic Press.

Lipowski, Z. J. 1979. Consultation-liaison psychiatry. General Hospital Psychiatry 1:3–9.

Nemiah, J. C. 1975. Hypochondriacal neurosis. *In* A. M. Freedman, H. I. Kaplan, and B. J. Sadock, eds.: Comprehensive Textbook of Psychiatry II. Baltimore: Williams and Wilkins; pp. 1273–1278.

Physicians' Desk Reference. 1981. 35th edition. (PDR) New Jersey: Medical Economics Company.

Weissman, M. M., J. K. Myers, and W. D. Thomson. 1981. Depression and its treatment in a U.S. urban community 1975–76. Archives of General Psychiatry 31:417–421.

Zung, W. W. K. 1965. A self-rating depression scale. Archives of General Psychiatry 12:63–70.

18

Psychosocial Perspectives on Depressive Disorders

Joseph Becker, Ph.D.,* John A. Chiles, M.D.,† and
Nicholas G. Ward, M.D.‡

Current evidence suggests that psychosocial therapy should be an integral part of treating most patients with diagnosible depressive disorders, regardless of their severity. In general, chemotherapy has its major effects on the biological symptoms of depression, whereas psychosocial interventions have their main effects on the psychological and interpersonal aspects of the disorder (Rounsaville et al., 1981; Weissman, 1979). Except for classical endogenous depressions (i.e., depressions without an adequate precipitant), most depressions seem to result from an inability to cope with stressors, particularly those involving loss. It is important to note that behavioral, cognitive, and neurochemical response systems are all affected by aversive events. If the adaptive process of coping does not tax these response systems excessively, psychopathological symptoms do not occur. However, unsuccessful attempts at adaptation may cause any or all of these response systems to go awry. For example, depletion or stimulation of amines or serotonin have negative feedback effects on cognitive–behavioral adaptation (Anisman and Zacharko, 1982). Thus an optimal treatment intervention could include measures designed to (1) modify neurochemical imbalances, (2) mitigate the secondary cognitive–behavioral effects of the neurochemical imbalances, (3) enhance the capacity to cope with the precipitating aversive events, and (4) reduce vulnerability to the aversive precipitants.

*Professor, Department of Psychiatry and Behavioral Sciences, University of Washington School of Medicine, Seattle, Washington.

† Associate Professor, Department of Psychiatry and Behavioral Sciences, University of Washington School of Medicine, Seattle, Washington.

‡ Associate Professor, Department of Psychiatry and Behavioral Sciences, University of Washington School of Medicine, Seattle, Washington.

There appears to be considerable variation in vulnerability to depression both among and within individuals over time. The precise causes of depression remain unknown. Nor do all depressives require a comprehensive treatment program like the one sketched above (Weissman et al., 1981). Some depressives, though thoroughly miserable, will manifest minimal biological symptoms; others with marked biological and psychosocial symptoms will respond adequately to either major treatment modality alone (Kovacs et al., 1981; Prusoff et al., 1980). But, in general, if biological and psychosocial dysfunctions are present, both types of intervention are advisable. Current research suggests that the application of several psychosocial treatments yields better results than any one alone (Rehm, 1981a, Chaps. 1–4).

Informed treatment of the psychosocial aspects of depression requires a broader apperceptive mass than a single technique-oriented chapter can convey. Complex reactions like depression typically have multiple determinants whose interactions and feedback loops are probably best reflected by a general systems approach (Bertalanffy, 1976). Stainbrook (1977) provided an excellent application of this approach to depression, though, with an information-processing emphasis.

Before presenting specific treatment perspectives, it may be useful to briefly discuss certain orienting attitudinal factors about depression that could influence the efficacy of any therapeutic efforts.

There is still some stigma attached to depression in our society. Males, especially, sometimes regard depression as an indication of weak character though even such stalwarts as Lincoln and Churchill often struggled with the "black dog" of depression. The capacity to experience depression appears to be tied to the capacity for meaningful attachments (Bowlby, 1980) to others. Human attachments entail social cohesiveness, sharing, and caring, which inevitably involve vulnerability to loss. Thus depressions that are not primarily due to genetically determined neurophysiological imbalances can be construed as an indication of psychosocial maturity, at least as compared with other psychopathological reactions which do not involve depression (Zigler and Phillips, 1961; Zetzel, 1965).

It is also useful to bear in mind that depression appears to be a basic affect (Izard, 1977) that presumably exists because it has provided survival value during the evolutionary process. Depression, like anxiety, optimally provides a signal function. It alerts the self to a sense of despair about fulfilling vital needs; ideally it mobilizes the individual to engage in coping behaviors designed to alleviate a sense of resignation and despair. Adaptive coping in response to depressive affect–cognitions can assume a multiplicity of forms, ranging from unavoidable submissive behavior in a primate dominance hierarchy, to eliciting succor from others, to actively seeking alternative sources of gratification in order to replace ones that are no longer available.

Obviously, the first necessity in treatment is to establish a working relationship with the patient. Sullivan's *The Psychiatric Interview* (1954) remains a useful guide for what to listen to and inquire about. Its value is measurably enhanced by repeated readings within the context of growing clinical experience.

In brief, one wants to know what the signs and symptoms of the depressive reaction are and have been, what are the apparent precipitants of the depressive episode(s) or of fluctuations in its course if the condition is chronic and what is the current life situation of the patient in terms of whatever is likely to be important to a person of his or her sex, age, social class, and ethnic and racial background. Factors such as interpersonal relations, health, vocational and academic achievement, and athletic or mechanical ability may be obvious candidates for exploration, depending upon the patient's demographic characteristics. In listening to the patient's account, it is extremely important for the practitioner to attend to indications of the loss or the anticipated loss of objects that are vital to the maintenance of the patient's self-esteem. Helping the patient to test the reality of assumptions about the nature and implications of his or her perceived helplessness and hopelessness is the core of most psychosocial treatments. Several studies have suggested that disturbance in a significant interpersonal relation, especially marital friction (Weissman and Paykel, 1974) is the commonest cause of depressive reactions.

Overview of the Psychosocial Perspective: Similarities and Differences

The principal psychosocial approaches to depression fall roughly into the psychodynamic and the cognitive–behavioral social learning perspectives (Becker, 1974, 1977). Psychoanalysis tends to focus more on early developmental or "distal" causal factors; it heavily weights the effects of infancy and early childhood on adult personality formation (Freud, 1917). According to this viewpoint adult depressions result largely from the reactivation of a sense of helplessness and hopelessness associated with early developmental vulnerabilities related to conflict, frustration, or deprivation (Bibring, 1953). Insight into these distal causes as well as into dynamically related current instigators to depression is considered essential for durable treatment results. Psychoanalytical theory is mostly derived from clinical observations obtained during psychoanalytical treatment.

In contrast to psychoanalysis cognitive–behavioral social learning theorists are more concerned with "proximal" here-and-now ways of behaving, interpreting, and anticipating events. Cognitive behaviorists typically have limited concern with the distal determinants of troublesome cognitions (cognitions include thoughts, dreams, reveries, fantasies, images) and behavior; rather, they emphasize awareness of and change in the proximal determinants or "contingencies" of thoughts and behavior and changes in the content of depressive thoughts and behaviors. Cognitive–behavioral theoretical speculations are often more closely tied to general behavioral theory and research than to extended clinical observation of depressives. Therapeutic approaches are more highly structured and their efficacy is more systematically evaluated. Theory is more responsive to relevant laboratory and clinical investigation. Both psychodynamicists (Rapaport, 1959) and cognitive behaviorists are concerned with observable behavior, but the former are more concerned with inferring or understanding the motivational "whys" of behavior, while the latter are more focused on direct efforts to change thought and behavior.

Undue interpersonal dependency is viewed as the central thread in the psychodynamic theory of depression (Hirschfeld et al., 1976). Hirschfeld et al. contended that self-esteem in depression-prone persons is so unduly regulated by dependency needs that alternative sources of self-esteem are relatively neglected. Interpersonal dependency refers to thoughts, feelings, and behaviors related to obtaining support from other persons. Dependency is a normal personality disposition that derives from the innate attachment–bonding tendencies of primates during infancy. Human infant primates are much more biologically helpless than species lower on the phylogenetic scale. As a result, mothers and infants are reciprocally "wired up" to be attentive and responsive to each other. Hunger and separation tend to be especially anxiety-fraught issues during infancy. Early interactions provide the matrix from which subsequent interpersonal and survival skills evolve. Interactions that repeatedly plunge the infant–child into states of helpless, hopeless despair are believed to be conducive to subsequent depressive vulnerability. Early psychodynamic writers stressed the tendency of predepressives to become fixated on very early ways ("oral") of experiencing and relating. This reputedly happened because the predepressive had intense, innate, or acquired needs for oral gratification that were either frustrated or overindulged, and usually the former. When stressed as adults, such individuals reputedly regress in part to these earlier modes of seeking and experiencing gratification of their self-esteem.

Many analysts (Sullivan, 1954) and personality theorists (Bem, 1972) assume that self-evaluative tendencies develop largely from the inferences one makes about the attitudes of important others toward oneself. Children learn to label their private events much as they do public ones. If the parental labeling of the child's value is largely negative, the child will apply such labeling to himself long before he is able to critically evaluate the validity of his parents' labeling of himself. Highly overlearned cognitions and behaviors tend to become automatic and unquestioned; repeated exposure to labeling seems to be all that is required for learning to occur (Harrison, 1977). The damaging effects of negative labeling, even in normal well-functioning adults, have been well demonstrated (Langer and Benevento, 1978).

Depressives are ten times as likely as the general population to have had a depressed parent. Studies of socialization practices of depressed parents suggest that they would be highly detrimental to healthy self-regard in their offspring (Becker, 1979). Depressed parents may oscillate between "murderous hostility" and extreme inhibition and withdrawal. They have great difficulty with limit setting, negotiation, and sustained interest. Indeed, the worst interpersonal relations depressed mothers have are typically with their children. Depressives are frequently very tense so that normal childhood activities and demands can be extremely irritating to them. The most consistent deficiency noted among depressives is their poor communication of their own needs (Weissman and Paykel, 1974). Guilt induction is commonplace in the socialization of depressives. As children, depressives were often taught that their prime concern should be to fulfill the needs of others, implicitly or explicitly the parent, though typically this is a futile endeavor (Hogan and Hogan, 1975). The result can easily be an unhappy mixture of concern for and hatred toward the parent, as well as derogation of the self. Not all of the children of depressed parents become depressed; in fact, only a minority do so. Some children are unscathed; others turn to antisocial acting out with drugs or sexual promiscuity; but some who become depressed report feelings of becoming exactly like the depressed parent, or "transmogrified," to use Anthony's (1975) graphic term.

Treatment

Psychodynamic Perspective

The only psychodynamic therapy whose efficacy with depressives has been tested is the so-called Short-Term Interpersonal Psychotherapy of Depression (IPT) (Klerman et al., 1979). As the name suggests, the approach is partly derived from Sullivan (1954). IPT is designed for use by experienced therapists with outpatient depressives.

Interpersonal therapy is generally concerned with the treatment of dysfunctional social role performances; it is especially concerned with troubled interpersonal relations with significant others that appear to be associated with the onset of depression. As Bowlby's (1980) exegesis of attachment theory has noted, the most intense human emotions are related to the formation, disruption, and renewal of affectional bonds. Disruption of such bonds has been repeatedly implicated as a major instigator and sustainer of depressive episodes (Brown and Harris, 1978; Henderson, 1977). Our society provides better training in forming relations than in terminating them.

IPT does not attempt to restructure the patient's personality, as is often true in conventional long-term psychodynamic therapy; rather, it attempts to reduce symptoms and improve interpersonal relations. Symptom reduction efforts are largely accomplished by supportive psychosocial interventions that are sometimes supplemented by medication. Four major sources of interpersonal dysfunction have been identified and treatment strategies evolved for each. Chief therapeutic reliance is placed upon improving reality testing and communication, and on providing reassurance and clarification; little effort is made to interpret unconscious material, intrapsychic conflict, or the developmental origins of difficulties. Therapy is brief, 12–16 sessions, and very much focused on here-and-now issues related to interpersonally defined conflicts, frustrations, anxieties, and wishes. The objective is to increase competent adaptation to current interpersonal realities in order to reduce social isolation and make existence more meaningful.

IPT is reputedly as effective as the antidepressant amitriptyline with *acute depressives*, though its principal effects are different. Medication chiefly affects vegetative depressive symptoms, while IPT has more effects on mood, suicidal ideation, work, and interests. The effects of amitriptyline occur more quickly than the 4–8 weeks required for IPT (DiMascio et al., 1979).

Therapy is initiated by an explicit review of symptoms with the patient within the context of the Hamilton (1980) the Research Diagnostic Criteria (Spitzer et al., 1978), or the DSM III criteria (American Psychiatric Association, 1980) so that the patient realizes that his or her difficulties fit a well-known clinical syndrome. Achievement of the latter objective is furthered by discussing the prevalence, prognosis, and treatment program with the patient.

Interpersonal problems associated with the onset of depression are categorized by the therapist under the rubrics of grief, interpersonal disputes, role transitions, and interpersonal deficits. An attempt is made to establish a consensus and contract with the patient regarding which problems will be addressed and how.

In normal grief, typical depressive symptoms occur for 2–4 months, but the bereaved person gradually regains the capacity to perform and to enjoy life (Siggins, 1966). IPT is used for delayed or distorted grief reactions. During initial history taking, data on the deaths of significant others and the patient's mourning reaction should be routinely obtained. The IPT manual provides detailed suggestions for identifying abnormal grief reactions and therapeutic techniques for alleviating them. Basically, treatment entails encouragement to discuss prior relationships with the deceased, as well as circumstances related to their deaths, and the patient's reactions to the loss.

All close enduring relations are occasionally marred by interpersonal disputes. Only those disputes that are thought to be relevant to the patient's depression are addressed in IPT; poor communication and demoralization typically accompany discussion of these disputes. Depressives sometimes fail to convey the existence of interpersonal disputes to therapists or even to other parties in the dispute. Furthermore, they tend to assume excessive responsibility for such difficulties. The nature of therapeutic intervention depends on whether the dispute between the principals is being negotiated, is at an impasse, or has reached a point where dissolution of the relationship is inevitable. Quite different interventions are proposed for these situations. However, exploration of discrepant expectancies, difficulties in communication, and decision-making analyses are shared in common by all of these interventions. Repetitive patterns of difficulty are sought, and their consequences and underlying assumptions explicated.

IPT is especially concerned with the frequent problem of depressions induced by role transitions that result from losses due to events such as divorce or death. As Klerman et al. (1979) noted, pathological grief is more often associated with loss of a role and an inability to deal adaptively with the loss than with grief over the lost object per se.

Interpersonal deficits often result in social isolation. Careful scrutiny of earlier successful or partially successful relations may provide helpful cues for enabling the patient to become more socially involved and effective. Many isolated patients respond to troubled relationships with avoidance rather than with efforts directed toward the resolution of difficulties. Such unadaptive measures are likely to occur within the patient–therapist relationship, which provides an excellent opportunity for the adoption of generalizable corrective measures.

In IPT the therapist functions as a relatively active patient advocate. Long silences and free associations are discouraged. Sessions are focused on several problem areas but are not as directed as in cognitive–behavioral therapy. While Sullivan (1954) sometimes gave homeworklike prescriptions, IPT therapists do not. IPT, like the cognitive–behavioral therapies, is designed to change the patient's ways of thinking, feeling, and acting, but always within the context of troubled interpersonal relations.

Several cautions are noteworthy within the IPT framework. Other psychodynamic therapists like Bonime (1976) regarded much of depressive behavior as highly manipulative. While the advocates of IPT do not deny that depressive behaviors may be sustained by secondary gains, they contend that seriously depressed persons show little evidence of conscious, deliberate manipulation of others by depressive behavior. Since loss figures prominently in many depressive episodes, termination of treatment can be a considerable problem with some depressives. It is recommended that termination be discussed three to four sessions before it occurs. These discussions should anticipate the possibility of some grief reaction and underscore the patient's enhanced autonomy and competence.

No other psychodynamic approach to depression is as well explicated as the IPT variety, and even as articulated as it is, its developers contend that extensive clinical training is required for its effective implementation. The only other psychodynamic treatment of depression that has been described in considerable detail is by Arieti and Bemporad (1978). Since the efficacy of this approach has not been formally assessed, it is not described. Nonetheless, familiarity with this theoretical and treatment perspective is strongly encouraged. The Arieti–Bemporad approach is also interpersonally oriented but, like Sullivan's, is more concerned with developmental issues than is true of IPT. The former is not a brief therapy and is more aimed at basic personality reorganization, and hence probably even less suited than IPT to adaptation by general practitioners.

A crucial difference between most psychodynamicists and cognitive behaviorists is the former's conviction that self-esteem is largely determined during the early years of life and is resistant to change. Cognitive behaviorists tend to be more sanguine about the modifiability of self-esteem. Analysts tend to believe that an extended corrective emotional experience in therapy is an essential requirement for durable increases in positive self-regard. Cognitive behaviorists are more inclined to try to change the depressive's unadaptive thinking and behavior directly. They assume that if the person functions better, they will also expect to do better; the resultant increase in feelings of competence or "self-efficacy" (Bandura, 1977; Bandura and Schunk, 1981) should enhance self-esteem.

Cognitive–Behavioral Perspectives

Most psychological therapies that are not psychodynamic or supportive can be characterized as multimodal social learning derivatives. Social learning theory and research (Bandura, 1977) attempts to integrate stimulus–response, operant, and cognitive approaches to the understanding and modification of personality development, structure, and function. Intrapersonal, behavioral, and environmental events interact and reciprocally determine each other. Some of these derivative therapies are more behaviorally oriented, while others are more cognitively focused.

Persons associated with a somewhat more behavioral than cognitive perspective are Lewinsohn and Ferster. Lewinsohn's (Lewinsohn and Arconad, 1981) basic tenets are that depressives have poor social skills, which result in their receiving a low rate of response-contingent positive reinforcement (RCPR) and/or experiencing a high rate of aversive experience (punishment). These conditions result in dysphoria and passivity. Other factors that may contribute to depression are the *unavailability* of positive reinforcers, the reduced potency of positive events, and the increased potency of negative events. Empirically, Lewinsohn and his associates found that severity of depression covaries systematically with rates of RCPR and of punishment. Depressives tend to be especially deficient in such rewarding experiences as social and sexual interaction, enjoyable outside activites, and a sense of being able to work effectively. The chief sources of punishing events are marital, social, and vocational troubles.

Lewinsohn's treatment approach attempts to increase the frequency, quality, and range of RCPR, and to decrease punishment; increased social interaction, more positive and realistic cognitions, and improved self-regulation are stressed. His objective is to tailor specific techniques to the specific needs and goals of the depressive; he does not believe that any single therapeutic method is universally applicable to depressives.

The widespread conception of depression as a biological disease that is best treated by the passive intake of antidepressants or as a deeply rooted psychogenic disorder requiring deep developmental insights can make for initial difficulties with implementing any action-oriented psychosocial interventions.

The first phase of Lewinsohn et al.'s interventions involve differential diagnosis and a functional analysis of relations between events and fluctuations in the patient's level of depression. Every effort is made to have the patient evolve a shared perspective with the therapist while construing himself as an active participant. Lewinsohn uses an extensive battery of measures, but the Research Diagnostic Criteria (RDC) (Spitzer et al., 1978) has become his chief diagnostic tool and his Pleasant Events and Unpleasant Events Schedules (PES and UES) as well as a home visit are the chief tools for a functional analysis of the patient's reinforcement experience. These schedules are rated for the frequency of occurrence of events and their subjective pleasurable or aversive qualities. Scoring patterns are used to formulate hypotheses about what is causing the depression and thus which interventions might be indicated. A daily activity schedule is also devised from these scores. The latter lists 80 of the most common pleasant and 80 of the most common aversive events; the patient monitors his daily encounters and reactions to these events. Likewise, the patient monitors and records is daily mood on the Depressive Adjective Check List (Lubin and Levitt, 1979) (ACL). On the basis of covariations between scores on the PES, UES, and ACL, therapy goals are pinpointed and a contract agreed upon that specifies these goals. The goals are to acquire skills that increase activities which are inversely related to depression and to decrease aversive activities. The contract also specifies the reinforcements to be self-administered for goal achievements. The time required to learn how to construct and fulfill these contingency contracts and the schedules that are designed to increase the amount of RCPR typically spans 12 sessions, which are spread over 1–3 months.

The particular interventions used depend on the particular goals set with the patient. Lewinsohn cited such examples as assertiveness training, parenting skills, communication skills, stress and time management, problem solving, and cognitive self-management, as well as teaching the family to reward nondepressed behavior and ignore depressed behavior. Skill training of patients involves didactics, modeling and coaching, and role-playing and rehearsal, as well as practice in the everyday world.

Lewinsohn's treatment program continuously stresses a problem-solving, educational rationale that is designed to pinpoint areas of difficulty and provide alternate coping tactics. This program has been least successful when therapist and patient have been unable to identify specific treatment goals for change. During the last several treatment sessions maintenance and prevention measures are discussed and therapist structure and support are gradually lessened.

Lewinsohn and his associates are also developing "course" materials for group treatment programs. As for overall efficacy, Lewinsohn et al. have repeatedly shown the superiority of their interventions to no-treatment control groups. However, the anticipated specific effects of particular treatments for particular difficulties has not been substantiated (Zeiss et al., 1979).

In an attempt to distill their thinking about the effective ingredients of this treatment program, Lewinsohn and Arconad (1981, pp. 62–63) seemed to implicitly modify their adherence to *conventional* social learning applications to depression. In effect, they emphasized the importance of indoctrinating the patient with the belief that he or she has sufficiently well grasped a meaningful rationale and skills to exercise substantially increased independent control over his or her life.

An excellent way to familiarize oneself with Lewinsohn's treatment approach would be to obtain a copy of *Control Your Depression* by Lewinsohn et al. (1978), which references most of the techniques and contains copies of most of the instruments referred to in this review.

Self-Control. Lewinsohn's model of depression derived from a Skinnerian concern with the environmental consequences of behavior. Rehm's (1981b) self-control model is derived from theoretical work on self-regulatory processes by Kanfer (Kanfer and Hagerman, 1981). Self-regulatory processes refer to behaviors that alter the probability of their recurrence despite the relative absence of environmental consequences. Loss or absence of expected reinforcers is said to instigate self-monitoring, self-evaluating, and self-reinforcement processes. Skill and experience determine the adaptiveness of these self-regulatory processes. According to Rehm, depressives typically exhibit two deficits in each phase of self-regulation. During the self-monitoring phase, depressives ostensibly focus on negative events to the exclusion of positive events, and on immediate consequences rather than on long-term consequences; in the self-evaluative phase, their standards are overly rigorous and they expect negative outcomes for which they blame themselves unduly; and in the self-reinforcement phase they self-administer insufficient rewards and excessive punishment. Their behavior is so controlled by negative reinforcement, that is, by escape and avoidance from aversive conditions, that inadequate efforts are made to attain desirable long-term goals. There is a fair amount of systematic research by a number of independent investigators that supports these contentions.

Therapy is designed to remedy these apparent deficits. Most treatment has been done in groups in 90-minute sessions lasting 4–6 weeks. Drawing on Lewinsohn's position, patients are instructed that participation in pleasurable activities results in positive moods, whereas a paucity of such activity and an excess of involvement in or preoccupation with escaping or avoiding unpleasant activities results in dysphoria. In subsequent sessions, the rationale and relevant skills for altering behavior are taught, homework is assigned, and periodic assessments of progress are administered. The components of the program are taught in modules from manuals in order to assure consistency.

Evaluations of treatment effectiveness in five replications essentially show superior results to no-treatment controls for the total program or for any of its components, regardless of whether treatment is extended from the usual 6 weeks to 12 weeks. By the end of a 1-year follow-up, differences between treated and nontreated patients were negligible, but a much higher proportion of nontreated patients had sought additional treatment. It is noteworthy that Rehm used patients who met criteria for a *major depressive disorder* by RDC criteria. They were solicited by newspaper ads and treated for the most part by relatively inexperienced though closely supervised graduate students.

As Rehm noted, although the theoretical rationales differ considerably among the various cognitive–behavioral therapies, the therapeutic techniques are very complex and overlap greatly; all contain cognitive and behavioral components. They share having explicit rationales, being highly structured, sequential, short-term, didactic, and requiring the patient's active efforts in dealing with current daily concerns. However, as Rehm stated (1981b), "we have little empirical evidence to pinpoint the essential ingredients of behavior therapy methods for depression" (p. 104). As he indicated, further work is required on nonspecific aspects (Frank, 1973) of therapy with depressives, and on the matching of specific techniques to particular depressives. The components of both depression and cognitive–behavioral treatment packages are multivariate, yet little effort has so far gone toward matching up particular depressive needs with particular treatment components. Lazarus' (1981) clinical efforts in this direction are interesting and look encouraging.

Multimodal Therapy. Lazarus has probably been the foremost expositor and conceptualizer of a broad-based or "multimodal" approach to psychotherapy. His assessment and treatment approach is reflected in the acronym BASIC ID (behavior, affect, sensation, imagery, cognition, interpersonal, drugs–biological) that describes his program. He pioneered some of the earlier unimodal behavioral approaches to depressives but became dissatisfied with their often initially impressive but transient impact. There has been no systematic comparison of his approach with others, but informal follow-up suggests a durable impact, even with characterological depressives (Fay and Lazarus, 1981). Lazarus viewed the seven components of BASIC ID as interactive components of personality that must be addressed if the whole person is to be treated.

After several assessment sessions, a multimodal profile assessment is generated and patients are provided with a large index card that contains instructions for modifying behavior in each BASIC ID category. For examples for depressives and a more extended exposure to this promising perspective, a reading of *The Practice of Multimodal Therapy* (1981) by Lazarus is highly recommended.

Cognitive Therapy. Among the reasons that Beck (1967) and his associates strongly advocated a cognitive therapy for depression is the refusal by many depressives of medication, and the failure of 35–40% who do accept medication to respond favorably. Beck's main assumption is that emotions are determined by the way people construe and evaluate their world. He contends that depressives develop a negative view of themselves, the world, and the future. These negative cognitive biases ostensibly account for the affective, behavioral, and motivational symptoms of depression. He contends that all functional psychopathology stems from systematic errors in thinking that involve aspects of undue overgeneralization, selective abstraction, and arbitrary inference. Reminiscent of the psychodynamic notion that stress triggers regressive reactivation of earlier modes of experiencing, Beck contends that stresses construed as losses to the self-reactive idiosyncratic "primitive, illogical" thoughts associated with earlier traumas. When the patient is not depressed, Beck contends that these cognitive biases are not operative.

In Beck's treatment approach, patients are first taught to observe associations between their thoughts and their feelings and behavior.

Instruction in techniques for recognizing and modifying thought distortions then follow.

With severely depressed patients, simple behavioral experiments that challenge their negative outcome expectancies are sometimes used. Emphasis is placed mainly on alerting the patient to his or her negative cognitive set rather than on success or pleasure per se as in conventional behavioral therapy. As Coleman and Beck (1981) noted, the cognitive distortions of depressives can easily diminish the impact of experience that deviates from their distorted expectancies unless the discrepancy is made the focus of therapeutic concern.

Many thoughts that shape mood and activity are so automatic as to be outside of focal awareness. Patients are taught to scrutinize their thoughts when they notice an affective change occurring; they are taught "experientially that perceptions of reality are not reality itself, that interpretation of reality is based on cognitive processes that are fallible, and that beliefs are hypotheses that are themselves not factual" (Beck and Bedrosian, 1980).

Beck et al. specifically stressed the importance of nonspecific factors like warmth, empathy, and genuineness in the delivery of cognitive therapy. They also cautioned against the common tendency of neophyte therapists to become depressed when working with depressives. Their volume *Cognitive Therapy of Depression* (Beck et al., 1979b) is rich in general clinical wisdom, regardless of the extent to which their particular perspective is accepted. This volume contains the most generally available exposition of their treatment approach.

Although there is a strong directive component in Beck's treatment, collaborative effort between patient and therapist is vital. The therapist acts as a guide in collecting and evaluating data, but the patient must contribute the data. Beck et al. cautioned against the therapist assuming an adversarial role. As they noted, the patient's beliefs have powerful internal consistency; the therapist's objective is to encourage the patient to examine their external validity.

Patients are initially provided with a brochure, "Coping with Depression," which explains the rationale, goals, and methods of cognitive therapy. In the first session, the patient's symptoms and presenting complaints are redefined within a cognitive framework that entails a problem-solving, hypothesis-testing orientation. Concrete behavioral and motivational issues are typically the initial concern. Later in treatment, the focus shifts to dysfunctional cognitions and their underlying assumptions. A therapy plan is outlined for the patient and each session has a jointly derived problem-focused agenda. Homework is regularly assigned and discussed in subsequent sessions. The homework mainly involves recording dysfunctional cognitions, testing their validity, and generating alternative thoughts and coping tactics.

In terms of specific behavioral techniques, flexible activity scheduling for observational purposes may be encouraged. Activities are rated for mastery and pleasurableness. Review of these schedules can yield rich data on such cognitive dysfunctions as perfectionistic tendencies. Patients are taught to break complex goals into subgoals and to evaluate their performances within the context of these subgoals rather than to retrospectively belittle their accomplishments.

Probably the main instrument for achieving therapeutic objectives is the so-called "triple column technique." Patients record events associated with affective changes and the automatic thought or image that intervened between the event and the dysphoric shift. Patients are trained to logically analyze these sequences: Does a thought jibe with reality? Are the alleged consequences of a belief tenable? On the same form, patients initially rate the strength of their original emotional response to the event, and then their emotional response to their alternative rational analysis of the event.

Some behavioral therapies are alleged to encourage unrealistic positive thinking. But in cognitive therapy, patients are strongly encouraged to explore the validity of negative cognitions; if they prove justified, a problem-solving remediation of deficits is encouraged. Particular effort is devoted to curbing tendencies to assume excessive responsibility. During the final phase of treatment, assumptions underlying automatic thoughts are increasingly examined; these are implicit rules such as "My value as a person depends on what others think of me." In dealing with suicidal tendencies, emphasis is usually placed on undermining hopelessness, which is often based on arbitrary, rigid conclusions; contradictory evidence for these conclusions is systematically sought for.

Beck and his associates have conducted several of the few studies that have compared the efficacy of cognitive or behavioral therapy with antidepressents (Kovacks et al., 1981). While reservations can be entertained about certain aspects of this work (Becker and Schuckit, 1978), the overall findings suggest that cognitive therapy is at least as effective as chemotherapy and that a combination of the two is no more effective than cognitive therapy alone. If these results are replicable, they are most encouraging, since, as indicated before, many patients are reluctant to take antidepressants, or antidepressants are contraindicted by adverse side effects.

Another cognitive perspective on depression has been provided by Seligman and his associates (Seligman, 1981). They stressed the depressogenic role of expected outcomes that have been generated by certain types of causal attributions for important adverse events whose outcomes were perceived as beyond the person's control. The greater the tendency to ascribe undue responsibility to oneself and to perceive the causes of uncontrollable aversive outcomes as long lasting and affecting broad spheres of one's behavior, the more severe and chronic the depressive reaction is likely to be and the greater its impact on self-esteem. Again, the depressogenic impact of these attributions reputedly stems from the expectancies they generate about future outcomes (Hollon and Garber, 1980). Beach et al. (1981) have explicated the therapeutic implications of Seligman's "learned helplessness" perspective, which is generating very substantial attention from a broad spectrum of social scientists (Garber and Seligman, 1980).

The learned helplessness model is not applicable to all depressions (Depue and Monroe, 1978). It relates primarily to those depressions in which the person feels helpless about his or her ability to control important outcomes, with resultant symptoms of passivity, a negative cognitive set, depressed affect, and low self-esteem.

The learned helplessness model implies that intervention can most fruitfully be applied by (1) reversing the patient's expectations of being unable to achieve significant goals, (2) shifting from unrealistic to more realistic goals, (3) decreasing the import of unreachable goals, and (4) increasing the depressive's reality testing of the ability of others to attain goals that he or she cannot attain. Beach et al. (1981) described the various cognitive–behavioral techniques that would be most suitable for intervening at each of these points. Most of the techniques are ones developed by Beck and his associates. Beach et al. concluded, with the appropriate caution, that while much theory and clinical application stresses the need to divest depression of negatively biased thinking in favor of more realistic thinking, a considerable body of research indicates that depressives may have more realistic thinking than nondepressives. The latter are prone toward self-serving positive biases that, if not overdone, are adaptive.

Eclectic Therapy. Liberman (1981) presented some eminently sound suggestions about implementing treatment with depressives as befits someone with an exceptionally broad range of clinical and therapy research experience. His experience is probably broader than any other writer's in the cognitive–behavioral depressive domain, with the exception of Beck Lazarus, and several of their associates.

As Liberman noted, many depressives respond quite well to the nonspecifics of several sessions of supportive therapy alone. Supportive treatment usually includes giving acceptance, encouragement, advice, and reassurance, conveying optimism, and providing information and an opportunity for the patient to freely express his concerns and feelings. Liberman's concept of supportive therapy extends considerably beyond a conservative supportive approach, however. He urges a strong problem-solving focus throughout this initial phase. Stressors and symptoms are viewed as challenging problems rather than as burdens. To the extent possible, causes and consequences of dysfunctions and symptoms are identified. Clarification is sought for which problems are most disruptive and/or responsible for sustaining the depression, and for what resources are available for terminating the depression and for how these resources can best be used. Goals are set, and alternative actions elicited and proposed. Only if these supportive procedures are not effective does Liberman recommend systematically implementing cognitive–behavioral techniques. Needless to say, before any treatment there is careful assessment to determine possible need for hospitalization. The latter would be especially advisable if the patient were acutely suicidal or severely depressed and without an adequate support system. The assessment and initial supportive phase should serve to identify crucial problem areas and thus the order in which various therapeutic techniques (or combinations thereof), including medication, should be applied. As noted before, these decisions are largely a product of judgment and intuition rather than objective indicators at this time. Assessment of the patient's condition and response is an ongoing process throughout treatment. Liberman has devised useful flow charts to illustrate his treatment principles.

An integral aspect of Liberman's problem formulation and goal setting is the use of so-called contingency management and self-control techniques. Contingency management refers to the therapist's use of approval and attention to reinforce adaptive behaviors and ignoring or disapproving unadaptive behaviors. His self-control techniques are essentially identical to those described previously (Rehm, 1981b) for self-monitoring, self-evaluating, and self-reinforcing.

In addition to early decisions about hospitalization and medication, a decision frequently is needed about involvement of the family or other components of the patient's social network. Liberman cited evidence that depressives are hypersensitive to criticism from significant others (Vaughn and Leff, 1976). Depending on the patient's treatment response and the ongoing assessment, additional modules designed to remedy social skill deficits, cognitive distortions, and anxiety problems may be employed in whatever sequence or degree needed; environmental manipulations may also be desirable. If resistance to treatment occurs, so-called strategic and paradoxical techniques are suggested (Haley, 1973).

Liberman very appropriately stressed that just as the type and dosage of medication must be individually tailored in clinical medicine, so must the application of treatment modules. Mechanical application of models is ill advised because of individual differences in causes, sustainers, and intra- and interpersonal and environmental resources. Tailoring should be guided mainly by the patient's and therapist's assessments of individual efficacy, as well as by data in the research literature.

It would be highly desirable if this section could conclude with specific recommendations about what subtypes of depressives would be most likely to respond best to what particular form of biological and/or psychosocial intervention. Regrettably, an able review of this scant literature on depressive outpatients by McLean (1981) concluded that no such experimentally validated knowledge exists as yet, though several studies have yielded somewhat promising leads.

Family Therapy

An allusion should also be made to the rapidly burgeoning use of family therapy in the treatment of depression. There has been little systematic evaluation of its efficacy and treatment protocols are not yet available. Nonetheless, some very useful source materials on this approach include work by Hinchliffe et al. (1978), Hogan and Hogan (1975), Liberman and Raskin (1971), and Liberman and Roberts (1976). The last two sources would probably be most adaptable by general practitioners.

Suicide Prevention

Anyone who undertakes the treatment of depression must be sensitive to the risks of suicide and of suicide attempts; the latter especially appear to be gradually increasing (Brown, 1979). The literature on the theory, research, assessment, and treatment of suicide and parasuicide (attempted suicide) has been ably reviewed by Linehan (1981).

What are the major characteristics of those who commit suicide and parasuicide? Usually they have recently experienced major emotional upsets and have inadequate social supports, their thinking tends to be rigid, they feel hopeless and powerless, and they are impulsive. There is considerable overlap between suicides and parasuicides, and a substantial proportion of parasuicides eventually commit suicide. The common notion that those who talk about suicide are unlikely to commit such behavior is incorrect. A total of 50–80% of those who engage in suicidal behavior communicate their intent beforehand; 48% of suicides see a physician within the week prior to death and 68% within 3 weeks. If the patient threatens suicide, it is important to clarify the nature and extent of suicidal plans. The Suicide Intent Scale, the Scale for Suicidal Ideation, and the Hopelessness Scale developed by Beck et al. (Beck et al., 1974a,b, 1979a) are useful resources for this purpose. Another bit of misguided folklore is that risk of suicide may be increased by inquiring about it. On the contrary, relief from suicidal impulses is more likely to occur and certainly the patient is likely to acquire an enhanced respect for the clinical competence of the interviewer. Patients rarely present with suicidal concerns as their major complaint.

There are no well-validated treatment strategies for dealing with suicidal behavior. A plethora of legal and ethical issues are inherent in suicide intervention. These issues have been discussed by Perlin (1975). If the therapist has serious reason to believe the patient may attempt suicide, it is extremely important that therapist and patient be as clear as possible about what actions the therapist would take if a suicide attempt is made or threatened. If feasible, these decisions should not be made amid a crisis. Alternatives that may or may not be acceptable could include involuntary hospitalization, notification of the police, family, and/or friends, lengthy phone involvements, or home visits. Follow-up contact with suicide attempters may not reduce the number of eventual suicides, but it does seem to reduce the number of subsequent parasuicides. However, data on this issue are scant. It appears that a high proportion of suicide attempters decline follow-up treatment, but occasional letters from would-be helpers that indicate unpressured continued interest seem to reduce the number of parasuicides.

In terms of treatment, the social isolation typical of suicide attempters makes it imperative that a trusting relationship be developed as rapidly as possible. Genuine concern is more likely to be helpful than an abundant display of superficial warmth. Since suicidal impulses usually reflect the patient's despair about resolving critical problems, treatment should be largely envisaged as training in how to cope with problems. Unrealistic expectancies should not be conveyed. In life, many problems can only be partially solved and some have to be endured while alternative gratifications are sought.

Specific interventions depend on the nature of the problem, the person, and the context; the instigators and reinforcers of suicidal tendencies need to be identified if possible. These are all highly individual matters.

Linehan (1981) summarized a number of additional helpful points in treating potential suicides. These include involving others who are significant in the patient's life in his/her care; assuring that not all treatment time is consumed in crisis intervention, as contrasted with basic long-term problem resolution; avoiding the assumption of undue responsibility for the patient's existence; being accessible when needed; giving the patient a "crisis card" with critical phone numbers for an emergency, including those of the therapist, hospital, crisis clinics, friends, and police; keeping addresses and telephone numbers important to the patient available in case of a crisis; making continuously renewed short-term antisuicide contracts with the patient; making clear that if the patient commits suicide, the therapist and others will be sad and disappointed, but will continue on with their living—the patient will be unable to witness any desired consequences of his or her act; and underscoring Mintz's (1971) maxim that "all forms of psychotherapy are ineffective with a dead patient."

Managing a suicidal patient can be very demanding. Periodic consultation with an experienced colleague is highly desirable.

In conclusion, formal training and consultation in the use of any of the modalities described in this chapter would be highly desirable. One of the easier to learn and best validated behavioral techniques is systematic desensitization, which is described in some detail in Chapter 19 on anxiety. Wolpe (1979) argued that many depressions result from chronic unresolved anxiety, and that desensitization of these anxiety instigators is often the method of choice. Unfortunately, no systematic data are yet available to support this contention. Both the assessment (Glazer et al., 1981; Hammen, 1981) and the treatment (Blaney, 1981) of depression are still in a formative, rapidly evolving, and promising phase of development. A growing appreciation of the inherent complexity of the problems involved (Hersen, 1981) is resulting in more appropriate, sophisticated, and diverse approaches (Coates and Wortman, 1980; Coyne et al. 1981).

References

American Psychiatric Association. 1980. Diagnostic and Statistical Manual of Mental Disorders, 3rd ed. (DSM III). Washington, DC: American Psychiatric Association.

Anisman, H., and R. M. Zacharko. 1982. Depression: The predisposing influence of stress. Behavioral and Brain Sciences.

Anthony, E. J. 1975. The influence of a manic-depressive environment on the developing child. In E. J. Anthony and T. Benedek, eds.: Depression and Human Existence. Boston, Massachusetts: Little, Brown; pp. 231–279.

Arieti, S., and J. Bemporad. 1978. Severe and Mild Depression: A Psychotherapeutic Approach. New York: Basic Books.

Bandura, A. 1977. Self-efficacy: Toward a unifying theory of behavioral change. Psychological Review 84:191–216.

Bandura, A., and D. H. Schunk. 1981. Cultivating competence, self-efficacy, and intrinsic interest through proximal self-motivation. Journal of Personality and Social Psychology 41:586–598.

Beach, R. H., L. Y. Abramson, and F. M. Levine. 1981. Attributional reformulation of learned helplessness and depression: Therapeutic implications. In J. F. Clarkin and H. I. Glazer, eds.: Depression: Behavioral and Directive Intervention Strategies. New York: Garland STPM Press; pp. 131–169.

Beck, A. T. 1967. Depression: Clinical, Experimental, and Theoretical Aspects. New York: Harper and Row.

Beck, A. T., and Bedrosian, R. C. 1980. Principles of cognitive therapy. In M. D. Mahoney, eds.: Psychotherapy Process: Current Issues and Future Directions. New York: Plenum Press.

Beck, A. T., D. Schuyler, and I. Herman. 1974a. Development of suicidal intent scales. In A. T. Beck, H. L. P. Resnik, and D. J. Lettieri, eds.: The Prediction of Suicide. Bowie, Maryland: Charles Press.

Beck, A. T., A. Weissman, D. Lester, and L. Trexler. 1974b. The measurement of pessimism: The hopelessness scale. Journal of Consulting and Clinical Psychology 42:861–865.

Beck, A. T., M. Kovacs, and A. Weissman. 1979a. Assessment of suicidal intention: The scale for suicide ideation. Journal of Consulting and Clinical Psychology 47:343–352.

Beck, A. T., A. J. Rush, B. F. Shaw, and G. Emery. 1979b. Cognitive Therapy of Depression. New York: Guilford Press.

Becker, J. 1974. Depression: Theory and Research. Washington, D.C.: Winston-Wiley.

Becker, J. 1977. Affective Disorders. Morristown, New Jersey: General Learning Press.

Becker, J. 1979. Vulnerable self-esteem as a predisposing factor in depressive disorders. In R. Depue, ed.: The Psychobiology of the Depressive Disorders: Implications for the Effects of Stress. New York: Academic Press.

Becker, J., and M. A. Schuckit. 1978. On the comparative efficacy of cognitive therapy and pharmacotherapy in the treatment of depressions. Cognitive Therapy and Research 2:193–197.

Bem, D. 1972. Self-perception therapy. Advances in Experimental Social Psychology 6:1–62.

Bertalanffy, L. 1976. General system theory and psychiatry. In S. Arieti, ed.: American Handbook of Psychiatry, Vol. 3. New York: Basic Books; pp. 705–721.

Bibring, E. 1953. The mechanism of depression. In P. Greenacre, ed.: Affective Disorders. New York: International Universities Press.

Blaney, P. H. 1981. The effectiveness of cognitive and behavioral therapies. In L. P. Rehm, ed.: Behavior Therapy for Depression: Present Status and Future Directions. New York: Academic Press; pp. 1–33.

Bonime, W. 1976. The psychodynamics of neurotic depression. Journal of the American Academy of Psychoanalysis 4:301–326.

Bowlby, J. 1980. Attachment and Loss, Vol. 3: Loss, Sadness and Depression. New York: Basic Books.

Brown, G. W., and T. Harris. 1978. Social Origins of Depression: A Study of Psychiatric disorder in Women. New York: Free Press.

Brown, J. H. 1979. Suicide in Britain. Archives of General Psychiatry 36:1119–1124.

Coates, D., and C. B. Wortman. 1980. Depression maintenance and interpersonal control. In A. Baum, J. Singer, and Y. Epstein, eds.: Advances in Environmental Psychology, Vol. 2. Hillsdale, New Jersey: Lawrence Erlbaum Associates, pp. 149–181.

Coleman, R. E., and A. T. Beck. 1981. Cognitive therapy for depression. In J. F. Clarkin and H. I. Glazer, eds.: Depression: Behavioral and Directive Intervention Strategies. New York: Garland STPM Press; pp. 111–131.

Coyne, J. C., C. Aldwin, and R. S. Lazarus. 1981. Depression and coping in stressful episodes. Journal of Abnormal Psychology 90:439–447.

Depue, R. A., and S. M. Monroe. 1978. Learned helplessness in the perspective of the depressive disorders: Conceptual and definitional issues. Journal of Abnormal Psychology 87:3–21.

DiMascio, A., M. M. Weissman, B. A. Prusoff, C Neu, M. Swilling, and G. L. Klerman. 1979. Differential symptom reduction by drugs and psychotherapy in acute depression. Archives of General Psychiatry 36:1450–1456.

Fay, A., and A. A. Lazarus. 1981. Multimodal therapy and the problems of depression. In J. F. Clarkin and H. I. Glazer, eds.: Depression: Behavioral and Directive Intervention Strategies. New York: Garland STPM Press; pp. 169–179.

Frank, J. D. 1973. Persuasion and Healing. Baltimore, Maryland: Johns Hopkins Press.

Freud, S. 1917. Mourning and melancholia. In J. Strachey, ed.: Collected Works of Sigmund Freud: The Standard Edition, Vol. 14. London, England: Hogarth Press (reprinted 1957).

Garber, J., and M. E. P. Seligman. 1980. Human Helplessness: Theory and Applications. New York: Academic Press.

Glazer, H. I., J. F. Clarkin, and H. F. Hunt. 1981. Assessment of depression. In J. F. Clarkin and H. I. Glazer, eds.: Depression: Behavioral and Directive Intervention Strategies. New York: Garland STPM Press; pp. 3–31.

Haley, J. 1973. Uncommon Therapy: The Psychiatric Techniques of Milton A. Erickson. New York: W. W. Norton.

Hamilton, M. 1980. Rating depressive patients. Journal of Clinical Psychiatry 41:21–24.

Hammen, C. L. 1981. Assessment: A clinical and cognitive emphasis. In L. P. Rehm, ed.: Behavior Therapy for Depression: Present Status and Future Directions. New York: Academic Press; pp. 255–279.

Harrison, A. A. 1977. Mere exposure. Advances in Experimental Social Psychology 10:40–86.

Henderson, S. 1977. The social network, support and neurosis: The function of attachment in adult life. British Journal of Psychiatry 131:185–191.

Hersen, M. 1981. Complex problems require complex solutions. Behavior Therapy 12:15–29.

Hinchliffe, M. K., D. Hooper, and J. F. Roberts. 1978. The Melancholy Marriage: Depression, Marriage and Psychosocial Approaches to Therapy. New York: Wiley.

Hirschfeld, R. M. A., G. L. Klerman, P. Chodoff, S. Korchin, and J. Barrett. 1976. Dependency, self-esteem, clinical depression. Journal of the American Academy of Psychoanalysis 4:373–388.

Hogan, P., and B. K. Hogan. 1975. The family treatment of depression. In F. F. Flach and S. C. Draghi, eds.: The Nature and Treatment of Depression. New York: Wiley; pp. 197–229.

Hollon, S. D., and J. Garber. 1980. A cognitive–expectancy theory of therapy for helplessness and depression. In J. Barber and M. E. P. Seligman, eds.: Human Helplessness: Theory and Applications. New York: Academic Press; pp. 173–197.

Izard, C. E. 1977. Theories of emotion and emotion–behavior relationships. In C. E. Izard, eds.: Human Emotions. New York: Plenum Press; pp. 19–42.

Kanfer, F. H., and S. Hagerman. 1981. The role of self-regulation. In L. P. Rehm, eds.: Behavior Therapy for Depression. New York: Academic Press; pp. 143–181.

Klerman, G. L., B. J. Rounsaville, E. Chevron, and C. Neu, and M. M. Weissman. 1979. Manual for Short-Term Interpersonal Psychotherapy (IPT) of Depression, unpublished manuscript, 4th revision.

Kovacs, M., A. J. Rush, A. T. Beck, and S. D. Hollon. 1981. Depressed outpatients treated with cognitive therapy or pharmacotherapy. Archives of General Psychiatry 38:33–39.

Langer, E. J., and A. Benevento. 1978. Self-induced dependence. Journal of Personality and Social Psychology 36:886–893.

Lazarus, A. A. 1981. The Practice of Multimodal Therapy. New York: McGraw-Hill.

Lewinsohn, P. M., and M. Arconad. 1981. Social learning and depression. In J. F. Clarkin and H. I. Glazer, eds.: Depression: Behavioral and Directive Intervention Strategies. New York: Garland STPM Press; pp. 33–68.

Lewinsohn, P. M., R. F. Munoz, M. A. Youngren, and A. M. Zeiss. 1978. Control Your Depression. Englewood Cliffs, New Jersey: Prentice-Hall.

Liberman, R. P. 1981. A model for individualizing treatment. In L. Rehm, ed.: Behavior Therapy for Depression. New York: Academic Press; pp. 231–255.

Liberman, R. P., and D. E. Raskin. 1971. Depression: A behavioral formulation. Archives of General Psychiatry 24:515–523.

Liberman, R. P., and J. Roberts. 1976. Contingency management of neurotic depression and marital disharmony. In H. J. Eysenck, ed.: Case Studies in Behaviour Therapy. London, England: Routledge and Kegan Paul; pp. 205–225.

Linehan, M. M. 1981. A social behavioral analysis of suicide and parasuicide: Implications for clinical assessment and treatment. In J. F. Clarkin and H. I. Glazer, eds.: Depression: Behavioral and Directive Intervention Strategies. New York: Garland STPM Press; pp. 229–295.

Lubin, B., and E. E. Levitt. 1979. Norms for the depression adjective check lists: Age, group and sex. Journal of Consulting and Clinical Psychology 47:192.

McLean, P. D. 1981. Matching treatment to patient characteristics in an outpatient setting. In L. P. Rehm, ed.: Behavior Therapy for Depression. New York: Academic Press; pp. 197–209.

Mintz, R. S. 1971. Basic considerations in the psychotherapy of the depressed suicidal patient. American Journal of Psychotherapy 25:56–73.

Perlin, S. (ed.). 1975. A Handbook for the Study of Suicide. New York: Oxford University Press.

Prusoff, B. A., M. M. Weissman, G. L. Klerman, and B. J. Rounsaville. 1980. Research diagnostic criteria subtypes of depression: Their role as predictors of differential response to psychotherapy and drug treatment. Archives of General Psychiatry 37:796–801.

Rapaport, D. 1959. The structure of psychoanalytic theory: A systematizing attempt. In S. Koch, ed.: Psychology: A Study of a Science, Vol. 3. New York: McGraw-Hill; pp. 55–184.

Rehm, L. P. (ed.). 1981a. Behavior Therapy for Depression: Present Status and Future Directions. New York: Academic Press.

Rehm, L. P. 1981b. A self-control therapy program for treatment of depression. In J. F. Clarkin and H. I. Glazer, eds.: Depression: Behavioral and Directive Intervention Strategies. New York: Garland STPM Press; pp. 68–111.

Rounsaville, B. J., G. L. Klerman, and M. M. Weissman. 1981. Do psychotherapy and pharmacotherapy conflict? Archives of General Psychiatry 38:24–33.

Seligman, M. E. P. 1981. A learned helplessness point of view. In L. P. Rehm, ed.: Behavior Therapy for Depression: Present Status and Future Directions. New York: Academic Press; pp. 123–143.

Siggins, L. D. 1966. Mourning: A critical survey of the literature. International Journal of Psychoanalysis 47:14–25.

Spitzer, R. L., J. P. Endicott, and E. Robins. 1978. Research diagnostic criteria. Archives of General Psychiatry 35:773–786.

Stainbrook, E. J. 1977. Depression: The psychosocial context. In G. Usdin, ed.: Depression: Clinical, Biological and Psychological Perspectives. New York: Brunner/Mazel.

Sullivan, H. S. 1954. The Psychiatric Interview. New York: W. W. Norton.

Vaughn, C. E., and L. P. Leff. 1976. The influence of family and social factors on the course of psychiatric illness. British Journal of Psychiatry 129:125–137.

Weissman, M. 1979. The psychological treatment of depression. Archives of General Psychiatry 36:1261–1269.

Weissman, M., and E. S. Paykel. 1974. The Depressed Woman: A Study of Social Relationships. Chicago, Ilinois: University of Chicago Press.

Weissman, M., B. Prusoff, and G. L. Klerman. 1981. In reply to: Drugs and psychotherapy in acute depression. Archives of General Psychiatry 38:115–116.

Wolpe, J. 1979. The experimental model and treatment of neurotic depression. Behaviour Research and Therapy 17:555–565.

Zeiss, A. M., P. M. Lewinsohn, and R. F. Munoz. 1979. Nonspecific improvement effects in depression using interpersonal skills training, pleasant activities schedules or cognitive training. Journal of Consulting and Clinical Psychology 47:427–439.

Zetzel, E. R. 1965. Depression and the capacity to bear it. In M. Schur, ed.: Drives, Affects, Behavior. Vol. 2. New York: International University Press; pp. 243–277.

Zigler, E., and L. Phillips. 1961. Psychiatric diagnoses and symptomatology. Journal of Abnormal and Social Psychology 63:69–75.

19

Anxiety and Insomnia
in Medical Practice

Nicholas G. Ward, M.D.,* Joseph Becker, Ph.D.† and
John A. Chiles, M.D.‡

While depression is the most common psychiatric diagnosis, anxiety and anxiety-induced insomnia are the most common psychological complaints in medical practice. People with anxiety-related problems represent approximately 30% of patients seeking help from primary care physicians (Pitts, 1971). Frequently, these patients complain about somatic symptoms related to anxiety—for example, heart racing, diarrhea, upset stomach—rather than about the anxiety itself. When both the patient and physician maintain a strictly somatic orientation, the underlying anxiety frequently goes unrecognized. In the following discussions it will be assumed that anxiety is not a unitary phenomenon but, rather, a complex and variable response involving cognitive and physiological reactions.

Normal Versus Pathological Anxiety

The presence of anxiety and anxiety-related symptoms does not automatically imply pathology. Anxiety in moderation can be and often is highly adaptive. Janis (1958) theorized that optimal learning and adaptation to a variety of problems occurs at moderate rather than high or low levels of anxiety arousal. This inverted-U relation between arousal and behavioral efficiency varies with task difficulty and complexity. Optimal functioning on simple tasks is found at moderately high levels of arousal,

*Associate Professor, Department of Psychiatry and Behavioral Sciences, University of Washington School of Medicine, Seattle, Washington.

† Professor, Department of Psychiatry and Behavioral Sciences, University of Washington School of Medicine, Seattle, Washington.

‡ Associate Professor, Department of Psychiatry and Behavioral Sciences, University of Washington School of Medicine, Seattle, Washington.

whereas complex, difficult tasks require moderately low, relaxed–attentive levels of arousal for optimum performance.

Studies in medical settings support this conclusion. In one study, surgical patients with moderate levels of preoperative fear showed the lowest levels of anger, complaining, and fear postoperatively, and recovered most rapidly, whereas the low-fear group had the poorest postoperative adjustment (Janis, 1971). This and other studies suggest that good postoperative adjustment requires some preoperative arousal. In addition to arousal, information about what to expect from and how to cope with the situation increases adaptiveness (Ley, 1977). Thus it is not necessarily appropriate for physicians to provide blanket reassurance or to emplore patients to "not worry."

While moderate levels of anxiety may be normal and adaptive, the ability to vary anxiety levels in response to different situations is also desirable. Most people have a characteristic range of anxiety responses that is relatively fixed and which can be viewed as a personality trait. This form is called trait anxiety (Spielberger et al., 1971). In clinical settings, when trait anxiety is uniformly high and maladaptive, it is called chronic anxiety. In contrast to trait anxiety, the anxiety response at a particular time and situation is called state anxiety. By definition, it is not fixed and is time limited. In clinical settings, when state anxiety is high and maladaptive, it is referred to as acute anxiety. As will be discussed later, acute anxiety may continue beyond the particular stressful situation and become chronic anxiety.

How then is pathological anxiety diagnosed? In diagnosing an anxiety syndrome, the presence of both psychological and physiological symptoms should be elicited (Davis et al., 1981). The psychological symptoms include apprehensive expectation or anticipatory fear either of unknown danger or out of proportion to known specific events. Hypervigilance, in which the person becomes hyperattentive to the point of distractability, irritability, or insomnia, is also frequently present. Physiological symptoms include motor tension (tremors, twitches, muscle aches, jitters) and autonomic hyperactivity (sweating, heart racing, frequent urination, diarrhea, dizziness, hot or cold spells). Making the diagnosis of anxiety can be difficult when the patient presents only with physiological symptoms, since each of these symptoms may represent a host of other medical disorders. For example, if patients complain only of headache or diarrhea, direct but supportive questioning may reveal additional symptoms of an anxiety syndrome that they have been reluctant to reveal.

Just eliciting the patient's report of anxiety-related symptoms is not enough. Many of these symptoms may exist with normal anxiety. Normal and pathological anxieties are quantitatively and not qualitatively different. In pathological anxiety, the anxiety is high and maladaptive. A person with an anxiety syndrome has decreased functioning because of the anxiety:

The physiological symptoms are distressing and disturbing normal functioning and/or the psychological symptoms are interferring with the individual's ability to cope. Even when complete information is available, diagnosing anxiety is not a simple task. There are no concrete or cardinal signs; rather, the physician will have to exercies considerable judgment, for example, when concluding that the patient's emotional reactions are out of proportion to the situation. Often the diagnosis will require negotiation with the patient as described by Rosen and Kleinman in Chapter 5.

Anxiety Secondary to Medical Problems

Normal or even acute anxiety may occur in response to or along with a medical problem. However, a variety of other conditions can present with anxiety as the chief complaint. The differential diagnosis of anxiety should rule out the medical syndromes described below (Dietch, 1981; Rakel, 1981). Fortunately, each of these other syndromes has relatively distinctive features that can help a clinician differentiate them from a pure anxiety syndrome.

1. Caffeine overuse. This is frequently not recognized by patients as the cause of their anxiety symptoms. For example, in the elderly, increased sensitivity to caffeine can precipitate a new anxietylike syndrome in a person who has maintained a constant intake over the years. Only a reduction in caffeine intake will relieve the symptoms.
2. Alcohol or sedative withdrawal. Frequently, the patient will not recognize this as a cause of anxiety but, rather, will see it only as a treatment of anxiety. Direct questioning about alcohol and sedative use is necessary, as many patients may try to conceal this. If the patient had been using long-lasting sedatives such as diazepam, withdrawal symptoms might not appear for 4–7 days following drug discontinuation.
3. Hyperthyroidism. In this syndrome, a fine tremor and heat intolerance usually accompany symptoms of anxiety.
4. Pheochromocytoma. This is a rare catecholamine-secreting tremor that produces marked episodic elevations of blood pressure and vasomotor lability in conjunction with acute exacerbations of anxiety.
5. Hypoglycemia. A constellation of symptoms including hunger, weakness, headache, sweating, and palpitations will accompany this anxiety, which can be reversed by glucose ingestion. Differentiating anxiety from hypoglycemia is somewhat complicated by the fact that anxiety can worsen glucose tolerance.

6. Cardiopulmonary disorders. (a) Recurrent pulmonary emboli produce repeated episodes of acute anxiety with hyperventilation or dyspnea in conjunction with decreased oxygen concentration in the blood. Functional anxiety is associated with slightly increased oxygen concentrations. (b) Paroxysmal atrial tachycardia starts with a sudden increase in heart rate and then, unlike anxiety syndromes, suddenly decreases. (c) Mitral valve prolapse, while diagnosed by auscultation and echocardiagram, is less clearly differentiated from anxiety syndromes. It occurs much more commonly in patients with anxiety but does not change after the anxiety is satisfactorily treated.
7. Organic brain syndrome secondary to delirium, head trauma, or temporal lobe epilepsy. Careful history taking is important.

Anxiety Secondary to Other Psychiatric Problems

Differentiating anxiety from depression is somewhat more difficult (Rakel, 1981). Since the frequency of these mixed anxiety depressions is perhaps as high as 50%, patients complaining mainly of anxiety who have definite symptoms of the depressive syndrome should be treated as having depression. Antidepressants have been shown to be more effective than antianxiety agents in this group. While these anxious depressives may not complain of depression, they usually do experience anhedonia, a distinct loss of pleasure in situations that were formerly enjoyable, along with other classic depressive symptoms, such as insomnia, anorexia, and fatigue.

The early paranoid schizophrenic with extensive anxiety is more easily diagnosed. He or she manifests disorganized thinking, will be suspicious and distrustful, and may appear to be emotionally remote, with very constricted affect.

It is very important for the physician to be able to recognize anxiety in patients who are not complaining of it. High levels of anxiety can exacerbate a wide variety of medical conditions, including gastric and duodenal ulcers, ulcerative colitis, asthma, hypertension, hives, hypoglycemia, and some seizure disorders. It may also be an important component in the aggressive, pressured type A cardiac personality, who is at increased risk for myocardial infarction (Rosenman, 1971).

What should be done when anxiety exists and it is not secondary to a medical condition or some other psychiatric condition? Because there are several forms of anxiety, the physician should obtain a clear description of the course and nature of the anxiety. The following are descriptions of the major types of anxiety syndromes, with outlines of their treatment (Sheehan, 1982). They rely on two main dichotomies, endogenous versus exogenous and acute versus chronic.

Acute Endogenous Anxiety

After determining that a patient has pathological anxiety, it is important to ask if there is any reason for the anxiety. If the physician determines that there is no adequate reason, that it came "out of the blue" with panic attacks, a diagnosis of acute endogenous anxiety can be made. Sheehan (1982) noted that many of these patients only acknowledge the somatic symptoms and do not complain of the psychological symptoms of anxiety. Contrary to earlier psychoanalytic formulations, this endogenous anxiety appears to respond best to pharmacological and behavioral approaches and analytic therapy accomplishes no more than placebo.

While depression is not often seen in the early stages of endogenous anxiety, the antidepressants—including tricyclic antidepressants such as imipramine, monoamine oxidase inhibitors such as phenelzine, and a newer benzodiazepine, alprazolam—all are capable of blocking endogenous panic attacks.

Acute Exogenous Anxiety: Situational Versus Phobic

Patients who identify specific stressors are considered to have exogenous anxiety. It should then be determined if the anxiety is out of proportion to the specific precipitant. If it is not out of proportion, it is called *situational or reactive anxiety*. If the anxiety appears to be out of proportion to the situation, it can be referred to as *phobic anxiety*.

For most cases of acute situational anxiety support and reassurance are sufficient. The physician should be a calm, warm, receptive listener in such situations. Most people find it reassuring to discuss their anxiety with an understanding person who remains calm and supportive. When the stressor is specific, as in post-traumatic stress disorder, repeated talking about the stressful event can be very therapeutic. In other cases, the stressor creating the anxiety may not always be obvious and straightforward. Searching for and finding the stressor(s) may help the patient begin to develop a sense of mastery over the situation. The physician should keep in mind that some anxiety is a normal part of living and that anxiety with an acute onset is usually of brief duration. Generally, the physician should share this information, as most patients find it reassuring to find that they are not alone in their misery and that the situation will not go on forever. This should be communicated in a caring, noncondescending manner. Patients are not reassured by suggestions that they "just have anxiety" and not a medical problem. The physician should indicate that they appreciate the degree of the patient's distress.

When should medication be considered in acute anxiety? If the patient is actually having trouble functioning and reassurance is not working, then medications may be helpful. As discussed previously, for some patients the anxiety not only is unpleasant but may significantly interfere with their ability to cope with situations that, in turn, may increase the anxiety further. The inability to cope needs to be carefully assessed. Frequently, very anxious people will feel that they cannot handle a situation, but in fact do quite well. To determine if this is a subjective experience or a reality, the physician should ask for specific examples of stressful situations and for the patient's approach to coping with them. Sometimes straightforward advice on other strategies may be helpful, but if the anxiety is paralyzing the patient's ability to act, medications may be in order.

Before prescribing medications, the physician should be aware that the placebo effect in acute situational anxiety is very great. More than 80% of patients with acute anxiety respond well to a placebo (Rickels, 1972). While talking with a physician helps many patients, others have the expectation that medication is the real source of help for them. If their anxiety is disabling and their belief in the medication firm, then medications certainly can help. In these cases, the patient can be given a prescription that takes maximum advantage of placebo effects. A time-limited prescription using very small multiple doses of a long-acting benzodiazepine may be especially helpful and yet minimizes the risk of tolerance, addiction, or side effects. Thus the small amount of "true" antianxiety effect may be immensely amplified by the placebo effect. However, if this fails, more usual dosing and administration of medication should be considered.

Behavioral approaches such as desensitization and relaxation training can also be helpful in acute reactive anxiety. These approaches are best suited for acute phobic anxiety, acute reactive anxiety with a well-defined precipitant, and, as will be discussed later, various aspects of chronic anxiety. The desensitization approaches take time and practice and so are better suited to reliable, conscientious patients and work best on mild to moderate levels of anxiety. Immediate, *in vivo*, if possible, mastery-oriented, counterphobic, and behavioral approaches are recommended for the acutely phobic patient. Each time the patient avoids the phobic situation, the phobic gains strength. Immediate interventions can prevent a chronic course.

Chronic Endogenous Anxiety

In some individuals anxiety symptoms become chronic, persist for more than 6 months, and do not appear to be directly related to specific stressors. A careful exploration of the clinical course of this anxiety reveals panic attacks or subpanic symptom attacks at the onset. The subpanic symptom attacks may consist of brief episodes of heart palpitation and/or hyperventilation, but without the entire constellation of panic symptoms. Unlike exogenous anxiety, in which there is no age group or sex at particular risk, endogenous anxiety usually begins between 20 and 30 years of age and 85% of those affected are women (Sheehan, 1982). If these patients are not treated immediately, they are at risk for a large and bewildering array of secondary symptoms and presentations.

People with panic attacks frequently progress to *hypochondriasis*. Their palpitations make them fear that there is something wrong with their heart and hyperventilation can make them fear that there is something wrong with their lungs. If the panic attack occurs in a particular situation, as on a bridge or in an elevator, a *single phobia* may develop. If the panic attack occurs in a social setting, a *social phobia* may develop. As more and more panic attacks occur in a wide variety of circumstances, a person may develop *multiple phobias* and *pananxiety*. To avoid these perceived dangers the same person may decide to stay at home and may be mislabeled as having *agoraphobia*, a fear of open spaces. As suffering continues, depression may ensue and the person will be labeled as having *atypical depression*.

Patients who have progressed to chronic endogenous anxiety usually need more than just medications that are recommended for acute endogenous anxiety. The secondary symptoms described above may become autonomous and persist after the panic attacks are relieved. Psychological and behavioral interventions are then generally required.

Chronic Phobic Anxiety. Phobias untreated in the acute stages can easily become chronic, persisting for more than 6 months. A person who avoids a phobic situation(s) will experience a decrease in anxiety upon performing this behavior. Thus the phobic behavior is rewarded and strengthened with each exposure. For example, if a man is afraid of elevators, he may become increasingly anxious as he gets closer to one. While he may be determined to use the elevator, if at the last minute he chooses to use the stairs, he will be rewarded with substantial relief from his anxiety. The next time he is confronted with the possibility of using an elevator it will be even easier to choose the stairs. Thus this elevator phobia strengthens rather than diminishes with time as a result of negative reinforcement.

Phobias that substantially affect the normal course of living are frequently accompanied by extensive secondary anxiety. An affected person may then begin to worry about phobic situations before they actually occur. While specific behavioral treatment for the phobia(s) is recommended first, the general anxiety that may accompany the phobia(s) may require more extensive psychotherapeutic work.

Chronic Situational Anxiety. In some individuals the "normal" anxiety associated with specific stressors does not diminish. This may occur either because the stressors themselves have not diminished or because a person has developed a maladaptive style in dealing with stressors. An example of the former situation would be working as an air traffic controller at a very busy airport or being poor in a threatening, high-crime neighborhood. An example of the latter situation would be a person with a "Chicken Little" approach to life, in which the sky is always falling.

Frequently chronically anxious people are catastrophizers, seeing the worst possibilities in relatively benign situations. They may then handle these situations so poorly as to make the worst possibilities come true. Others may have ongoing conscious or unconscious conflicts that continue to produce anxiety. For example, a person who wants to be seen as likable all of the time may experience considerable anxiety on a chronic basis. In this person the threat of not being liked may be consciously or unconsciously present, and unacceptable feelings such as anger may exacerbate the anxiety still further.

Because the mechanisms maintaining chronic anxiety are often complex and initially unclear, its treatment is usually difficult. While medications may be transiently effective in relieving anxiety symptoms, there is a risk that they then will be taken on a chronic basis, with the attendant problems of tolerance, physical and psychological dependence, and addiction. Simple reassurance and a problem-solving approach as recommended in the treatment of acute anxiety are seldom sufficient for the chronically anxious patient. Such patients need more extensive treatment, with the occasional judicious use of medication.

When and how should medications be used in chronic anxiety? As with acute anxiety, the physician should decide if the anxiety is dysfunctional. Some patients, particularly those prone to alcoholism and drug addiction, may believe that life should be lived with no anxiety and that any anxiety experienced is unacceptable. Psychotherapy and counseling, not anti-anxiety medication, should be considered for these patients. Patients who have chronic anxiety may have episodes of acute exacerbation during which functioning is quite impaired. Medications can be considered in these patients, but strict limits should be made. A definite time limit on the use of the medications should be agreed on in advance. Periods between 1 and 5–6 weeks are generally used. During this time the patient should also be receiving psychotherapeutic help in order to break out of the chronic pattern. Frequently patients will push to extend the prescription further. In many cases this will be counterproductive, as the patient ultimately will have to learn how to manage chronic anxiety without medication.

Occasionally there is an indication for prolonged use of medication. Some chronically anxious patients obtain significant relief from antianxiety agents and will not engage in psychotherapeutic approaches or get little or no benefit from them. It seems reasonable and fair to consider these patients for long-term treatment with medications. In such cases, careful safeguards and surveillance should be established. The patient should be seen regularly and evaluated for efficacy of treatment and for the development of problems.

Treatment of Chronic Anxiety. Treatment of chronic undifferentiated anxiety tends to be most effective if pharmacotherapy is combined with some form of psychotherapy (Luborsky et al., 1975). Medication alone will alleviate the somatic aspects of anxiety, but it is often ineffective in alleviating the cognitive–emotional aspects of the disorder (Freedman et al., 1981). There are variants of psychotherapy, but there is no clear evidence yet as to which is most effective. The optimal approach has to be tailored to the needs of the individual.

Effective psychotherapeutic intervention first requires an assessment and the formulation of some hypotheses about what especially threatens the patient. Even though the conditions surrounding the onset of the patient's chronic anxiety may be vague, it is usually possible to get useful information about contexts that significantly increase or lessen the anxiety over time. Some patients will claim that they are always highly anxious, but persistent, low-keyed, nonthreatening inquiry and encouragement to reflect more carefully frequently yields a much more differentiated affective history. Identification of current and past conditions under which the patient functioned with least anxiety and greatest efficacy can provide valuable therapeutic leads.

Low self-esteem, social skill deficits, and threats to significant relationships frequently contribute to chronic anxiety and ultimately to depression. People with low self-esteem are easily threatened by a wide variety of their own impulses (thoughts, feelings, desires, expectancies) and by their perceptions of their external circumstances. Mediocre social skills often accompany this low self-esteem, resulting in inadequate and tenuous social support systems. If a significant relationship is threatened, anxiety with its mobilization of fight or flight responses may actually be a favorable sign. Depression with the attendant resignation and the despair suggests a poorer prognosis.

Sometimes anxiety is clearly secondary or reactive to skill deficits, in which case it makes more sense to focus initially on the skill deficit. For example, if a patient is objectively as well as subjectively socially inept and hence acutely anxious about social situations, treatment may progress more rapidly by social skill training that involves rehearsing performances in imagination and in practice. However, if the anxiety associated with social context is so high as to impede skill acquisition, it makes better sense to deal with the anxiety first. Likewise, if the patient has adequate skills that are inhibited by anxiety, it makes good sense to address the anxiety initially. The desensitization techniques described in the following sections on simple phobias may be especially helpful techniques for alleviating situationally specific anxieties.

Transient improvement is not uncommon with the application of relatively simple cognitive–behavioral techniques to delimited aspects of the patient's difficulties; however, follow-up suggests that a substantial proportion of relapses occur unless patients experience improved self-esteem and social skills, as well as a change in their perspectives on living. Because relationships with significant others are often a major source of anxiety, this person(s) should be involved in the treatment process.

Several studies indicate that about two-thirds of patients with diagnosible anxiety neuroses who seek treatment show considerable improvement upon follow-up, whether they were treated or not (Noyes et al., 1980). Most studies find that chronic anxiety states without phobic symptoms respond better to treatment. The chief risk with inadequately treated or untreated chronic anxiety appears to be the development of secondary depression, with its attendant suicidal risk.

Behavioral Treatments: Phobias

Systematic desensitization is one of the most effective and best validated cognitive–behavioral methods for treating relatively specific phobias and situational anxieties. This method involves training the patient to relax deeply and then to visualize in sequence a hierarchy of items related to his or her fears. The items in the hierarchy are ranked in order of increasing anxiety elicitation. Consider the example of the patient who fears bridges. During the first several sessions the physician should get a detailed account of the history and nature of the fear, including the patient's fantasies about what are the most frightening things that could happen in the situation. If the patient's thoughts or fantasies reveal some strong suicidal tendencies that the physician has reason to believe might be acted upon, he may well choose to refer the patient to a mental health professional. If no such life-threatening material or underlying psychopathology is elicited, the physician will want to accomplish three objectives during the first several sessions.

The first step is to instruct the patient in the rationale for systematic desensitization. Essentially, the patient is told that fears are learned or conditioned and can be unlearned or counterconditioned. It is impossible to be tense and relaxed at the same time. By training the patient to be deeply relaxed while visualizing a series of items that are ordered from least to most anxiety provoking, his or her anxiety will gradually be counterconditioned. The whole procedure is carried out in a warm, supportive manner.

The second step is to train the patient in progressive relaxation. This procedure may initially require 20–35 minutes but diminishes very rapidly thereafter. Recordings are available for this purpose (advertised in behavioral therapy journals) or the specific methods are detailed in most volumes on behavioral therapy (e.g., Paul, 1966). The patient should be instructed to practice desensitization at home several times a day between sessions.

The third task during these initial sessions is either to instruct the patient on how to generate a 10- to 15-item hierarchy or to jointly construct one with him. Various kinds of stimulus dimensions might be used in our case example, for example, spatial or temporal proximity to the bridge or the structural similarity of bridges to a particularly feared bridge (see Wolpe and Lazarus, 1966, for detailed instructions).

Once the patient seems able to relax reasonably well, desensitization to the feared stimuli begins. First the patient is encouraged to visualize a particularly pleasing and relaxing scene of his choice. After about 10 seconds the patient is told to stop visualizing and additional relaxation instructions are given for 30–45 seconds. The patient is told that if anxiety reoccurs at any time he should raise his right index finger without speaking as as not to disrupt this relaxed state. Treatment then proceeds by starting with the least anxiety-provoking item in the hierarchy. As each item is presented, the patient signals whether or not he is experiencing anxiety. When anxiety occurs, the patient is instructed to concentrate on relaxation. If the item is too acutely provoking, it may have to be placed higher in the hierarchy or transitional items may have to be interpolated into the hierarchy. A session should never end on an item that is still evoking anxiety. If necessary, the therapist should end by returning to an earlier successful item. Patients are brought back to a fully alert status from deep relaxation by the numerical method of trance termination, in which the patient is told that he will count from 1 to 4 and gradually move additional specified parts of his body until achieving full alertness.

While systematic desensitization appears to be a relatively simple procedure, it would be wise to obtain consultation in initial cases and periodically thereafter. Capably used, it is a versatile and highly effective tool. Marks' (1969) *Fears and Phobias* contains a very readable yet scholarly account of psychological perspectives on situationally or object-specific irrational fears.

Insomnia. Difficulty falling asleep (onset insomnia) commonly occurs with anxiety, whereas difficulty staying asleep (middle and late insomnia) occurs more commonly with depression. Frequently patients present with insomnia rather than with anxiety or depression. While often wedded to anxiety or depression, it should be explored as a problem in itself. At any given time 30% of the population will complain of insomnia and over the age of 60 the prevalence of insomnia increases to 60%. Besides age, other risk factors include lower socioeconomic status and being female (Karacan et al., 1976).

While the psychological factors of anxiety or depression may lead to insomnia, there are also situational and physical causes of insomnia that should be considered (Regestein, 1976). The need for sleep decreases with age. People who once needed 8 hours of sleep per night may only need 6 or 7 hours of sleep when they are older. The most effective approach to this problem is education and reassurance. Elderly patients should be informed of this change in sleep need and told to schedule fewer hours in bed. Napping, which will further decrease the need for nighttime sleep, should be discouraged in an older patient insistent on sleeping as much as possible during the night.

Other physical causes of insomnia include the following.

1. Pain, as nocturnal angina or arthritis.
2. Itching.
3. Hypermetabolic states, particularly hyperthyroidism.
4. Pregnancy, owing to discomfort, hypermetabolism, and frequent urination.
5. Involuntary movements such as restless legs syndrome, nocturnal cramps, and myoclonus.
6. Nocturia, which is frequently seen in diabetes, congestive heart failure, and urinary tract infections.
7. Chemical causes, for example, alcohol or sedative/hypnotic withdrawal or stimulant ingestion.

In addition to physical causes of insomnia, there are several situational or environmental causes of insomnia:

1. Change of normal bedtime, which is particularly severe in people who work variable shifts.
2. Change of sleep location.
3. Vigorous exercise near bedtime.
4. Discomfort such as a lumpy bed, noise, heat, and humidity.

While many of these physical and situational causes for insomnia may seem obvious, patients may only complain of insomnia and not associate the problem with these causes. The physician should carefully explore possible causes for insomnia. Many cases of insomnia can be managed best by treating these underlying problems.

Cognitive–Behavioral Problems in Insomnia. Many insomniacs have a particular approach to sleeping that exaggerates their problem. It begins with a belief that the need for a good night's sleep is all important. Because of this belief, they worry more about not sleeping and try harder to sleep, thus resulting in further insomnia. They then will try to compensate for a poor night's sleep by spending more time in bed. If they only need 7 hours of sleep a night, as many people do, increasing the time spent in bed to 9 or

10 hours guarantees at least 2 to 3 hours of wakefulness. Worrying about this time of wakefulness may worsen the quality of the sleeping time. A vicious cycle develops and the bed takes on the overtones of a battle zone. It becomes a place in which to be awake and to fret and not sleep.

Behavioral Approaches to Insomnia. There are two major tasks in helping patients with this cycle. The first is to begin to change the bed back to being a cue for sleep and not wakefulness, and the other is to diminish the belief that a good night's sleep is all important. The patient should attempt to use the bed only for sleeping. Reading, doing paper work, watching television, and so on, should not be done in bed. Sex is the only exception to this rule. If a person wakes up and stays awake, then he or she should get out of bed and do something else for a while.

Patients with insomnia also need to examine their ideal of a good night's sleep. They should examine how many hours of sleep they really need. While they often have slept poorly for years, many still believe that unless they get a good night's sleep, they will not be able to function adequately the next day. Certainly there have been occasions when they have functioned adequately after these nights of insomnia. These (often numerous) exceptions in the patient's experience can be examined to help them change their beliefs. They should be encouraged not to look at the clock so they cannot then calculate the number of hours of sleep they have missed. Patients should be assured that developing a relaxed attitude toward sleeping is a slow gradual process.

If a patient has primary insomnia or insomnia secondary to chronic anxiety, several behavioral approaches might be considered before medication (Regestein, 1976).

1. Relaxation. The deep muscle relaxation methods discussed in the treatment of chronic anxiety can be successfully used in bed prior to going to sleep. The patient should be warned that this method requires regular practice and will not work immediately (Borkovec et al., 1975).
2. A metronome. Some research has shown that a metronome set at 60 beats per minutes can be used as successfully as deep muscle relaxation in helping people fall asleep (Pendleton and Tasto, 1976).
3. Sex. Sexual intercourse, when it is pleasurable, can decrease sleep latency. However, if there is sexual conflict, then sex may actually worsen insomnia.
4. Decreased stimulation prior to bedtime. Developing a quiet, low-stimulation bedtime ritual can be helpful. Rapid transition from energetic conversations, arguments, or highly suspenseful movies will usually be accompanied by onset insomnia.

5. Vigorous daytime exercise. Heavy exercise more than 4 hours before bedtime promotes better sleep. Not only is sleep latency decreased, but the quality of sleep is improved. Vigorous exercise increases stage 4 sleep, the deepest stage of sleep.

6. Tryptophan. There is some sleep laboratory evidence indicating that 500–1000 mg of tryptophan, an essential amino acid, will promote sleep, particularly in the first 4 hours of the night (Hartmann, 1977). While milk is relatively high in tryptophan, it would take almost three glasses to equal a 500-mg dose of tryptophan. Tryptophan tablets, while safe, are quite expensive.

Medication for Anxiety and Insomnia: The Benzodiazepines. The most acceptable medications for the treatment of anxiety and insomnia are the benzodiazepines (for an excellent discussion, see Hollister 1980). They are significantly less toxic and addicting than other sedative–hypnotics (i.e., barbituates and carbamates). Because of their high therapeutic index, the lethal dose of benzodiazepines is many times that of the sedative–hypnotic dose. The benzodiazepine sleeping medications disturb normal sleep architecture less, develop tolerance more slowly, and do not cause rebound insomnia. The benzodiazepines can have sedative, antianxiety, and muscle relaxation effects. Each of these three effects is somewhat independent of the others.

In prescribing benzodiazepines, a working knowledge of their pharmacokinetics is essential. They differ in half-life and some have active metabolites that in turn differ in half-life. The effective duration of action will affect the necessary frequency of pill taking and the intensity of possible drug withdrawal reactions. Many benzodiazepines (diazepam, chlordiazepoxide, chlorazepate, prazepam, flurazepam) have a duration of action well in excess of 24 hours. Clinically, this means they only need to be given once a day and, with regular administration, plasma levels will keep increasing for 1–2 (or more) weeks. This also means that there will be a gradual decline in plasma level after the medication has been discontinued. Thus withdrawal symptoms should be relatively mild and may not appear until 4–7 days after abstinence.

If significant antianxiety effects are not seen in 1–2 weeks, it is unlikely that any will be seen later. Maximum improvement is seen in 4–6 weeks. When medication is continued beyond 4–6 weeks, for 6 months no further decline or improvement is noted. Because of their long half-life, benzodiazepines must be used very cautiously in elderly patients, who may be more sensitive to the drugs and metabolize them more slowly. In some instances drug administration every other day is preferred in the elderly to prevent dangerous drug accumulation. Similarly, extreme caution must be used with patients with liver disease, as drug metabolism of the longer acting benzodiazepines is mainly accomplished in the liver.

Some of the benzodiazepines are specifically used for insomnia. Flurazepam has been shown to be highly effective and continues to work well for 4 weeks. Because it has a very long half-life (greater than 48 hours), it typically works better on the second and third nights, after plasma levels have accumulated. Temazepam with similar efficacy, has only a 10-hour half-life and therefore may produce less morning drowsiness or plasma level accumulation. Lorazepam may have similar advantages. Oxazepam, with its short half-life, can be used as a suitable hypnotic for people with only onset insomnia or for geriatric patients. All of these shorter acting agents take over 2 hours to develop peak plasma levels and so are not indicated on a PRN basis and should be given at least 2 hours before bedtime. Triazolam, a newer agent, may be particularly suitable for insomnia because it has only a 2–3 hour half-life and is quite lipid soluble with peak plasma levels often occurring in less than 1 hour (Settle, 1983). One nonbenzodiazepine, chloral hydrate, is rapidly effective, but tolerance to it develops after 1 week.

Conclusion

Anxiety is first and foremost a complex behavioral phenomenon that under normal circumstances may be adaptive and beneficial. It includes component behaviors of subjective emotional distress, cognitive expectations and appraisals involving failure and danger, and the physiological reactions of stress. It can facilitate performance on tasks and anxiety is a common accompaniment of medical conditions, particularly acute ones. Moderate amounts of anxiety will facilitate recovery from surgery.

Anxiety that occurs to excessive degrees or durations, however, may interfere with performance. When the patient focuses primarily on the physical symptoms, anxiety will frequently be presented as a medical complaint. If may be secondary to other physical or psychological disorders or be a primary complaint in various forms. Differential diagnoses of these various forms of anxiety are essential. Differing treatments have proven effective for each category of anxiety. For example, behavioral interventions are the treatments of choice for specific phobias but are ineffective unless combined with medication for other kinds of anxiety.

Insomnia is a frequent and complicating aspect of anxiety. Insomnia may be a cause of normal anxiety, which in turn may exacerbate the anxiety, or secondary to the emotional disorder. The insomnia may require direct intervention itself. Again, consideration of both biomedical and behavioral interventions is warranted.

Diagnosing and assessing anxiety is unfortunately subjective and will require careful judgment on the part of the physician. The frequency of anxiety and anxiety-related complaints demands that physicians exercise that judgment continually. Careful history taking and attention to the full range of components (cognitive, situational, subjective, and physiological) are the keys to adequate assessment and eventually treatment.

References

Borkovec, T. D., D. G. Kaloupek, and M. Slama. 1975. The facilitative effect of muscle tension-release in the relax treatment of sleep disturbance. Behavior Therapy 6:301–309.

Davis, J. M., S. Nasr, N. Spira, and C. Vogel. 1981. Anxiety: Differential diagnosis and treatment from a biological perspective. Journal of Clinical Psychiatry 42:4–14.

Dietch, J. T. 1981. Diagnosis of organic anxiety disorder. Psychosomatics 22(8):661–669.

Freedman, A. M., R. L. Dornbusch, and B. Shapiro. 1981. Anxiety: Here today and here tomorrow. Comprehensive Psychiatry 22:44–54.

Hartmann, E. 1977. L-Tryptophan: A rational hypnotic with clinical potential. American Journal of Psychiatry 134:366–370.

Hollister, L. M. 1980. A look at the issues. Psychosomatics 21:4–8.

Janis, I. L. 1958. Psychological Stress: Psychoanalytic and Behavioral Studies of Surgical Patients. New York: Wiley.

Janis, I. L. 1971. Stress and Frustration. New York: Harcourt Brace and Janovich.

Karacan, I., I. Thornby, M. Anch, C. Holzer, G. J. Warheit, and J. J. Schwab. 1976. Prevalence of sleep disturbance in a primarily urban Florida county. Social Science and Medicine 10:239–244.

Ley, P. 1977. Psychological Studies of Doctor–Patient Communication. In S. Rachman, ed.: Contributions to Medical Psychology, Vol. 1. Pergamon Press, London; pp. 9–42.

Luborsky, L., B. Singer, and L. Luborsky. 1975. Comparative studies of psychotherapies. Archives of General Psychiatry 32:995–1008.

Marks, I. 1969. Fears and Phobias. New York: Academic Press.

Noyes, R., Jr., J. Clancey, P. R. Hoeuk, and D. J. Slymen. 1980. The prognosis of anxiety neurosis. Archives of General Psychiatry 37:173–179.

Paul, G. L. 1966. Insight Versus Desensitization in Psychotherapy: An Experiment in Anxiety Reduction. Stanford, California: Stanford University Press.

Pendleton, L. R., and L. Tasto. 1976. Effects of metronome-conditioned relaxation, metronome-induced relaxation, and progressive muscle relaxation on insomnia. Behavior Research and Therapy 24:165–166.

Pitts, F. M. 1971. Biochemical factors in anxiety neurosis. Behavior Science 16:82–91.

Rakel, R. E. 1981. Differential diagnosis of anxiety. Psychiatric Annals 11:11–14.

Regestein, Q. R. 1976. Treating insomnia: A practical guide for managing chronic sleeplessness, circa 1975. Comprehensive Psychiatry 17:517–526.

Rickels, K. 1972. Predictors of response to benzodiazepines in anxious outpatients. In S. Gavattini, E. Mussini, and L. O. Randall, eds.: The Benzodiazepines. New York: Raven Press; pp. 257–281.

Rosenman, R. H. 1971. Assessing the risk associated with behavior patterns. Journal of the Medical Association, Georgia 60:31–34.

Settle, E. C. 1983. Triazolam: The latest FDA approved hypnotic. International Drug Therapy Newsletter 18(1):1–4.

Sheehan, D. V. 1982a. Current perspectives in the treatment of panic and phobic disorders. Drug Therapy (September), pp. 49–60.

Sheehan, D. V. 1982b. Current concepts in psychiatry: Panic attacks and phobias New England Journal of Medicine (July 15), pp. 156–158.

Spielberger, C. D., R. E. Lushene, and W. G. McAdoo. 1971. Theory and measurement of anxiety states. In R. B. Cattell, ed.: Handbook of Modern Personality Theory. Chicago: Aldine.

Wolpe, H., and A. A. Lazarus. 1966. Behavior Therapy Techniques: A Guide to the Treatment of Neuroses. New York: Pergamon Press.

20

Behavioral Aspects
of Drug Misuse and Abuse

Albert S. Carlin, Ph.D.* and Nicholas G. Ward, M.D.†

Congressional committees, local citizens boards, and newspaper headlines regularly decry our society as one that is "overmedicated" and point the finger of blame at physicians and pharmaceutical manufacturers. Regardless of the truth of these accusations, physicians have been held morally as well as legally responsible for diagnosis and treatment of drug misuse and its complications (Lennard et al., 1971; Wesson and Smith, 1978). The factors that underlie drug misuse are to a large extent the content area of the behavioral sciences. In addition to pharmacology, the variables that must be considered in coming to an understanding of drug misuse include learning and conditioning theories, personality and psychopathology, the cultural context of the person, and socioeconomic factors. This chapter will not focus only on the use of illicit substances, which too frequently has been the primary concern of drug abuse workers and policy; it will instead address a basic set of concepts that underlie misuse of many substances, including licit pharmaceuticals as well as street drugs.

Although most people think they know what drug abuse is on some intuitive basis, it is difficult to articulate. All too frequently the first set of intuitive definitions provided are superficial, ambiguous, and can be easily challenged. A wife periodically uses her husband's prescribed Dalmane when she cannot sleep; he borrows her Percodan to ease a twisted knee. A couple of friends share a joint of marijuana before dinner. A young woman occasionally takes Quaalude before a party. A young executive drinks six to eight cups of coffee a day. All of these behaviors are viewed as benign

*Associate Professor, Department of Psychiatry and Behavioral Sciences, University of Washington School of Medicine, Seattle, Washington.
†Associate Professor, Department of Psychiatry and Behavioral Sciences, University of Washington School of Medicine, Seattle, Washington.

by some and as drug abuse by others. These differences in opinion may exist even within a group of professional drug abuse workers. The difficulty in actually defining drug abuse is the result of several coexisting independent definitions. Definitions range from a chronicity/frequency notion that implies that some drug abuse is acceptable, but "too much" is abuse, to the belief that any nonprescribed use of mind- or mood-altering substances is abuse. Most of these definitions can be characterized within three basic types.

Drug abuse may be defined as any pattern of drug use that is frowned upon by society. Society's concerns may well be independent of risk of negative consequences. For example, drinking alcohol, even to the point of mild intoxication, is generally accepted, whereas consumption of short-acting barbiturates for their intoxicating effects is frowned upon. Certain religious groups tolerate the use of coffee and tea, but not alcohol, while others abjure the use of these substances as well (Blum, 1969; de Roop, 1976). Some social groups tolerate marijuana use, whereas others view the use of cannabis as a sine qua non of drug abuse.

The social definition of drug abuse is not only based upon the substance consumed but also considers the usual route of administration. Drugs administered via familiar routes such as inhaling, drinking, or eating are frequently viewed to be less destructive than substances that are sniffed or injected.

The societal concerns are strongly correlated with the concepts of "hard drugs" and "soft drugs," a distinction that fails to meet any logical test. There does not exist anything akin to the Mohs scale of hardness for psychoactive substances. The hardness of minerals can be determined by what substance scratches which, but such distinctions are inapplicable to pharmaceuticals. Heroin is the quintessential "hard drug," while "pills" are usually seen as a "soft drug." The media portrays heroin withdrawal as frightening and unimaginably evil; but few know that withdrawal from barbiturate drugs or alcohol can be fatal, while heroin withdrawal has no major medical consequences. Lethality and likelihood of deleterious consequences are at least partially independent of concepts such as "hard drugs." Although not empirically established, it appears as if hard drugs are those the classifier and his friends would never seriously consider using, while soft drugs remain a distinct possibility.

The legal definition of drug abuse considers any pattern of use that violates statutory regulation as abuse. Frequently a behavior becomes legally defined as drug abuse following a societal concern. The definition represents an eventual effort to control or limit the use of drugs that society believes have a potential for abuse. The legislation may also represent attempts to control a segment of the population that uses that substance. The early testimony for legislation regulating cocaine dealt at length with the impact of that drug on black males' behavior toward white women (Musto, 1973, 1974). Early coffeehouses in England were regulated not out of concern about the impact of the beverage, but because persons who frequented coffeehouses were political troublemakers (Wellman, 1961).

Societal concerns can be somewhat more mercurial than legal status. An example of this lag in the legal system exists in attitudes and legislation surrounding marijuana. The drug was not seen as a problem in the 1920s until a rash of magazine articles appeared in the 1930s describing bizarre criminal activities and immoral acts carried out under the influence of cannabis (Anslinger and Cooper, 1937). Legislation soon followed. The great prevalence of cannabis in the late 1960s and early 1970s softened public concern, yet legislation frequently maintained a draconian approach.

The final definition is the one that is of greatest utility to physicians and others in the health professions. It is a functional definition based on a pattern of drug use or use of substances that jeopardize the user's health or psychological, social, or fiscal functioning. Such a definition is based on the likelihood or actual presence of deleterious consequences for the individual, not the substance per se, nor chronicity and/or frequency, nor social reputation. For example, a person who episodically consumes LSD with no apparent consequences would not be considered a drug abuser, whereas a person who uses the same drug with the same frequency but whose use each time results in a depressive episode and suicidal preoccupation would. Societal and legal definitions are ephemeral; deleterious consequences maintain a degree of constancy.

The actual substance abused is frequently less the issue than is the pattern of use in the development of deleterious consequences. Over time people have attempted to alter their mental functioning with any purported psychoactive substance, including mothballs. These subtances have been smoked, chewed, snorted, and injected into various orifices in a effort to "get high." Use eventually focuses on substances that have certain properties in common: a relatively short latency of onset and the ability to produce disinhibition and/or euphoria.

An abusable drug is one that changes thinking or mood quickly enough to be recognized by the user. The change in feeling is one that allows the person to feel better or at least to feel less bad. Disinhibition/euphoria is, of course, the equivalent of being "high" or "drunk." Although drugs (once again, including alcohol as a drug) are necessary to achieve this state, they are not necessarily a sufficient cause. Everyone who drinks alcohol has had the experience of merely becoming sleepy after a drink or two taken in a subdued setting, and of also becoming giddy, expansive, or disinhibited in a party setting. Carlin et al. (1972) and Jones (1971) provided data that demonstrate the imporance of setting and expectation in facilitating or attenuating the effects of marijuana. Carlin et al. (1974) also found that marijuana intoxication is a learned phenomenon. Naive marijuana smokers experienced as many symptoms as did experienced users after exposure to marijuana, but failed to identify their state as intoxication. Some symptoms (stimulus preoccupation and enhanced eating behavior) were influenced by the presence of others modeling these behaviors. Thus drugs may provide a physiological basis for disinhibition/euphoria, but its occurrence is dependent upon the user's expectations and experiences, as well as the setting in which the drug is used.

An example of the addicting properties of a substance that is relatively free of any social opprobrium but which nonetheless demonstrates the dynamics of addiction is decongestant nasal spray. Although it does not produce a psychic effect akin to disinhibition/euphoria, the rapid decongestant effect is pleasurable to the congested. Tolerance develops and the careless user soon ignores the package directions and increases the frequency of use. Eventually a rebound effect that can be considered to be analogous to tissue dependence occurs. To the now addicted decongestant user it appears as if the "cold" were lingering and he were chronically congested and using the substance regularly. Only "cold turkey" withdrawal will reveal that the cold has since passed and an addiction exists.

Manifestations of dysfunctional drug use include physiological, behavioral, and social effects. It is useful to think of dysfunctional effects as consequences, as opposed to effects. For example, tachycardia is a common effect of marijuana use, whereas pulmonary disease may be a consequence of chronic use. Consequences of dysfunctional use may include the following.

Panic Reactions. Panic reactions, most frequently associated with use of hallucinogens and stimulants, consist of behavioral untoward effects ranging from mild dysphoria lasting only a few hours to certain conviction that you have witnessed your own death or are witnessing the destruction of the world. Anxiety attacks are more common than transient psychosis, but both may emerge as a function of the content of the experience, the context of use, or fear of loss of control. For the most part panic reactions are transitory and responsive to the passage of time (excretion of the substance from the body), reassurance that the experienced effects are drug related and not a function of the person "losing his or her mind," reduced environmental stimulation, and, if indicated, antianxiety agents (Heaton, 1975).

Obsessive concern about flashbacks is also an example of panic reactions. Flashback refers to the spontaneous reoccurrence of drug effects some time (even weeks) after its ingestion. Research indicates that the phenomenon is not the result of a pharmacological "dragon in the blood," but is psychological. Heaton (1975) studied experienced psychedelic drug users, some of whom had experienced flashbacks and some of whom had not, and found that he was able to create flashbacks in both groups via manipulation of expectancy. Subjects were given either ephedrine or placebo, placed in an environment likely to enhance flashback occurrence or not, and told to expect flashbacks or not. Those who expected flashbacks were more likely to experience them than those not told to expect them. The expectancy effect was far more powerful than the drug or situation effect.

Toxic effects. Toxic effects may manifest themselves as an acute brain syndrome or as a psychosis that is different from a panic reaction. Chronic use of high dosages of amphetamines and other stimulants, including cocaine, may result in a paranoid psychosis that resolves rapidly within a drug-free state (Ellinwood, 1967). Phencyclidine (PCP) use may create a more lasting psychotic state similar to schizophrenia, but one that is resistant to neuroleptic drugs (Luisada, 1978). The toxic effects of sedative hypnotic drugs and narcotics are those seen in overdose—sedation, coma, and respiratory depression (Greene and DuPont, 1975; Reed et al., 1952). Psychological test data suggest that chronic abuse of sedative hypnotics, narcotics,and alcohol may be associated with cognitive deficits similar to those observed in brain-damaged persons (Grant et al., 1978).

Tolerance. Chronic use of some psychoactive drugs calls forth a compensatory or homeostatic response in the body and continued effects then require increased dosage. The mechanisms of tolerance are not clearly understood but are thought to be partly due to more rapid degradation of the substance owing to increased enzyme production and/or compensation at a cellular level (pharmacodynamic tolerance). In addition to this physiological tolerance, persons can develop a psychological tolerance. This may be a learned compensation for drug effects or a seeking of an increased change in psychological status.

Physical Dependence. Owing to a variety of changes in the body in response to the chronic presence of drugs and associated with the development of tolerance, the sudden interruption of the drug may result in the emergence of physical symptoms. The avoidance of these symptoms is a powerful motivation for continued drug use. Sedative hypnotic drug withdrawal is marked by (in order of increasing severity of withdrawal) anxiety, tachycardia, hypertension, tremulousness, postural hypotension, hyperpyrexia, delerium, seizures, and death. Narcotic withdrawal is evidenced by anxiety, tremulousness, chills, piloerection, diaphoresis, and muscle cramps. A forthright heroin addict who had experienced "cold turkey" withdrawal on several occasions likened the withdrawal to severe flulike symptoms, but added that drug craving and the knowledge that a "fix" could alleviate the symptoms somehow intensified their unpleasantness. Controversy exists over whether the fatigue and depression associated with stimulant withdrawal should be characterized as evidence of tissue dependence.

Withdrawal from sedative hypnotic drugs and narcotics is treated via gradual reduction, using long-acting substances as the withdrawal agent. The patient is given a sedative dose of the drug to which he or she is addicted hourly until symptoms of intoxication are observed. The total challenge dosage then is prescribed in divided doses over the next 24 hours. Then it is reduced by approximately 10% per day until the last dose is given. The bedtime dose is the last to be reduced and withdrawn. The drugs used for withdrawal are typically phenobarbital or chlordiazepoxide for sedative hypnotic drugs, and methadone for narcotic drugs. The object of the scheduled withdrawal is to prevent the emergence of physical symptoms, not the provision of psychological comfort during withdrawal. The challenge method is used to empirically determine the starting point of the withdrawal schedule. This empirical determination is a more reliable index of present level of addiction than patient history. Some patients are embarrassed by their addiction and underreport their usage, while others overreport in an effect to obtain more drug during their withdrawal.

Psychological Dependence. This concept addresses the learned aspects of drug-seeking behavior. A difficulty with this powerful dysfunctional manifestation of drug abuse is its universality. Almost any reinforcing behavior can create a psychological dependence: Gambling, sex, and even nail biting, among others, can create a volitional disorder. It is a meaningful and powerful aspect of addiction but requires more specific definition if it is to be usefully applied.

Psychosis. A psychosis in response to use of psychoactive drugs here is differentiated from a toxic psychosis, as is observed, for example, with stimulants. Usually if a psychosis emerges, it is in conjunction with the use of hallucinogenic drugs, among which marijuana should be included. In most cases the emergence of a psychosis is a correlate of premorbid psychiatric vulnerability interacting with drug effects rather than pure pharmacological effects. Evidence suggests that the incidence of such psychosis is a function of the individual's and the culture's previous experience with the substance (Becker, 1967). Prior to the explosion of marijuana use in the late 1960s and early 1970s, marijuana psychosis seemed more frequent among users than at present. Similarly, the frequency of LSD psychosis seems also to be diminishing. Perhaps increasing familiarity with a drug's ability to produce peculiar thoughts, behaviors, and sensations leads one to attribute these to the drug rather than one's self, and hence not to view these as alien behaviors. The recent concerns about PCP-related psychosis may be a function of the drug's relative novelty. However, there is also some suggestion that the substance may create a unique toxic psychosis.

Physical sequellae. Many physical complications may emerge from patterns of chronic drug abuse. Some of these are expected and obvious, whereas others are more subtle. Physical sequellae are a function of substance, route of administration, and personal exposure to other risk factors. Automobile accidents, falls, and fractures are a frequent accompaniment of drug use brought on by impaired attention, coordination, or judgment. Injury and death associated with fire is not uncommon among those who both smoke and use substances that are sedating. Decubitis ulcers have been observed when persons have been unconscious for prolonged periods of time following drug overdose. Those who use the intravenous route of administration are at risk for absesses, vasculitis, hepatitis, and other complications resulting from nonsterile injection techniques. Poor technique may result in the person injecting drugs into an artery rather than a vein, resulting in circulatory crisis, gangrene, and even loss of the effected limb.

This discussion has for the most part addressed general issues of substance abuse independently of the drugs involved. The specific risks associated with particular drugs are listed in Tables 1–4 below.

Although smoking is usually not thought of as abuse of a drug, it is clearly an addiction and nicotine is a powerful drug. The addictive properties of smoking tobacco cigarettes are illustrated by the relapse rate of smokers, which exceeds that of heroin addicts. Commercial programs designed to rid smokers of their habit are immensely popular and profitable, as were the patent medicines of 60 years ago that also promised to rid the victim of his habit. A consideration of this powerful addiction is

Table 1. Sedative Hypnotics: Sleeping Agents and Anxiolytics

Consequences	Secobarbital	Valium	Meprobamate	Dalmane	Phenobarbital
Panic reaction	—	—	—	—	—
Toxicity	+++	+	++	+	++
Tolerance	+++	+	+	+	++
Physical dependency	+++	+	+	+	++
Psychological dependency	+++	++	++	+	+
Psychosis	—	—	—	—	—
Physical sequellae	DDRA[a]	DDRA	DDRA	DDRA	DDRA
Disinhabition	+++	+++	+++	+	+

[a]Dependent on the dose and route of administration.

Table 2. Analgesics: Opiates and Synthetics

Consequences	Heroin	Dilaudid	Codeine
Panic reaction	—	—	—
Toxicity	++	++	+
Tolerance	+++	+++	+++
Physical dependency	+++	+++	++
Psychological dependency	++++	+++	+
Psychosis	—	—	—
Physical sequellae	DDRA[a]	DDRA	DDRA
Disinhabition	++++	+++	+

[a]Dependent on the dose and route of administration.

Table 3. Hallucinogenic Drugs

Consequences	Cannabis	LSD	PCP
Panic reaction	+	++	+++
Toxicity	—	+	++
Tolerance	?	—	?
Physical dependency	?	?	?
Psychological dependency	+	+	+
Psychosis	?	+	++
Physical sequellae	?	?	?
Disinhabition	++	++	++

Table 4. Stimulants: Amphetamines, Ritalin, and Cocaine

Consequences	Stimulant
Panic reaction	++
Toxicity	++, psychosis
Tolerance	++++
Physical dependency	?
Psychological dependency	++++
Psychosis	Toxic psychosis
Physical sequellae	Dependent on the dose and route of administration

useful in highlighting the complex and intimate relation between pharmacological and psychological dependence.

The physiological function served by smoking is not clear; nicotine
seems to both facilitate and then diminish synaptic transmission, and it is
associated with cortical arousal and increased perception of weak stimuli.
Smokers claim that smoking relaxes them, that they smoke when anxious,
that it helps them to work, that it stimulates them and gives them
something to do with their hands, and so on (Tomkins, 1968). Schachter
(1980) reported a number of studies that examined the relation between
stress and smoking. Smokers who smoked high-nicotine cigarettes during a
study tolerated more painful electric shocks than did smokers who
smoked low-nicotine cigarettes, who in turn tolerated more shock than did
smokers not allowed to smoke during the study. Nonsmokers tolerated as
great a shock level as did smokers allowed to smoke high-nicotine
cigarettes. In a study of irritability, smokers allowed to smoke high-
nicotine cigarettes were similar to nonsmokers in response to annoying
stimuli; both these groups were less irritable than smokers who smoked
low-nicotine cigarettes or no cigarettes at all. Smokers who were switched
to low-nicotine cigarettes seemed to guard their level of nicotine intake by
increasing the number of cigarettes smoked. The amount smoked was also
affected by manipulations of urinary pH; acidic urine is associated with
faster excretion of nicotine, and alkaline urine with slower excretion.
Schachter reported that smokers given sodium bicarbonate smoked less
even under stress than smokers given a placebo. The evidence would
suggest that smokers smoke to maintain a given level of nicotine that they
find optimal. It is less clear as to what sets that level. Is it based on
experience, chronicity/frequency, or an organismic variable? All of this
seems to be independent of any interpretation based personality, be it of
dependent personality, frustrated oral cravings, or risk taking.

In addition to this physiological aspect of addiction to nicotine, a
number of social factors are important in initiating and maintaining the
smoking habit. One's first experience with tobacco is usually aversive,
made up in part of nausea and choking. Yet the behavior is repeated partly
in response to internal images of Marlboro men, Bogie, Bette Davis, or the
high school hood or fox. Once the behavior is learned, it becomes
associated with environmental cues that will elicit smoking. A smoker who
quit over the summer and who by August was free of cravings found
himself automatically reaching into his shirt pocket for a cigarette when his
regular poker group reconvened in the fall. The situation in which he had
never experienced not smoking reevoked his smoking set. A habit
practiced 20–40 times a day will be resistant to extinction.

The material discussed above is based on the pharmacology and
psychopharmacology of psychoactive drugs and represents the more
straightforward aspects of the substance abuse problem. The material

below discusses frequently less well conceptualized areas of the problem of substance abuse: Who does it, and why?

When Gertrude Stein wrote, "Rose is a rose is a rose," she was correct both botanically and appellatively; however, the statement is not true for drug abusers. Man's desire to bring about an altered state of consciousness is ubiquitous. Meditation, fasting, vigils, and manipulation of sensory input reflect nonchemical modes of changing mental status. Drugs, including alcohol, have been used from ancient times as a reliable means of altering consciousness. Increased efficacy through the technology of pharmacology has allowed more precise and powerful effects, but also greater problems. Drugs are used and misused by a wide variety of people and for a wide variety of reasons. An addict personality does not exist. Events and contingencies can shape a similar complex of behaviors in any of us. The vulnerability of persons to addiction is situational as well as personal. A terminally ill person in severe pain can be shaped to display "junkie" behavior in an effort to increase frequency and dosage of pain medication.

Cohen (1981) has enumerated variables that are associated with the initiation of abuse drug use as well as those which are implicated in the perpetuation of drug use. He believes that the social–developmental factors associated with adolescence are also associated with the onset of drug use: the search for novel stimulation and exploration, vulnerability to peer modeling and influence, and increased risk taking accompanied by incompletely developed impulse control. Additional external factors include available of drugs and reduced opportunities for social and academic mastery.

Drug use is perpetuated by the pleasurable "rush" associated with the short latency of onset of drugs taken intravenously or by inhalation, avoidance of the unpleasant effects of withdrawal, and the pleasure of disinhibition/euphoria. These pharmacological phenomena combine with subculture identification, social setting, and availability in increasing the likelihood that drug use will be continued. The experience with heroin addiction among American troops in Vietnam demonstrated the importance of nonpharmacological factors in addiction. The widespread heroin use among American military personnel, coupled with the experience of marked resistance of that addiction to treatment, should have resulted in continuation of that pattern of drug use in the United States and hence a major increase in the prevalence of heroin addiction. An American heroin epidemic did not, however, emerge. Differences in drug availability, social setting, and reduction of stress levels all contributed to the discontinuation of heroin use once troops returned to the United States.

The diversity of users and patterns of use does not preclude the usefulness of seeking common characteristics in an effort to determine the existence of homogeneous subgroups. It does suggest that traditional groupings by personality or substance may be less useful than classification by more relevant variables.

We have found it useful to classify drug abusers with a 2-by-2 classification system in which one dimension describes the social identification of the user and the other the function drug use serves the person (Carlin and Stauss, 1978). The descriptive dichotomy classifies the person as "streetwise" or "straight." Streetwise persons are those who identify with the youth street drug cultures and who manifest this identification through their manner of dress, grooming, place of residence, and knowledge of the street cant and jargon. A streetwise person, operationally defined, is one who can be dropped off on the corner of First and Pike in Seattle (Times Square in New York City, or any local street scene) with $100 and the instructions to appear 24 hours later "high" or with an appropriate amount of drugs in his or her possession. The person who succeeds is "streetwise"; the person who does not is "straight."

The functional dichotomy classifies drug use as motivated by "social recreational" factors or as "self-medication." The former is demonstrated by a pattern of drug use in which the drug is consumed with other people, used in binges, used intravenously, and consumed in large doses short of toxicity. Self-medication use is marked by solo use, regular use, oral administration, a fixed dose that escalates slowly with the development of tolerance, and care exerted to maintain a future supply.

Social recreational use does not imply merely avocational drug use free of consequences but, rather, a primary motivation of "getting high" to achieve euphoria and novel psychological states. Factors of tissue dependence, tolerance, and psychological dependence can come into play to bring about frank addiction. Self-medication is an effort to acquire "chemical comfort" for anxiety, depression, or even psychosis. For most, this effort results in a journey to dependence owing to the nature of the drugs available. Depressed persons may use depressants because initially the disinhibition/euphoria and sedation provided alleviates the dysphoria of depression. The long-term result is increased depression. Similarly, if they choose stimulants, the buildup of tolerance and the eventual "rebound" can only produce further depression. Anxiety treated only by anxiolytic agents may eventually result in increased anxiety owing to initial factors underlying anxiety now synergized by withdrawal.

The typologies described above are independent of the drug of choice. Pharmacologically a drug will be abused if it meets the minimal criteria of short latency of onset and the ability to produce disinhibition/euphoria. Beyond these factors choice is frequently a function of availability and fashion. Methaqualone, a sedative–hypnotic drug, became a recreational drug of abuse among young adults in the Midwest, an alleged "rock and roll" drug (silver replicas of which were advertised in the classified section of *Rolling Stone*), while in Seattle it became a recreational drug popular in the homosexual male community. Similarly, methylphenidate was a major street drug of abuse in Seattle among heroin addicts and other streetwise users, but was little abused elsewhere until more recently. Social contagion is a major mechanism by which abuse of a particular substance is transmitted.

Studies of which drugs are abused by whom have revealed the presence of four major clusters of drugs (Braucht et al., 1978). A major cluster revealed that persons who abuse cocaine are also likely to abuse methaqualone, illegal methadone, and opiates and synthetic narcotics. Those who abuse inhalants (glue, paint, Pam, toluene, etc.) are equally likely to abuse codeine and nonnarcotic analgesics. A third cluster contained marijuana, amphetamines, and hallucinogenics. Barbiturates and minor tranquilizers comprised a fourth cluster. User groups can be attributed to these drug clusters. The first represents a group of streetwise illicit drug users; the second cluster is used by street persons without the financial or social resources to acquire any but the most readily available and cheap subsances. It takes less skill and resources to shoplift a can of spray paint or to score codeine cough syrup than to illicitly acquire hydromorphone or methadone. The third cluster is made up of drugs that can be considered as recreational or "tripping drugs." The fourth cluster consists of drugs that would be highly used by straight persons who are attempting to medicate themselves in an effort to cope with depression and anxiety. Alcohol and heroin form two additional clusters whose meaning is straightforward.

The emergence of these clusters and the utility of the streetwise–straight and self-medication–social/recreational dichotomies indicates the need to maintain a flexible orientation in both the diagnosis and treatment of drug misuse. The diagnosis must rely on more than superficial factors of appearance and grooming and treatment must take into account not only the substance involved but also the function served by the pattern of use. Drug treatment programs aimed only at the youth–street–drug subcultures, the mental health counselor or psychiatrist who assumes that all problems are a function of psychiatric deficits and who ignores drug and alcohol use, and the physician who assumes that anyone asking for Valium is a weakling are all operating from stereotypes which will interfere with their ability to provide appropriate treatment.

Learning about the dynamics of drug misuse is also useful in allowing the physician to avoid inadvertently addicting his patients to psychoactive drugs. Physician-induced addiction is a prime example of iatrogenic disease and one that is avoidable. The ability to minimize iatrogenic addiction also allows the physician to be a more effective agent in the alleviation of chronic pain. If one were to set out with the paradoxical intent of addicting a patient iatrogenically, a better understanding of how to avoid such an unfortunate outcome could be achieved.

There are several ways in which physicians can avoid the risk of iatrogenic addiction in their patients. They can avoid drugs that have a high addictive potential: those that rapidly produce disinhibition/euphoria or significant relief from distress (pain, anxiety) or those which are short acting, with a fast offset and uncomfortable withdrawal symptoms. They then can prescribe medications in such a way as to further decrease addictive risk. PRN (as needed) administration can ensure that patients are taking medication when they are maximally uncomfortable and will then have dramatic improvement followed by uncomfortable withdrawal. Patients on this schedule quickly associate pill taking with relief and not taking pills with discomfort. These problems can be avoided by prescribing long-acting medications with a fixed dosage schedule. For example, many benzodiazepines have a half-life greater than 24 hours and can be prescribed for anxiety on a once-a-day basis. Patients then can have relatively uniform antianxiety effects, minimum withdrawal effects during administration, and need to take pills less frequently. In some circumstances, it may be necessary to use certain highly effective pain medications with short half-lives (4–6 hours). These can become addictive either with PRN administration or with a fixed dosage schedule with administration too widely separated so that the patient continualy relapses into pain. For example, if the medication lasts 5 hours and is prescribed every 6 hours, the patient will go through a continual pain relief–pain exacerbation withdrawal cycle. Prescribing the medication every 5 hours will reduce the risk of addition, because the patient will have continuous analgesic effect and not associate taking pills with dramatic relief.

There are also certain patients who have increased risk of addiction. Any patient who has previously had an addiction to drugs or alcohol obviously is more likely to become addicted again. People who are antisocial, impulsive, and irresponsible and who have little insight into their own behavior are more likely to become addicted. For them, pills may represent a fast external solution to their problems that does not require them to examine their own behavior and patiently seek solutions through personal change.

People who are already addicted can become quite skillful at "conning" prescriptions from physicians. There are several ways that physicians can protect themselves from being used. They should try to determine if the patient is a high addiction risk. If there is any suspicion at all, the physician should get the names of other physicians who have treated the patient and try to contact them. Pain complaints should be assessed to see if they are acute and medically plausible.

After extensive screening, the physician still may decide that a prescription is warranted in a potentially risky patient. Treatment for a definite time-limited period should be negotiated. In writing the prescription, numbers of pills and renewals should be written out. Zeros can be added after numbers to increase by 10- or 100-fold the intended prescription. Narcotic license numbers should not be printed on the prescription pad but, rather, should be added in longhand. Pads with numbers printed on them are quite valuable on the street. Refills should not be given without further contact with the patient and the pharmacy. Through all of this the physician should maintain a helpful but firm professional manner and not succumb to a condescending or punitive style.

As physicians you will have responsibilities as "gatekeepers" for psychoactive drugs. In addition, you will have been attributed a great deal of wisdom about the morality and ethics of drug use. Parents will request consultation about their child's drug use; PTAs will ask you to speak about drug and alcohol use; you will be required to diagnose and treat drug abuse in your patients. We hope that you will be aware that the issues are complex and require an awareness of more than pharmacology. Knowledge of drugs, the person, and his social context are required if you are to make informed decisions about this problem.

References

Anslinger, H., and C. Cooper. 1937. Marihuana; assassin of youth. American Magazine (July).

Becker, H. 1967. History, culture and subjective experience: An exploration of the social basis of drug induced experiences. In C. Hollander, ed.: Background Papers in Student Drug Involvement. Washington, DC: United States National Student Association; pp. 69–85.

Blum, R. 1969. Society and Drugs. San Francisco, California: Jossey-Bass.

Braucht, G. N., M. W. Kirby, and G. J. Berry. 1978. An empirical typology of multiple drug abusers. In D. Wesson, A. Carlin, K. Adams, and G. Beschner, eds.: Polydrug Abuse: The Results of a National Collaborative Study. New York: Academic Press, pp. 129–147.

Carlin, A. S., C. B. Bakker, L. Halpern, and R. D. Post. 1972. Social facilitation of marihuana intoxication. Journal of Abnormal Psychology 80:132–40.

Carlin, A. S., R. D. Post, C. B. Bakker, and L. Halpern. 1974. The role of modeling and previous experience in facilitation of marihuana toxication. Journal of Nervous and Mental Disease 159:275–281.

Carlin, A. S., and F. F. Stauss. 1978. Two typologies of drug abusers. In D. Wesson, A. Carlin, K. Adams, and G. Beschner, eds.: Polydrug Abuse: The Results of a National Collaborative Study. New York: Academic Press; pp. 97–127.

Cohen, S. 1981. Substance abuse: Initiation and perpetuation. Drug Abuse and Alcoholism Newsletter 10 (entire issue).

Ellinwood, E. H., Jr. 1967. Amphetamine psychosis: A description of individuals and the process. Journal of Nervous and Mental Disease 144:273.

Grant, I., K. M. Adams, A. S. Carlin, P. M. Rennick, L. L. Judd, and K. Schoof. 1978. Neuropsychological effects of polydrug abuse. In D. Wesson, A. Carlin, K. Adams, and G. Beschner, eds.: Polydrug Abuse: The Results of a National Collaborative Study. New York: Academic Press; pp. 223–261.

Greene, M. H., and R. L. DuPont. 1975. The treatment of acute heroin toxicity. *In* P. G. Bourne, ed.: A Treatment Manual for Acute Drug Abuse Emergencies. Rockville, Maryland: National Institute on Drug Abuse Information; pp. 23–32.

Heaton, R. 1975. Subject expectancy and environmental factors as determinants of psychedelic flashback experience. Journal of Nervous and Mental Disease 161:156.

Jones, R. T. 1971. Marihuana induced "high": Influence of expectation, setting and previous drug experience. Pharmacological Review 23:359–369.

Lennard, H. L., A. Bernstein, and C. Epstein. 1971. Mystification and Drug Misuse: Hazards in Using Psychoactive Drugs. San Francisco, California: Jossey-Bass.

Luisada, P. V. 1978. The phencyclidin psychosis: Phenomenology and treatment. *In* R. Petersen and R. Stillman, eds.: Phencyclidine (PCP) Abuse: An Appraisal. Rockville, Maryland: National Institute on Drug Abuse; pp. 241–253.

Musto, D. 1973. The American Disease: Origins of Narcotic Control. New Haven, Connecticut: Yale University Press.

Musto, D. 1974. Early history of heroin in the United States. *In* P. G. Bourne, ed.: Addiction. New York: Academic Press; pp. 175–185.

Reed, C. E., M. F. Driggs, and C. C. Foote. Acute barbiturate intoxication: A study of 300 cases based on a physiologic system of classification of the severity of the intoxication. Annals of Internal Medicine 37:290.

Roop, de, R. S. 1976. Drugs and the Mind. New York: St. Martin.

Schachter, S. 1980. Non-psychological explanations of behavior. *In* L. Festinger, ed.: Retrospectives in Social Psychology. New York: Oxford University Press; pp. 131–157.

Tomkins, S. 1968. A modified model of smoking behavior. *In* E. F. Borgatta and R. R. Evans, eds.: Smoking Health and Behavior. Chicago, Illinois: Aldine; pp. 165–186.

Wellman, F. L. 1961. Coffee: Botany, Cultivation and Utilization. New York: Interscience Publishers.

Wesson, D. R., and D. E. Smith. 1978. Barbiturates: Their Use, Misuse and Abuse. New York: Human Sciences Press.

21

Alcohol Abuse
in Medical Practice

James W. Smith, M.D.* and Ruth E. Little, S.C.†

The World Health Organization (1952) describes alcoholics as "those excessive drinkers whose dependence upon alcohol has attained such a degree that it shows a noticeable mental disturbance or an interference with their bodily and mental health, their inter-personal relations and their smooth social and economic functioning or who show the prodromal signs of such development." The Criteria Committee of the National Council on Alcoholism (NCA) (1972) defines alcoholism as "a pathological dependence on alcohol."

Alcoholism is one of the most commonly encountered diseases in medical practice. The Fourth Special Report to Congress on Alcohol and Health (United States Department of Health and Human Services, 1981a) revealed that one out of ten Americans who drink are alcoholic (and 66% drink; therefore 6.6% are alcoholic). In 1977 there were over 95,000 alcohol-related deaths (United States Department of Health and Human Services, 1981b), which constituted the third leading cause of deaths (United States Department of Commerce, 1979). Males appear to become alcoholic more frequently than females. A total of 15% of adult male drinkers and only 3.9% of adult female drinkers report consuming 120 or more drinks per month (United States Department of Health and Human Services, 1981a); 5% of males and 2% of female drinkers report experiencing three or more symptoms of alcohol dependence (United States Department of Health and Human Services, 1981a). Physicians as a

*Clinical Associate Professor, Department of Psychiatry and Behavioral Sciences, University of Washington School of Medicine, Seattle, Washington. Present address: Medical Director, Schick-Shadels Hospital, Seattle, Washington.

† Director, Alcoholism and Drug Abuse Institute, University of Washington School of Medicine, Seattle, Washington.

group have a higher than average rate of alcoholism. Of all physicians, 10% are reported to be alcoholic (not just 10% of those who drink) (Halenar, 1979).

Approximately 1 out of every 20 patients seen by a family physician is alcoholic (Ewing, 1978), so that in most practices at least one should be seen every day. However, only about one alcoholic in ten is appropriately diagnosed and treated (Whitfield and Williams, 1977), making it one of the most poorly diagnosed of the common illnesses.

This anomaly seems to stem primarily from the fact that relatively few medical students received specific alcoholism education and training in medical school (an approach that can only be described as bizarre when applied to the number 3 killer in the United States).

Fortunately, this situation can be relatively easily corrected, since the diagnosis of the disease is both simple and straightforward. Getting the patient to accept the diagnosis and undertake appropriate treatment is a little more difficult in some cases, but no more difficult than in many other chronic illnesses (e.g., diabetes, hypertension, and emphysema). These latter issues will be dealt with later in this chapter.

Etiology

Theories of causation of alcoholism generally fall into three categories: psychogenic, genetic, and biochemical.

For years alcoholism was viewed as a symptom of some underlying psychiatric problem that, once the problem(s) was successfully resolved, would disappear. A great deal of effort was put into attempting to find the "alcoholic personality type" and/or a specific type of psychiatric or social disorder underlying this "symptom." These attempts have proved frustrating and fruitless. It is not possible to specify a personality type, social/ personality disorder, or psychiatric illness that is consistently associated with alcoholism (Imboden and Urbaitis, 1978). All types of people with a variety of personalities may become alcoholics. To be sure, some of them have psychiatric or personality disorders, just as some nonalcoholics do.

One part of the problem is in assuming alcoholism to be a single entity. Many in the field now prefer to speak in terms of the "alcoholisms" rather than "alcoholism" in the singular. Jellinek (1960) categorized alcoholics into five "species" of alcoholism, which he labeled with the Greek letters α through ε. His γ alcoholic is common in the United States. γ Alcoholics are described as having a problem with "control," so that once they begin drinking, they are usually unable to stop until some external force (e.g., health problem, financial depletion, family or legal intervention) prevents the continuation of the "bender." Once the "bender" is terminated, however, the alcoholic may be able to totally abstain for variable periods of time. This type contrasts markedly with the δ alcoholic commonly seen in

France, who can control the amount consumed at any one time but who cannot "abstain"; that is, the person is rarely intoxicated, but rarely completely free of alcohol.

A potentially more useful way to categorize the "alcoholisms" is to divide them into primary and secondary alcoholisms.

Primary Alcoholism

The primary alcoholic has no diagnosable psychiatric disorder associated with his or her alcoholism. In these cases when alcohol is completely eliminated, the person tends to function normally in all areas of life (except where physical damage from the prolonged drinking interferes). In these relatively uncomplicated cases, the outlook for success following appropriate treatment is good.

Secondary Alcoholism

The secondary alcoholic has a psychiatric disorder, usually either a primary affective disorder (depression or manic-depressive disorder) or sociopathy. Women secondary alcoholics are more likely to have a depressive disorder. Schuckit et al. (1969) found that 25% of a group of women alcoholics had significant depression prior to the onset of their alcoholism or during an extended period of abstinence. Winokur and Clayton (1967) confirmed this finding in women but noted only 3% of male alcoholics with affective disorder.

Alcoholism and depression tend to run together in families. Winokur and Clayton (1967) reported that as many as 30% of mothers and sisters of alcoholic women met research criteria for the diagnosis of depression. In a later study Winokur et al. (1971) found that 16% of sisters of female alcoholics but only 7% of sisters of male alcoholics were themselves alcoholic. The authors also noted that 32% of daughters of male alcoholics and 74% of daughters of female alcoholics had an affective disorder (depression). It is important to distinguish between depression and the transient state of sadness or "alcoholic depression" that is seen in the majority of alcoholics in the immediate postwithdrawal state. It tends to be a relatively benign state of mild depression, perhaps related to alcohol-induced derangement of neurotransmitter metabolism. It is self-limited and usually disappears within 5–14 days. The primary affective disorder of depression may occur before the onset of alcoholism and the symptoms are present even during a prolonged period of abstinence from alcohol. In addition to the dysphoric mood, somatic disturbances in one or more systems and altered sleep patterns are usually present (Woodruff et al., 1974).

Male secondary alcoholics usually demonstrate sociopathy. Schuckit et al. (1969) reported that approximately 25% of a group of male alcoholics met the criteria for the diagnosis of sociopathy (antisocial personality); in contrast, only 8% of a group of women alcoholics met the same criteria. They had a history of serious antisocial life-styles antedating their alcohol abuse (Schuckit et al., 1969) and demonstrated major problems in all major spheres of their life (family, peers, police, and school) before age 16 (Goodwin, 1979).

The course followed by secondary alcoholics tends to mirror that of the underlying psychiatric disorder. For example, if the depression is adequately controlled, the alcoholism responds to treatment much like it does in the primary alcoholic. If the depression is not adequately treated, the results of the alcoholism intervention are usually poor. Sociopathic alcoholics, like sociopathic nonalcoholics, tend to respond poorly to any type of treatment. Those under age 40 almost universally abuse drugs other than alcohol and the alcoholism may in some ways be the least of the problems of their disordered lives.

Genetic Factors

The fact that alcoholism tends to run in families has been known since ancient times. Aristole warned that drunken women "bring forth children like themselves" and Plutarch declared that "one drunkard begets another" (Goodwin, 1976). When either male or female alcoholics are studied, the rate of alcoholism in their male relatives ranges from 25 to 50%, and that among their female relatives from 5 to 8% percent (Goodwin, 1976). These rates are at least fivefold what would be expected in the general population.

Genetic marker studies were among the first efforts to link alcoholism with genetic factors. An association of alcoholism with characteristics known to be inherited would offer support for a biological factor in the etiology of alcoholism. Nordmo (1959) reported a high degree of association of alcoholism with blood group A in a series of 939 alcoholics in Colorado. Achte (1958) in Finland and Swinson and Madden (1973) in Great Britain failed to confirm this association. However, Camps and Dodd (1967) and Swinson and Madden (1973) found a highly significant correlation between alcoholism and nonsectors of salivary ABH blood group substances, particularly in persons of blood group A. In a study conducted at the Oslo City Hospital in Norway, Bell and Nordhagen (1972) found an association between alcoholic liver disease with cirrhosis and tissue type HLA-BW 40. Bailey et al. (1976) reported on another series of patients with alcoholic liver disease and found an increased incidence of HLA-B8. Black alcoholics, but not black nonalcoholic controls or white alcoholics or controls, have elevated red blood cell levels of the enzyme cupro-zinc superoxide dismutase (Del Villano et al., 1979).

Peeples (1962) found that alcoholics include a significantly greater percentage of nontasters of phenylthiocarbamide (PTC) than do controls (PTC taste response is inherited as an autosomal dominant trait). Varela et al. (1969) reported an association between color blindness (yellow–blue discrimination instead of the more common red–green variety) in male alcoholics and their female first-degree nonalcoholic relatives. They believed that this indicated an association between alcoholism and sex-linked recessive genes. However, Smith and Layden (1971) reported that alcoholics tend to have decreased color discrimination of all hues that returns to normal when alcohol use is discontinued, leaving a residuum of color blindness no greater than that seen in nonalcoholics.

Twin studies showed a much higher concordance for alcoholism in monozygotic ("identical") twins (54%) than in dizygotic ("fraternal") twins (28%) (Kaij, 1960). The latter showed no more concordance for alcoholism than any other sibling, although the incidence of alcoholism in any sibling of an alcoholic proband is higher than in the general population (10% of drinkers in the United States).

The reaction of the brain to alcohol also appears to be genetically determined (Propping, 1978). In twins, high heritability was noted in electroencephalogram (EEG) amplitude and distribution of frequencies. The EEGs of monozygotic twins tended to become still more similar after alcohol (Propping, 1978). Although the data are limited, there is also information to confirm that there is increased concordance for alcoholism in monozygotic twins reared apart (Shields, 1962).

Adoption studies carried out in Denmark (Goodwin et al., 1973) and in the United States (Cadoret et al., 1980) show that children of alcoholic biological parents adopted into nonalcoholic families and raised without knowing they had an alcoholic biological parent were much more likely to develop alcoholism than were comparable adoptees from nonalcoholic biological parents. In fact, the adopted sons of alcoholic parents did not differ in any significant respect from sons of alcoholics who were *not* adopted out (Goodwin et al., 1974). Confirming information also comes from half-sibling studies (Schuckit et al., 1972), which show that subjects were more likely to become alcoholic if their biological parent was alcoholic than if their surrogate parent was alcoholic.

There is remarkable unanimity in these studies showing what appears to be the heritability of some degree of susceptibility to the development of alcoholism once drinking (e.g., "social drinking") begins. Precisely what this heritable factor may be is not yet known.

Biochemical/Constitutional Factors

In an attempt to determine what may predispose an individual to the development (or lack of development) of alcoholism, a great number of biochemical and other constitutional factors have been investigated. These observations have been carried out in animals (alcohol-preferring versus alcohol-avoiding strains), as well as in humans. Human studies have included active alcoholics and recovered alcoholics, as well as non-alcoholics; they have also included studies on high-risk but not yet alcoholic groups (e.g., sons of alcoholics, native Americans, persons of northern European extraction) and those of lower risk (e.g., sons of nonalcoholic drinkers, persons of Mediterranean or Oriental ancestry). Some interesting but inconclusive differences have been noted.

One marked racial difference in response to alcohol is the striking facial flushing and increased pulse pressure observed in the majority of Orientals soon after ingestion of even small amounts of alcohol. Similar amounts of alcohol ingested by American Caucasians have no noticeable effect (Wolff, 1972). The response is noted as early as the neonatal period and is therefore not conditioned by previous use of alcohol. Ewing (1974) showed that this higher incidence of flushing in persons of Oriental extraction was the result of elevated blood acetaldehyde levels. Von Wartburg et al. (1975) reported that these findings coincide with racial differences of human liver alcohol dehydrogenase. The "atypical" enzyme is present in about 85% of Orientals and is responsible for producing the higher acetaldehyde levels. It is speculated that the slightly aversive symptoms experienced with flushing may help explain the low incidence of alcoholism among Orientals. The response is compared to a "mini-Antabuse reaction": Antabuse (disulfiram) blocks the enzyme aldehyde dehydrogenase and leads to a markedly uncomfortable acetaldehyde accumulation after alcohol ingestion.

On the other hand, Schuckit and Rayses (1979) found that nonalcoholic male first-degree relatives of alcoholics had a significantly elevated blood acetaldehyde concentration after a dose of alcohol compared to matched controls. First-degree relatives of alcoholics have a higher (not lower) risk of developing alcoholism, thus casting some doubt on the "mini-Antabuse reaction" explanation of the low alcoholism rate among Orientals. A similar pattern of elevated postalcohol acetaldehyde levels is seen in abstinent alcoholics (Korsten et al., 1975).

As a matter of fact, the elevated acetaldehyde levels may in some cases change the state of intoxication, perhaps making it more pleasant (rewarding). It might result in the formation of condensation products with monamine metabolites (neurotransmitters), with the production of addicting morphinelike alkaloids. Myers has shown that dopamine-related condensation products (tetrahydroisoquinolines, or TIQs) introduced directly into the brain of rats will induce a marked increase of voluntary alcohol consumption, even in rats that normally reject alcohol. This change in alcohol preference appears to be lifelong, since it was noted as long as 6 months after a single series of infusions (Myers and Melchior, 1977). In this respect, it resembles the permanent "crossing over the invisible line" of human alcoholics (Myers, 1978). Elevated TIQ levels have been found in human alcoholics after a dose of alcohol (Collins and Num, 1979).

Still other biochemical constitutional factors has been noted. Olson et al. (1960) reported that alcoholics demonstrate a defective conversion of the amino acid tryptophan into serotonin even after prolonged abstinence from alcohol.

In a series of tests of endocrine and autonomic nervous functions in drinking alcoholics, abstinent alcoholics (no alcohol for 2 or more years), and nonalcoholic controls, Kissin and his associates (1959a,b, 1960) and Kissin and Haukoff (1959) found a series of abnormalities in such functions as adrenal function, regulation of blood pressure, and metabolism of glucose. These differences, the authors believed, were constitutional characteristics of the alcoholics rather than the effects of alcoholism, because the abnormalities were still present more than 2 years after alcohol intake had been stopped. It might be argued that these changes could be the result of some permanent physiological derangement produced by heavy alcohol intake over many years in the past; however, even if this were true, perhaps the most interesting finding was that the intake of even small doses of alcohol by the alcoholics tended to restore these functions toward normal. That is, the alcoholics tended to be physiologically more normal with alcohol in their system than without alcohol. This may offer some clues into the phenomenon of alcohol "craving" experienced by alcoholics. Unfortunately, this "normalizing" effect does not mean that alcohol is "good" for alcoholics. It does suggest that there is a strong biochemical factor in maintaining alcoholism. These phenomena are supported by animal studies of alcohol consumption and alcohol effects.

Animal studies suggest that constitutional factors, perhaps, secondary to genetic variability, may influence the susceptibility to alcoholism. Marked differences in alcohol preference are found between inbred strains of mice (Rodgers et al., 1963). In fact, there are often substantial differences between the alcohol preferences of individual animals from the same litter (Schlesinger et al., 1967). In some cases, certain metabolic differences have been noted between alcohol-preferring and alcohol-avoiding animals (Iida, 1960).

Differences occur not only in alcohol metabolism, but also with quantitative and qualitative differences in the response of the brain to alcohol (Vogel and Matulsky, 1979). These results suggest that alcohol-related genetic differences and other constitutional differences between humans should also be sought at two levels (in alcohol metabolism and in influence on brain physiology).

Causing test animals to experience vitamin deficiencies or certain other deficiency states has been shown to increase the amount of alcohol they voluntarily consume (Mirone, 1959). Also, causing liver damage by chemical means (e.g., carbon tetrachloride) has been shown to be able to convert normal non-alcohol-preferring mice into alcohol-drinking mice (Iida, 1960). A somewhat similar phenomenon was reported in humans in which nonalcoholic drinkers of many years standing abruptly turned to an alcoholic drinking pattern following an episode of severe liver damage (e.g, carbon tetrachloride poisoning or severe viral hepatitis) (O'Hollaren, 1960). Although these studies are of great theoretical interest, at present we still have only some tantalizing glimpses of the "real" cause(s) of alcoholism.

These findings strongly suggest that alcohol consumption in the alcoholic is dependent upon physiological processes. While the specific processes are not well understood, it appears that motivation to consume alcohol, as well as the reinforcing effects of doing so, may depend upon biological processes. This relation may explain the apparent inability to identify an "alcoholic personality." Furthermore, these findings suggest that any attempts to change the drinking behavior of alcoholics will have to succeed in spite of such physiological processes. Most clearly, alcoholism is more complex than an explanation based upon lack of "will power" would imply.

Whatever the biological factors that may be involved in determining susceptibility to developing alcoholism, they can never act without some modulation by the environment and by the individual's psychological and emotional status. At the most basic level, it is required that alcohol be available in the environment and that the person be willing to initially consume some of it.

Some people find themselves in occupational or social settings where alcohol consumption is highly encouraged, whereas others have entirely different environmental settings. These factors cannot be ignored, no matter what the biological degree of susceptibility is.

Expectation also plays a role. Marlatt and Rohsenow (1980) have demonstrated that in a "taste-testing" task, the amount consumed depends on the subject's belief that the beverage contains alcohol. Both alcoholic and nonalcoholic subjects drink more if they believe that the beverage contains alcohol than if they believe it does not. These differences occur even when the beverage does not actually contain alcohol.

In any given individual there may be a complex interplay of a variety of environmental, psychological, hereditary, and other biological factors that ultimately determine whether or not that person becomes an alcoholic.

Diagnosis

Making the diagnosis of alcoholism is usually not exceptionally difficult once the possibility is considered. There are a number of clinical clues that, although not diagnostic in themselves, should alert one to the possibility of the diagnosis. Alcoholism is one disease that produces measurable damage in every system. Alcoholics will frequently present with a host of medical problems in different organ systems (but may never mention their drinking). Therefore transient symptoms in various systems should make one suspicious.

Before the patient even enters the physician's office, some clues may be present. When a spouse makes an appointment for his or her partner for a routine physical examination (and this is not a part of a long-established pattern of regular examinations) and no specific complaints are elicited in the history, one should think of alcoholism. This is particularly true if the patient is rather sulky during the process. In the hospital the patient who soon after admission begins to raise loud and unwarranted complaints over minor irritations and finally leaves in a huff, against medical advice, is also a likely candidate.

During the history-taking process several clues may be observed. When the drug history is taken, one must be alert to the phraseology of each response. When asking about alcohol use, an unusually long pause to "think up the right answer" or the opposite, the "too quick" response (one that has been planned out well ahead of time), should be alerting. Vague or distracting responses are also significant. Significant phrases are, "Alcohol is no problem for me"; "I can take it or leave it"; "I only drink beer"; "One or two ordinarily"; "I only drink socially"; "I only drink moderately." Some of these phrases are sufficiently elastic to include a fifth of whiskey per day. The average social drinker will usually give a few moments thought and then respond with a rather precise answer ("About once or twice a week I have a martini before dinner and one or two glasses of wine with dinner").

One way to increase the likelihood of getting a more responsive answer is to ask the questions in a somewhat less threatening and obviously logical order. One may begin by explaining that one is going to take a history of recent drug use—both prescription and nonprescription drugs—and that it is extremely important to be as accurate as possible about the kinds and amounts of drugs because of the possibility of interactions between one drug and some other drug that may later be prescribed, or interactions that may occur between a drug taken in the past and certain laboratory tests that may be done. Following this, one may then begin by asking what drugs have been taken in the last 2 months that were prescribed by a physician. This question is readily understood and nonthreatening. When it is answered, one may next ask what drugs have been taken in the last 2 months that have been prescribed by a pharmacist. This question is often not as easily understood and one may suggest that perhaps the patient has had a cold and was given some nonprescription nose drops or cough syrup by the neighborhood pharmacist. When this question is answered, one may then ask what drugs have been taken in the last 2 months that have been prescribed by the patient himself. At this point, one may explain that nicotine is a drug, as is alcohol, marijuana, cocaine, and so on. This progression of drug questioning is not foolproof, but it tends to produce less defensiveness than some more direct approaches.

The social and family history also holds many clues. A person who is functioning at a considerably lower job level than that for which he was trained (e.g., an engineer working as a clerk) is suspicious. A history of alcoholism in close blood relatives (alcoholism in a parent increases the likelihood of alcoholism in the patient fivefold) (Goodwin, 1976) or a history of child or spouse abuse is also suggestive (approximately 70% of beaten children are from alcoholic homes) (Bates, 1979).

During the physical examination itself, any or all systems may show clues.

Skin

In the skin some of the more obvious suggestive findings are spider angiomata, acne rosacea, or jaundice. However, one should also be suspicious of multiple bruises of differing ages, particularly at coffee table height (ankles and shins) and kitchen table or counter height (hips). It takes approximately 10 days for a bruise to progress from purple to yellow; therefore, a person with both purple and yellow bruises has acquired them at different times.

Also, particularly in men, cigarette burns—again of differing ages—and/ or the "mahogany finger syndrome" (brown fingers from cigarette tobacco tar) are all highly suggestive findings.

In women two or more horizontal "oven burns" on the forearms (again of differing ages) are also suspicious. The general principle is that anyone can be a little clumsy once in a while, but, if they make it a career, think of alcoholism.

Orthopedic System

The orthopedic system is also a fertile ground for clues. Vaguely explained fractures, particularly of the wrist, nose, legs, or skull, are suspicious (often referred to facetiously by emergency room personnel as "alcoholic bone disease"). Between the ages of 20 and 60 approximately 50% of home falls resulting in a fracture are due to alcoholism (Bates, 1979). This percentage rises to nearly 100% if the patient delays significantly in seeking treatment for the fracture (e.g., waits until the following day or two, when more sober).

Other clues are moderate muscle wasting of the proximal muscle groups of the upper and lower extremities (from chronic alcoholic myopathy), Dupuytren's contracture, and aseptic necrosis of the head of the femur in an adult without history of antecedent trauma.

Cardiovascular System

Almost any of the cardiac arrhythmias may be seen in alcoholics. Alcoholics frequently complain of palpitations, particularly in the acute withdrawal phase. It is almost axiomatic that the person who has his first episode of paroxysmal atrial tachycardia as an adult is an alcoholic until proved otherwise. Other common arrhythmias seen are ventricular premature contractions and paroxysmal atrial fibrillation.

Alcoholism should also be considered in the patient with an extremely erratic hypertensive course, one in which the physician is extremely frustrated trying to control it; one day the pressure may be up and the next day it may be too low.

Gastrointestinal System

The gastroingestinal system also shows many clues of alcoholism. Esophagitis, gastritis, pancreatitis, fatty liver (a palpably enlarged liver in an adult means alcoholism until proved otherwise), and cirrhosis are all diagnoses that have long been associated with alcoholism. Epidemiological data indicate that a 70-kg man who drinks approximately 210 g/day of alcohol for 20 years has a 50% risk of developing cirrhosis (Lelbach, 1974). Alcohol intake, rather than dietary protein or other nutrient content, is the primary factor here (Lieber et al., 1965).

More subtle clues than these are available, such as poor dental hygiene, with early loss of teeth, carcinoma of the upper gastrointestinal tract, heartburn, and intractible peptic ulcer (in alcoholism treatment facilities, next to the appendectomy scar, the most frequently encountered abdominal surgical scar is the gastrectomy scar). Recurrent diarrhea and various episodic "malabsorption" syndromes are also frequently seen in alcoholics.

Neurological System

The neurological system also contains many suggestive signs and symptoms. The typical "morning-after shakes," where it takes two hands to hold a glass of water, is highly suggestive, as is the classic picture of peripheral neuropathy (the tremor of age and Parkinson's disease is present at rest but improves with movement, while the tremor of alcohol withdrawal gets worse with movement). Less obvious to the uninitiated are the somewhat vaguely described "memory lapses," which are actually periods of amnesia that occur while the person has an elevated blood alcohol level. These are generally referred to as "alcoholic blackouts." During the "blackout" the person may be functioning completely normally (on the other hand, he may have a complete change of personality and describe himself as a Dr. Jekyll and Mr. Hyde when drinking). The next day all or a portion of that time is a complete blank in the memory, a blank that never gets filled in with reminding, hypnosis, returning to the scene of action, or any other technique yet tried.

The neurological examination conducted the "morning after" may show vertigo and nystagmus (a very early withdrawal symptom) that gradually clears during the day. Insomnia is also often listed as the complaint that first brought the alcoholic to the attention of his personal physician.

Alcohol withdrawal seizures 24–48 hours after the last drink are a relatively common occurrence. A first grand mal seizure after the age of 20 should cause one to consider alcoholism in the differential diagnosis.

Hematopoietic System

The hematopoietic system may also offer clues. One of the most common is macrocytosis, which is not associated with megaloblastosis or anemia. A mean cell volume of over 95 cubic microns should be considered suspicious. Other routine laboratory screening tests may offer additional clues. Alcoholics relatively often show disturbed glucose metabolism with either hyperglycemia or hypoglycemia. Elevations of lactic dehydrogenase, serum glutamic pyruvic transaminase, serum gamma-glutamic transaminase, and serum glutamic oxaloacetic transaminase may be noted, as well as hyperlipidemia, especially hypertriglyceridemia. Alcoholics may also show slight to moderate elevations in blood uric acid levels (in the absence of a history of gout).

Genitourinary System

Alcholics often show transitory evidence of renal damage with mild degrees of proteinuria after a drinking episode. Impotence is often the presenting complaint that first brings the alcoholic to the attention of a physician. It may occur first during an acute episode of intoxication but, in the chronic alcoholic, may be present during periods of abstinence from alcohol. The condition results from long-term, alcohol-mediated gonadal damage and endocrine derangement.

The fetal alcohol syndrome (FAS) is a significant risk for alcoholic women in the childbearing years. The family physician may first be alerted to the alcoholic woman's problem upon seeing an affected child. Such children are small for their gestational age, with a head size that is unexpectedly small even in relation to their reduced length. Their eyes are relatively undersized, so that the palpebral fissures are comparatively short. The midface is small, resulting in a rather flat lateral facial contour. The brain tends to be small and mental deficiencies from mild to severe may be observed (Smith, 1977). The risk of FAS in the offspring of severely alcoholic women has been estimated to be as high as 33% and the risk of mental deficiencies is approximately 50% (Jones et al., 1974).

None of these "clinical clues" are diagnostic in themselves. However, when one or more raise the possibility of the diagnosis of alcoholism, further exploration of that possibility should be carried out and the findings compared to the critieria for the diagnosis of alcoholism. Since denial is a major factor in alcoholism, if is often appropriate to question the spouse or some other family member. However, it is well known that denial is a major factor in alcoholism, it is often appropriate to question the patient, so that the physician must not dismiss his clinical impressions, even with a negative history from the family.

Making the diagnosis of alcoholism is only the first step in helping the alcoholic. The next and often most crucial step is presenting the diagnosis to the patient and getting his or her acceptance of it and a commitment to pursue treatment.

Timing is important in approaching the patient. Perhaps the most effective time is in the early postwithdrawal state ("the sick, sad, and sorry stage"). At this point the alcoholics's rationalization and excuses are often in a tattered state and it may be possible to "get through" most effectively at this time. If one delays even a day or two, however, the "impenetrable shields" are put back into place and it may not be possible to get the point across until after the next drinking episode. When approaching an alcoholic patient with his diagnosis, the physician should have the attitude and demeanor that he or she does in dealing with any other diagnosis. The slightest hint of a critically superior attitude or an accusatory approach will immediately reactivate all defenses.

Since the diagnosis is based on certain diagnostic criteria, it seems logical to start with these. Point out the positive findings the patient exhibits and tell what they mean. It is often helpful to have available a listing of the diagnostic criteria (e.g., the NCA criteria) to show the patient in order to avoid the argument that it is simply the physician's "biased opinion" prompted by an "unreasonable spouse" rather than a diagnosis based on generally accepted criteria.

When the patient's observable problem drinking behavior is described, it must also be emphasized that the drinking is the *source* of the problem, not the result. One must also monitor the patient's hostility and be ready to "titrate" it so that it does not result in premature termination of the doctor–patient relationship. The primary goal is to provide help. This cannot happen if the relationship is ruptured. This, however, does not mean that the physician should accept or discuss excuses or rationalizations for drinking. Like any other disease, when the diagnosis is discussed with the patient, a plan of therapy should also be discussed. It is important to convey to the patient that alcoholism can be treated successfully.

Treatment

Despite the physician's best efforts, the alcoholic patient often continues his or her posture of denial. The patient may stoutly maintain that he or she can "take it or leave it alone." At this point, rather than spending time in a fruitless argument, it is often useful to enter into a "therapeutic contract" (in writing) for self-diagnosis. To do this, ask the patient to specify the exact number of drinks he or she would feel comfortable with as a daily limit. The number of ounces of liquor in each "drink" must also be specified. When this amount is agreed upon (e.g., three drinks of 1½ oz. of whiskey per day), the period of time for limited drinking must also be agreed upon (e.g., 3 weeks). Then an agreement is made for the patient to return for another visit at the end of this specified time to discuss his or her experience with limited drinking.

It is a rare alcoholic who can limit his or her drinking for that length of time. Alcoholics may be able to abstain completely for that period, so it is important to have them agree to drink the specified amount each day—no more and no less.

If the patient is unsuccessful at "controlled drinking" but is still resistant to accepting alcoholism treatment, the physician may choose to set up an alcoholism intervention plan. The goal of the intervention is to break through the rationalizations and denials of the alcoholic by the force of a number of meaningful persons presenting, in a loving way, *specific* data on how his or her drinking is affecting their relationship and how those persons feel about it.

Treatment Options

Detoxification

Detoxification may be required if the patient presents in an intoxicated state or if the drinking history indicates that significant alcohol withdrawal reactions are likely to occur once drinking stops. When determining a detoxification plan, seven decisions must be made.

The first decision is whether to make the detoxification an inpatient or outpatient procedure. In determining the need for hospitalization, the physician must consider not only the present state of the patient, but also the expected severity of the withdrawal symptoms. For example, the patient who has been drinking a pint of whiskey daily for 2–10 days is likely to show only tremulousness on withdrawal; however, if he or she has been drinking that amount or more for a substantially longer period, delirium tremens or other serious withdrawal reactions may occur (Johnson, 1961). Other factors such as concurrent illness (peptic ulcer, pancreatitis, heart or liver disease) must also be evaluated. They, in themselves, may be indications for hospitalization or the added stress of alcohol withdrawal may adversely affect them.

Generally accepted criteria for outpatient withdrawal are the following:

1. Low volume and duration of drinking.
2. Previous successful efforts to withdraw as an outpatient.
3. Relative youth and general good health.
4. Good motvation.
5. Properly supportive home or other care-taking setting.

The second decision concerns how the alcohol should be withdrawn. In most settings, it should be withdrawn abruptly, rather than attempting to "taper off." This is particularly true in the outpatient setting, since one of the classic symptoms of alcoholism is loss of control over the total intake after the first two or three drinks. In the hospital setting with properly trained staff, the alcohol can be withdrawn either gradually over two or more days or abruptly. In the latter case, the patient must receive adequate supplemental sedation to control symptoms.

The third decision relates to fluid and electrolyte balance. The patient may be dehydrated or overhydrated; he or she often is depleted in potassium and/or magnesium. The patient's status must be determined and a decision made as to what, if any, treatment is required. In most cases allowing normal homeostatic mechanisms to return the patient to normal is appropriate. Providing free access to fluids and food is sufficient in these cases. In other cases, with more severe derangement of the fluid and electrolyte balance, appropriately tailored parenteral fluids must be administered.

The fourth decision concerns whether or not nausea and/or vomiting must be treated. Alleviation of nausea and vomiting, when present, is important in minimizing further fluid and electrolyte depletion. It also reduces the likelihood of additional complications such as ruptured esophageal varices, hemorrhage from alcoholic gastritis, or Mallory–Weiss syndrome. If the patient has a high blood alcohol level or significant blood levels of other sedatives, caution is required in the administration of antiemetic medications, since most are themselves sedating and may lead to a dangerous level of sedative depression. When a less sedating drug is desirable, trimethobenzamide (Tigan) is often used. When sedation as well as an antiemetic effect is desired, one of the phenothiazines [e.g., prochlorperazine maleate (Compazine)] is frequently used.

The fifth decision relates to the need for sedation. Sedation may be life saving in some cases. Anxiety states, insomnia, psychomotor agitation, tremors, and delirium tremens are the usual indications for sedation. One commonly used "withdrawal routine" is to substitute for the alcohol a long-acting drug that has cross-tolerance and cross-addiction with alcohol (e.g., one of the benzodiazapine tranquilizers). This longer-acting drug is then gradually withdrawn over a period of 2–4 days (or longer if the symptoms require it) (Kissin, 1977). The key point is to achieve *adequate* sedation. This, at first, may require a much larger dose of medication than the physician is used to prescribing; however, it is essential that adequate control be gained over the severe symptoms in order to prevent life-threatening complications such as delirium tremens. On the other hand, it must be remembered that alcoholics become addicted to sedative drugs relatively easily and care must be taken to discontinue those drugs as soon as possible. Drugs with properties of cross-tolerance and cross-addiction to alcohol are generally not suitable candidates for long-term use with alcoholics (although they are often useful for a short period of time during detoxification).

The sixth decision concerns whether or not anticonvulsant medication should be used during withdrawal. Alcohol withdrawal seizures are common during the first 24–48 horus. Without treatment one or more grand mal seizures may occur during this time. Untreated, the seizure rate in hospitalized alcoholics is as high as 20% (Nielsen, 1956). When a benzodiazapine tranquilizer is used for sedation, it also gives considerable anticonvulsant protection. Diphenylhydantoin (Dilantin) is also frequently used and is effective in controlling seizures (Sampliner and Iber, 1974).

The seventh decision concerns how and when to return the patient to normal nutrition. It is especially important to ensure a high vitamin intake, particularly of the B complex vitamins. Deficiencies of these vitamins can result in neurological complications. Even without overt signs of peripheral neuropathy or Wernicke's syndrome, the alcoholic is likely to be at least relatively depleted in thiamine (Smith, 1968). The vitamins should be given parenterally at first in order to ensure complete absorption. Later an oral preparation can be used. As soon as possible, the patient should be placed on a well-balanced diet, unless specific medical complications (e.g., liver failure) dictate dietary modifications.

Definitive Alcoholism Treatment

Detoxification is not treatment for alcoholism; it simply renders the patient ready to undertake treatment. The physician must then decide what definitive course of action to take. A major decision to make is whether to refer the patient to an inpatient treatment program or attempt to treat him or her in an outpatient setting. Inpatient treatment programs offer a number of advantages. A major one is that the patient is physically removed from his previous environment, one that often tends to support his drinking, and is instead "cloistered" in an alcohol-free setting. This helps to guarantee freedom from alcohol intake for a period of time long enough for healing to begin and/or alcohol-disordered thinking to return toward normal. In addition, spending 24 hours a day in a treatment facility allows the patient to focus intensely on the drinking problem. The educational, counseling, and other treatment processes do not have to compete with a host of other daily pressures and distractions related to job and family activities. This allows more rapid progress in achieving the therapeutic goal. The inpatient setting also allows a more integrated and structured treatment process to occur.

Many inpatient treatment programs involve 28 days of treatment (postdetoxification). These programs often contain the flexibility to continue the inpatient phase for 6–8 weeks or even longer if needed. The treatment plan, ideally, is individualized, but is generally multimodal and includes a physical and laboratory assessment, assessment of the patient's specific drinking pattern and its consequences in all spheres of life (health, family, social, employment/financial, spiritual).

Individual and group therapy sessions are held that usually deal with education about the disease concept of alcoholism and its consequences, drug-free coping strategies, and specific problem-solving strategies for the patient's individual situation. Many treatment facilities also include Alcoholics Anonymous (AA) indoctrination and meetings during the treatment phase and use AA as their primary aftercare support system. The treatment programs also generally focus on the family and usually invite family members or "significant others" to participate in at least the educational portion of the program and in the aftercare plan. Some programs also prescribe disulfiram (Antabuse) as part of the therapeutic regimen.

These programs vary widely in the degree of medical supervision and participation. They also vary widely in the degree to which they use other degreed personnel (masters of social work, registered nurses, psychologists) and "nondegreed professionals" such as recovered alcoholics with or without credentials as "certified alcoholism counselors" (most accrediting bodies now require that nondegreed counselors undergo specific training and appropriate certification).

The treatment goal of these programs is for the patient to live a drug-free life. To this end, it is emphasized that alcohol in all forms must be avoided permanently. The programs also emphasize the potential danger of becoming addicted to tranquilizers or other sedative drugs.

Baekeland et al. (1975) reviewed 401 references of these treatment approaches. They concluded that patient characteristics tend to play an even greater role in outcome than do kinds of treatment. Patients with higher socioeconomic status, higher motivation, and higher social stability have the best prognosis. Outpatient programs were reported to have slightly higher improvement rates (41.6%) than inpatient programs, but this finding is distorted by the substantially higher drop-out rate (36.9% versus 17%). The authors endorse a multimodal approach.

Aversion Conditioning

A more medically intensive type of inpatient treatment program emphasizes behavior modification treatment modalities in addition to counseling, education, medical evaluation, and aftercare. These facilities use aversion conditioning to pair the sight, smell, and taste of alcoholic beverages with an aversive stimulus (e.g., nausea). The purpose is to eliminate the craving for alcohol as rapidly as possible and to break down "conditioned reflexes to drink" (Smith, 1982).

One group of alcoholism hospitals also uses "pentothal interviews" in addition to aversion conditioning. This procedure is intended to assist the staff in gaining psychiatric diagnostic material and to monitor the development of aversion. These facilities use a multimodal treatment approach in addition to aversion conditioning and "pentothal interviews." They report long-term abstinence rates between 60 and 70% (Smith, 1966). In addition to having somewhat higher success rates, these programs are typically shorter in duration. The initial postdetoxification treatment period is usually about 10 days. This may be of advantage to patients who find it difficult to remain away from work for 28 or more days.

Outpatient Treatment

Physicians may elect to treat the alcoholic in their office alone or with the help of one or more outside agencies, depending upon their level of familiarity and skill in dealing with alcoholism. This approach allows the physician to deal with any alcohol-related physical/medical complications. Physician counseling with the patient and family may also be carried out. This is often combined with referral to one or more local agencies for additional alcohol education and/or alcohol counseling. The agencies may include formally organized alcoholism facilities and/or Alcoholics Anonymous (AA). For a detailed discussion of AA, see Leach and Norris (1977). Referral may also be made to other specific support or treatment agencies for related problems, for example, marriage counseling and job retraining.

The physician may also elect to administer disulfiram (Antabuse) as an adjunct to treatment. Disulfiram blocks the action of aldehyde dehydrogenase (the second step in alcohol metabolism) so that ingestion of even small amounts of alcohol leads to an accumulation of acetaldehyde. The patient then develops unpleasant symptoms of flushing, pounding headache, nausea, and vomiting. Severe life-threatening reactions may occur, with tachycardia, arrhythmias, hyperventilation, syncope, cardiovascular collapse, and even death. (The physician should familiarize himself thoroughly with the prescribing literature before using disulfiram. It is essential to be aware of the contraindications, potential side effects, and adverse reactions, as well as interactions that may occur with other drugs.) Although disulfiram does not eliminate the craving for alcohol, it may aid a motivated patient to resist a momentary impulse to drink. Alcohol–disulfiram reactions may occur for up to a week or more after the last dose. Therefore a patient on the drug who decides to return to drinking should be deterred from doing so for at least a week because of fear of having a severe reaction. During this interval he may change his mind about drinking and continue taking the drug. In this way alcoholics are protected from sudden urges to drink; however, they can always plan ahead for drinking and stop taking disulfiram for a week or more before they drink. Simply offering disulfiram to a patient is often a good test of motivation. The well-motivated patient will usually readily accept the offer, with the statement that he wants to do anything that might help. The patient who declines, perhaps with some lofty statement that he does not want to rely on a "crutch," can generally be expected to drink again soon (and does not want anything to interfere with his next planned binge). It is also imperative to warn family members not to give disulfiram to an alcoholic without his knowledge, since it might result in a life-threatening alcohol–disulfiram reaction.

In treating the alcoholic patient, the physician should keep in mind that alcoholism is a disease that is often associated with relapse. It is important to view alcoholic relapse with the same equanimity one views exacerbations of arthritis or diabetic ketoacidosis. One should always work to avoid relapses completely, but if they occur they should not be viewed as a sign of failure on the part of the physician or the patient. Efforts should be directed toward eliminating, or at least minimizing, relapse and prolonging abstinence from alcohol.

The goal should be for the patient to live a productive, satisfying, and drug-free life. Great care must be taken to avoid developing one or more other drug dependencies. Of particular danger for alcoholics are barbiturates, meprobamate, and benzodiazipine tranquilizers. These drugs share cross-tolerance and cross-addiction with alcohol. It is easy to become addicted to one of these drugs if they are prescribed for sedation after alcohol treatment. Also, simply taking one of the drugs may again stimulate the craving for alcohol. It has been the general experience in the alcoholism field that the relapse rate for alcoholism is substantially increased in patients who take these drugs regularly. Patients must also be cautioned against inadvertently taking alcohol in the form of medications (elixirs) or food (e.g., cherries jubilee). Some patients date the return of alcohol craving to such experiences.

With relatively nonspecific supportive office treatment such as that described above the remission rate can be expected to be approximately 33% (Schuchit, 1978). The alcoholic who is socially stable and free of major psychopathology is most likely to be successful in an outpatient program. If a major psychological problem is present, then referral to appropriate psychiatric treatment is indicated. Alcoholics whose lives have been totally disrupted so that they no longer have a family, job, or other stable social support system do not do well in outpatient programs (Kissin, 1980).

References

Achte, K. 1958. Correlation of ABO blood groups with alcoholism. Duodecim 74(1):20–21.

Baekeland, F., L. Lundwall, and B. Kissin. 1975. Methods for the treatment of chronic alcoholism: A critical appraisal. In R. J. Gibbons and Y. Israel, eds.: Research Advances in Alcohol and Drug Problems, Vol. 2. New York: Wiley; pp. 247–327.

Bailey, R. J., N. Krasner, A. L. W. F. Eddleston, et al. 1976. Histocompatibility antigens, antibodies, and hemoglobulins in alcoholic liver disease. British Medical Journal 2:727–729.

Bates, R. C. 1979. The hidden alcoholic clinical and behavioral signs of alcoholism. Diagnosis. 1:33–39.

Bell, H., and R. Nordhagen. 1972. Association between HLA-BW40 and alcoholic liver disease with cirrhosis. British Medical Journal 1:822.

Cadoret, R. J., C. A. Cain, and W. M. Grove. 1980. Development of alcoholism in adoptees raised apart from alcoholic biologic relatives. Archives in General Psychiatry 37:561–563.

Camps, F. E., and B. E. Dodd. 1967. Increase in the incidence of nonsecretors of ABH blood group substances among alcoholic patients. British Medical Journal 1:30–31.

Collins, M. A., and W. P. Num. 1979. Dopamine-related tetrohydroisoquinolines: Significant urinary excretion by alcoholics after alcohol consumption. Science 206:1184–1186.

Del Villano, B. C., et al. 1979. Cupro-zinc superoxide dismutase: A possible biologic marker for alcoholism (studies in black patients). Alcoholism (New York) 3:291–296.

Ewing, J. A. 1978. Recognizing, confronting and helping the alcoholic. American Family Physician 18:107–114.

Ewing, J. A., B. A. Rouse, and E. D. Pellizzari. 1974. Alcohol sensitivity and ethnic background. American Journal of Psychiatry 131:206–210.

Goodwin, D. W. 1976. Is Alcoholism Heredity? New York: Oxford University Press, 1976; p. 45.

Goodwin, D. W. 1979. Genetic determinants of alcoholism. *In* J. H. Mendelson and N. K. Mello, eds.: The Diagnosis and Treatment of Alcoholism. New York: McGraw-Hill; pp. 59–82.

Goodwin, D. W., F. Schulsinger, L. Hermansen, et al. 1973. Alcohol problems in adoptees raised apart from alcoholic biologic parents. Archives of General Psychiatry 28:238–243.

Goodwin, D. W., F. Schulsinger, N. Moller, et al. 1974. Drinking problems in adopted and nonadopted sons of alcoholics. Archives of General Psychiatry 31:164–169.

Halenar, J. F. 1979. Drinking and drugs: Behind the hard numbers. Medical Economics. Special issue 1:109–119.

Iida, S. 1960. Experimental studies on the craving for alcohol, III: The relationship between alcoholic craving and carbohydrate metabolism. Japanese Journal of Pharmacology 10:15–20.

Imboden, J. B., and J. C. Urbaitis. 1978. Practical psychiatry in medicine: Part 9: Alcoholism. Journal of Family Practice 6:685–691.

Jellinek, E. M. 1960. The Disease Concept of Alcoholism. New Haven, Connecticut: College and University Press.

Johnson, R. B. 1961. The alcohol withdrawal syndrome. Journal of Studies on Alcohol Supplement 1:66–76.

Jones, K. L., D. W. Smith, P. A. Streissguth, and N. C. Myrianthopoulos. 1974. Outcome in offspring of chronic alcoholic women. Lancet 1:1076–1078.

Kaij, L. 1960. Studies on the Etiology and Sequels of Abuse of Alcohol. Lund, Finland: Department of Psychiatry, University of Lund.

Kissin, B. 1977. Medical management of the alcoholic patient. *In* B. Kissin and H. Begleiter, eds.: The Biology of Alcoholism, Vol. 5. Treatment and Rehabilitation of the Chronic Alcoholic. New York: Plenum Press; pp. 53–103.

Kissin, B. 1980. Should All Physicians Be Trained to Treat Alcohol and Drug Abuse in Medical Education? U.S. Department of Health, Education and Welfare Publication No. (ADM) 79-891; p. 87. Washington DC: U.S. Government Printing Office.

Kissin, B., L. Hankoff. 1959. The acute effects of ethyl alcohol on the Funkenstein Mecholyl response in male alcoholics. Journal of Studies on Alcohol 20:696–703.

Kissin, B., V. Schenker, and A. C. Schenker. 1959a. The acute effects of ethyl alcohol and chlorpromazine on certain physiological functions in alcoholics. Journal of Studies on Alcohol 20:480–492.

Kissin, B., V. Schenker, and A. C. Schenker. 1959b. Adrenal cortical function and liver disease in alcoholics. American Journal of Medical Science 344–353.

Kissin, B., V. Schenker, and A. C. Schenker. 1960. The acute effect of ethanol ingestion on plasma and urinary 17-hydroxycorticoids in alcoholic subjects. American Journal of Medical Science 239:690–705.

Korsten, M. A., S. Matsuzaki, L. Feinman, and C. S. Lieber. 1975. High blood acetaldehyde levels after ethanol administration: difference between alcoholic and nonalcoholic subjects. New England Journal of Medicine 292:386–389.

Leach, B., and Norris, J. L. 1977. Factors in the development of Alcoholics Anonymous (AA). *In* B. Kissin and H. Begleiter, eds.: The Biology of Alcoholism. Volume V of the Treatment of the Chronic Alcoholic. New York: Plenum Press.

Lelbach, W. K. 1974. Organic pathology related to volume and pattern of alcohol use. *In* R. J. Gibbins, Y. Israel, H. Kalant, R. E. Popham, W. Schmidt, and R. G. Smart, eds.: Research Advances in Alcohol and Drug Problems, Vol. I. New York: Wiley; p. 136.

Lieber, C. S., D. P. Jones, and L. M. De Carli. 1965. Effects of prolonged ethanol intake: Production of fatty liver despite adequate diets. Journal of Clinical Investigation 44:1009–1021.

Marlatt, A. M., and D. J. Rohsenow. 1980. Coginitive processes in alcohol use: Expectancy and the balanced placebo design. *In* N. K. Mello, ed.: Advances in Substance Abuse: Behavioral and Biological Research, Vol. I. Greenwich, Connecticut: JAI Press.

Mirone, L. 1959. Water and alcohol consumption by mice. Journal of Studies on Alcohol 20:24–27.

Myers, R. D., and C. L. Melchior. 1977. Alcoholic drinking: Abnormal intake caused by tetrahydropapaveroline in brain. Science 196:554–555.

Myers, R. D. 1978. Tetrohydroisoquinolines in the brain: The basis of an animal model of alcoholism. Alcoholism (New York) 2:145–154.

National Council on Alcoholism. 1972. Criteria Committee: Criteria for the diagnosis of alcoholism. American Journal of Psychiatry 129:127–135.

Nielsen, J. M. 1956. The neurology of alcoholism. *In* G. N. Thompson, ed.: Alcoholism. Springfield, Illinois: Charles C. Thomas; p. 444.

Nordmo, S. H. 1959. Blood groups in schizophrenia, alcoholism and mental deficiency. American Journal of Psychiatry 116:460–461.

O'Hollaren, P. 1960. Differential diagnosis of problem drinkers. Northwest Medicine 59:639–643.

Olson, R. E., D. Gursey, and J. W. Vester. 1960. Evidence for a defect in tryptophan metabolism in chronic alcoholism. New England Journal of Medicine 263:1169–1174.

Peeples, E. E. 1962. Taste Sensitivity to Phenylthiocarbamide in Alcoholics. Master's thesis, Stetson University, Deland, Florida.

Propping, P. 1978. Pharmacogenetics. Review of Physiology, Biochemistry, and Pharmacology 83:123–173.

Rodgers, D. A., G. E. McClearn, E. L. Bennett, and M. Herbert. 1963. Alcohol preference as a function of its caloric utility in mice. Journal of Comparative and Physiological Psychology 56:666–672.

Sampliner, R., and F. L. Iber. 1974. Diphenylhydantoin control of alcohol withdrawal seizures: Results of a controlled study. Journal of the American Medical Association 230:1430–1432.

Schlesinger, K., E. L. Bennett, and M. Herbert. 1967. Effects of genotype and prior consumption of alcohol on rates of ethanol-1-^{14}C metabolism in mice. Journal of Studies on Alcohol 28:231–235.

Schuckit, M. A. 1978. The disease of alcoholism. Postgraduate Medicine 64:78–84.

Shuckit, M. A., and V. Rayses. 1979. Ethanol ingestion differences in blood acetaldehyde concentrations in relatives of alcoholics and controls. Science 203:54–55.

Schuckit, M. A., E. N. Pitts, Jr., T. Reich, et al. 1969. Alcoholism I: Two types of alcoholism in women. Archives of General Psychiatry 20:301–306.

Schuckit, M. A., D. W. Goodwin, and G. Winokur. 1972. A study of alcoholism in half siblings. American Journal of Psychiatry 128:1132–1136.

Shields, J. 1962. Monozygotic Twins Brought up Apart and Brought up Together. London, England: Oxford University Press.

Smith, D. W. 1977. Fetal alcohol syndrome: A tragic and preventable disorder. *In* N. J. Estes and M. Heinemann, eds.: Alcoholism: Development, Consequences, and Interventions. St. Louis, Missouri: C. V. Mosby; pp. 144–149.

Smith, J. W. 1966. Conditioned reflex aversion treatment of alcoholism. Western Medicine Medical Journal, December.

Smith, J. W. 1968. Medical mangement of acute alcoholic intoxication. General Physician 38:89–93.

Smith, J. W. 1982. Aversion conditioning hospitals. *In* E. Kaufman and E. M. Pattison, eds.: The American Encyclopedic Handbook of Alcoholism. New York: Gardner Press.

Smith, J. W., and T. A. Layden. 1971. Color vision defects in alcoholism, II. British Journal of Addiction 66:31–37.

Swinson, R. P., and J. S. Madden. 1973. Blood groups and the secretion of ABH substance in alcoholism. Quarterly Journal of Studies on Alcohol 34:64–70.

United States Department of Commerce. 1979. Statistical Abstract of the United States, 100th ed. Washington DC: Bureau of the Census; p. 76.

United States Department of Health and Human Services. 1981a. National Institute on Alcohol Abuse and Alcoholism. *In* J. R. DeLuca, ed.: Fourth Special Report to the U.S. Congress on Alcohol and Health from the Secretary of Health Human Health Services. Rockville, Maryland: U.S. Dept of Health and Human Services, NIAAA.

United States Department of Health and Human Services. 1981b. Statistical Compendium on Alcohol and Health, 1st ed. Rockville, Maryland: NIAAA. p. 81.

Varela, A., L. Rivera, J. Mardones, and R. Cruz-Coke. 1969. Color vision defects in non-alcoholic relatives of alcoholic patients. British Journal of Addiction 64:67–73.

Vogel, F., and A. G. Matulsky. 1979. Human Genetics: Problems and Approaches. New York: Springer-Verlag; p. 514.

Von Wartburg, J. P., D. Berger, M. N. Rio, and P. Tabakoff. 1975. Enzymes of biogenic aldehyde metabolism. *In* M. M. Gross, ed.: Alcohol Intoxification and Withdrawal: Experimental Studies, II. 59:119–138. New York: Plenum Press.

Whitfield, C. L., and K. Williams. 1977. The Patient With Alcoholism and Other Drug Problems: Medical Aspect for Physicians and Other Helpers, 3rd ed., Wisconsin: Medical College of Wisconsin Medical Education Program.

Winokur, G., and P. Clayton. 1967. Family history studies, II. Sex differences and alcoholism in primary affective illness. British Journal of Psychiatry 115:973–979.

Winokur, G., J. Rimmer, and T. Reich. 1971. Alcoholism, IV: Is there more than one type of alcoholism? British Journal of Psychiatry 118:525–531.

Wolff, P. H. 1972. Ethnic difference in alcohol sensitivity. Science 175:449–450.

Woodruff, R. A., Jr., D. W. Goodwin, and S. B. Guze. 1974. Affective Disorders in Psychotic Diagnosis. New York: Oxford University Press.

World Health Organization. 1952. Expert Committee on Mental Health. Alcoholism Subcommittee: Second Report: World Health Organization Technical Report Series, No. 48. Geneva, Switzerland: WHO.

22

Problems of Aging
in Medical Practice

Burton V. Reifler, M.D., M.P.H.* and Suzanne Wu, Ph.D.†

The Elderly Patient

Older patients are at greater risk to receive inadequate health care than younger persons, in part because of myths and sterotypes held by health service providers. Among the common myths that intefere with appropriate management are the beliefs that the elderly are in poor health and do not wish diagnosis and treatment, that diagnosis and treatment would not help anyway because the problems are incurable, and that no clinical problem really exists because the symptoms are an inevitable part of the aging process (Goodstein, 1980). A classic story relates the conversation of a 104-year-old man who went to see his physician because of a painful left knee. When the physician began to remark, "Well you know, at your age you must expect . . . ," the patient retorted, "My right knee is 104 too. It doesn't hurt—just fix up the other one."

In contrast to these stereotypes are research findings that show that older persons have fewer acute illness than do younger individuals. Such acute illnesses, however, last about 25% longer than for younger patients (Estes, 1969). Chronic illnesses, on the other hand, affect up to 80% of the elderly (Filner and Williams, 1981), but they do not usually prevent the person from doing his or her daily activities. Since the ability to live independently is a measure of health, it is important to note that less than 10% of those 75 and over live in nursing homes (Shanas, 1969).

It is still a controversial point as to whether there are age-related changes, independent of diagnosable illness, in the cognitive and intel-

*Associate Professor, Department of Psychiatry and Behavioral Sciences, University of Washington School of Medicine, Seattle, Washington.
† Instructor, Department of Psychiatry and Behavioral Sciences, University of Washington School of Medicine, Seattle, Washington.

lectual functioning of the elderly. As Eisdorfer (1969) reported, mental response are heavily influenced by social and psychological factors. When older people are given more time to respond, learning improves, whereas when time pressures are emphasized, they tend to withhold responses. There may be differences in performance due to situational factors, but ability may remain unimpaired.

In a thorough review of research concerning the elderly and their families, Stuart and Snope (1981) concluded that families care for their older members and do not abandon them. Brody (1977) has estimated that 80% of the support services the elderly receive are provided by families. Studies from the United Kingdom show that family neglect plays a negligible role in admissions to geriatric units (Issacs, 1971). Relatives willingly accept the care of impaired elderly upon discharge from a geriatric facility, even when the staff questions the relative's ability to provide the required home care (Lowther and Williamson, 1966).

Exposure of these stereotypes as myths has crucial implications for the practicing physician, since many physicians have an unfavorble bias toward the elderly patient (Ford and Sbordone, 1980). If a physician sees an 80-year-old dejected, mildly confused man and regards this patient as simply showing manifestations of old age, then he or she is unlikely to think of potentially reversible problems. And even if physicians perform complete assessments, they set goals for treatment that are too limited and which may not reflect what *is* normal for the elderly; to be active and among friends and family.

Goodstein (1980) recommended some practical guidelines in working with elderly patients, since the physician's style in treating the elderly can have a significant impact on the doctor–patient relationship. At the initial meeting the physician should indicate respect for the patient and sensitivity to the older generation's values and expectations by addressing the patient by his or her title and last name (e.g., Mr. Smith or Mrs. Jones), rather than by the first name. As the relationship develops, the salutations may become less formal, at the request of the patient.

When talking with a patient in a hospital setting, it is preferable to sit in a chair next to the patient's bed, giving the patient enough distance to feel comfortable, but close enough to allow him or her to see and hear. Often physicians will talk to patients while standing by their bedside, conveying to the patient that the physician is pressed for time. Since older men tend to inhibit responses when a time limit is emphasized (Eisdorfer, 1969), this will often reduce the exchange of information. Similarly inappropriate is the physician who sits on the patient's bed during the initial visit, implying a familiarity that may be viewed as presumptous. Although the elderly tend to accept the authority of physicians more than younger persons do (Haug, 1979), it is important to allow all patients some sense of control in decision making, given the correlation between absence of power and feelings of helplessness and depression (Schain, 1980).

The medical assessment of patients, particularly older ones, should be comprehensive and not just symptom oriented. It is important to determine the patient's social, financial, emotional, cognitive, and self-care status, as well as medical condition. For example, is the patient cognitively intact enough to take his medications as prescribed? The elderly are often overmedicated with different drugs prescribed by multiple physicians, which causes confusion for the patient. This confusion may result from conflicting information and from toxic effects of several medications. A good way to assess the patient's medication intake is to have him or her bring all medications when visiting the physician. When an adequate history is unobtainable from the patient, it is important to get information from family members or friends. History taking should address common psychological issues with which the elderly are concerned but may be afraid to express voluntarily, for example, fears of sexual dysfunction, dependency, memory loss, and death.

A study by Williamson and his colleagues (1964) investigated the unreported medical needs of older persons (aged 65 and over) in the community. These patients were randomly selected from elderly patients in three general medical practices. Since the practices were chosen partly because of the cooperation and willingness of the general practitioners, the quality of medical care was probably above average. Nevertheless, the most striking finding was the frequency of multiple disabilities. Men had a mean of 3.26 disabilities, of which 1.87 were unknown to the family doctor; women had a mean of 3.42 disabilities, of which 2.03 were unknown to the family doctor. Disabilities identified involved many different systems, including respiratory, circulatory, alimentary, nervous, genitourinary, and locomotor systems. A variety of psychiatric disorders had also gone undetected. Most of the unknown disabilities were slight or moderately severe, although a few were in the severe range.

The study has implications for general practitioners. Clearly, the unmet need for general medical attention was high. The fact that most of the unknown disabilities were mild or moderately severe suggests that older persons do not report their problems to their physicians until the condition is advanced. Thus a medical practice based on the self-reporting of illness may underserve the needs of the elderly.

Other problems include noncompliance with treatment recommendations, which may be particularly problematic with elderly patients but which can be corrected in several ways. Waiting time should be kept to a minimum because of greater susceptibility to fatigue. Offices should be designed with the physical capabilities of the older patient in mind, stairs should be avoided, rooms and hallways should be well lit, and handrails should be installed in bathrooms. Treatment recommendations, including medication dosages and side effects, should be written down for the patient in large, legible print. Instructions should be given slowly, and the patient tactfully asked to paraphrase the instructions to ensure comprehension.

Mental Illness in the Elderly

Cognitive Functioning in the Elderly

One of the most pervasive stereotypes concerning elderly patients concerns senility. It is often assumed that senility is common and even inevitable for those who reach an advanced age. In fact, some of the apparent senile dementia may be at least partly caused by reversible conditions.

A compilation of three studies on a total of 222 patients who had documented dementia (Wells, 1977) shows that 51% received a final diagnosis of Alzheimer's disease. Other diagnoses included vascular disease (8%), normal pressure hydrocephalus (6%), alcohol-related dementia (6%), intracranial masses (5%), Huntington's chorea (5%), depression (4%), drug toxicity (3%), and Creutzfeld–Jacob disease (1%). A wide variety of other diagnoses, such as hypothyroidism, pernicious anemia, and subarachnoid hemorrhage, made up the balance.

Some patients with dementia may have a reversible disease, whereas others will at least have a reversible component to their cognitive impairment. In a series of 76 patients seen at Geriatric & Family Services in Seattle, Washington, 47 had a previously undetected problem that was potentially treatable and 20 of these showed unequivocal improvement when such treatment was given (Table 1).

A brief discussion is warranted on Alzheimer's disease, which, as noted above, accounts for about half of all cases of irreversible dementia. A term once reserved for individuals with onset of dementia prior to age 60, the definition of Alzheimer's disease has now been expanded to include patients of any age with a slow, gradual deterioration due to neuronal degeneration. It is a diagnosis of exclusion, made after other causes have been ruled out, and can be confirmed only through examination of brain tissue, such as at autopsy. Although the cause is unknown, current theories include a viral origin and destruction of central nervous system cells that play a role in the production of the neurotransmitter acetylcholine (Growdon and Corkin, 1980). Alzheimer's disease does not seem to be due to blood vessel disease nor to a lack of oxygen supply to the brain (Lassen and Ingvar, 1980). A popular belief is that most dementia is due to "hardening of the arteries," but, as noted above, dementia due to vascular

Table 1. Treatable Illnesses Detected During Medical or Psychiatric Examination ($n = 76$)

Diagnosis	Number detected	Unequivocal motor or cognitive improvement on follow-up visit
Depression	16	10
Folate deficiency	10	1
Parkinson's disease	5	2
Urinary tract infection	5	0
Drug toxicity	4	4
Myxedema	1	1
Rheumatoid cerebral vasculitis	1	1
Metastatic breast carcinoma	1	0
Temporal lobe epilepsy	1	0
Metastatic carcinoma of colon	1	0
Subdural hygroma	1	1
Subarachnoid cyst	1	0
	47	20

disease accounts for but a small proportion of cognitive impairment. When present, this is called multi-infarct dementia and can be diagnosed only if there is good evidence for previous strokes or a history of transient ischemic attacks (TIAs), which are periods of neurological deficit lasting up to several hours.

While research indicates that loss of cognitive functioning is not an inevitable consequence of aging, a major problem for the physician is accurately assessing both the presence and degree of dysfunction, when it does occur.

Dementia, or the progressive deterioration of cognitive functioning, is a symptom complex, not a specific disease, which affects about 10–15% of people over 65 (Gurland et al., 1980). Useful guides to establishing the presence of dementia are the DSM III (American Psychaitric Association, 1980) criteria (Table 2) or the test developed by Pfeiffer (1975) (Table 3). Physicians cannot rely on their casual impressions of the patient to determine if dementia is present and should incorporate those questions proposed in Table 3 (or equivalent tests) into their routine examinations. Many patients will be well groomed and able to make pleasant small talk, but their deficits will appear with formal mental status examination, which can be tactfully prefaced by a comment such as, "You seem well oriented to your surroundings, but I'd like to ask you a few routine questions that I ask everyone."

Table 2. Diagnostic Criteria for Dementia[a]

A. A loss of intellectual abilities of sufficient severity to interfere with social or occupational functioning.

B. Memory impairment.

C. At least one of the following:

   1. Impairment of abstract thinking, as manifested by concrete interpretation of proverbs, inability to find similarities and differences between related words, difficulty in defining words and concepts, and other similar tasks.
   2. Impaired judgment.
   3. Other disturbances of higher cortical function, such as aphasia (disorder of language due to brain dysfunction), apraxia (inability to carry out motor activities despite intact comprehension and motor function), agnosia (failure to recognize or identify objects despite intact sensory function), "constructional difficulty" (e.g., inability to copy three-dimensional figures, assemble blocks, or arrange sticks in specific designs).
   4. Personality change, i.e., alteration or accentuation of premorbid traits.

D. State of consciousness not clouded (i.e., does not meet the criteria for delirium or intoxication, although these may be superimposed).

E. Either one of the following:

   1. Evidence from the history, physical examination, or laboratory tests of a specific organic factor that is judged to be etiologically related to the disturbance.
   2. In the absence of evidence such as in (1), an organic factor necessary for the development of the syndrome can be presumed if conditions other than organic mental disorders have been reasonably excluded and if the behavioral change represents cognitive impairment in a variety of areas.

---

[a]From the American Psychiatric Association Diagnostic and Statistical Manual, 3rd Ed.

If a patient manifests dementia, a thorough examination is required to determine the cause. Wells (1977) has described the fundamentals of the history and physical examination and has outlined a series of ancilary procedures (Table 4) that will identify virtually all of the reversible causes of dementia.

Cognitive Testing in the Elderly Adult

Cognitive evaluation through psychological testing in the older patient can provide useful adjunctive information when incorporated as part of a complete assessment (interview, historical data, physical examination, laboratory and radiological data). Most frequently, psychological testing is a useful aid in (1) differential diagnosis, (2) establishment of baseline measures from which to compare future levels of cognitive function (either decline or improvement), and (3) formation of treatment plans by assessing the patient's cognitive strengths and weaknesses.

A number of brief tests have been developed to screen for dementia. One of the better known is Pfeiffer's (1975) short portable mental status

Table 3. Short, Portable Mental Status Questionnaire[a]

Instructions: Ask questions 1–10 in this list and record all answers. Ask question 4b only if the patient does not have a telephone. Record the total number of errors based on ten questions.

+	−	
		1. What is the date today? _____ Month Day Year
		2. What day of the week is it? _____
		3. What is the name of this place? _____
		4a. What is your telephone number? _____
		4b. What is your street address? _____ (Ask only if patient does not have a telephone.)
		5. How old are you? _____
		6. When were you born? _____
		7. Who is currently the president of the United States?
		8. Who was president just before him? _____
		9. What was your mother's maiden name? _____
		10. Subtract 3 from 20 and keep subtracting 3 from each new number you get, all the way down.

For purposes of scoring, three educational levels have been established: (1) persons who have had only a grade-school education, (2) persons who have had any high school education or who have completed high school, and (3) persons who have had any education beyond the high school level, including college, graduate school, or business school.

For white subjects with at least some high school education, but not more than high school education, the following criteria have been established:

0–2 errors	Intact intellectual functioning
3–4 errors	Mild intellectual impairment
5–7 errors	Moderate intellectual impairment
8–10 errors	Severe intellectual impairment

Allow one more error if subject has had only a grade school education; allow one less error if subject has had some college education or better; and allow one more error for any black subject, using identical education criteria.

[a]From Pfeiffer (1975).

Table 4. Ancillary Diagnostic Procedures for Evaluating Dementia Believed Due to Diffuse Brain Disease[a]

Test	Rationale
Blood tests	
Complete blood count	Anemia (megaloblastic or hypochromic), infection
Serological test for syphilis (STS)	Syphilis
Drug levels (barbiturates, bromides, etc.)	Drug intoxication
Electrolytes (sodium potassium, chloride, carbon dioxide, calcium)	Pulmonary dysfunction, renal dysfunction, endocrine dysfunction
Urea nitrogen	Renal dysfunction
Liver function tests (bilirubin, enzymes, ammonia)	Hepatic dysfunction
Serum thyroxine by column (CT4)	Thyroid dysfunction
Vitamin B_{12} and folate levels	Vitamin B_{12} and folate deficiency
Urinalysis	Renal disease, hepatic disease
Electroencephalogram	Unsuspected focal lesion or diffuse cerebral dysfunction
Chest x ray	Infectious process, primary or metastatic tumor, chronic lung disease
Skull x ray	Unsuspected focal lesion, pineal shift, evidence of increased intracranial pressure, disordered calcium metabolism
Computerized axial tomography	Focal or diffuse cerebral atrophy, intracranial masses, hydrocephalus
Brain scan	Unsuspected focal lesion
Isotope cisternography	Impaired spinal fluid flow and absorption
Psychological testing	Focal or diffuse cerebral dysfunction

[a]Adapted from Wells (1977).

questionnaire (SPMSQ). It consists of ten questions that investigate the patient's orientation, short-term and long-term memories, knowledge of current events, and serial mathematical ability (Table 3). It was designed primarily for use with an outpatient geriatric population and takes into account the patient's race and educational background when determining the degree of dementia. Performance is categorized into four groups: intact intellectual functioning, mild intellectual impairment, moderate intellectual impairment, and severe intellectual impairment.

Another popular brief screening instrument is the "mini-mental state" (MMS) developed by Folstein et al. (1975). The MMS includes 11 questions that evaluate orientation, short-term memory, serial mathematical ability, naming of common objects, reading, writing, following commands, and constructional apraxia.

The primary advantages of screening tests such as the SPMSQ and MMS are their brevity (5–10 minutes to administer), their easy incorporation into a regular outpatient history and physical, and their simplicity. The major disadvantage is that they are not sufficiently sensitive to mild dementia and false negatives may be quite common.

Other, more detailed, more accurate, and more standardized tests are available for thorough assessment of cognitive abilities. These include the Wechsler adult intelligence scale, the Halstead–Reitan battery, and tests of discrete cognitive functions such as the Inglis paired associate learning test and Wechsler memory scale. These tests, however, must be used by appropriately trained and specialized psychologists. They may be particularly helpful for accurate differential diagnosis and quantification of cognitive deficits.

Depression

A recent study by Blazer and Williams (1980) indicated that 15% of elderly living in the community had significant dysphoric symptomatology and 4% had symptoms of a major depressive disorder. Another well-designed study (Gurland et al., 1980) suggested that 10% of people over 65 have "pervasive depression," that is, depression severe enough to require the attention of a health care professional. The generally accepted criteria for depression are those found in DSM III for a major affective disorder (Table 5).

There are many possible explanations for depression in the elderly, including loss of control over one's life and loss of self-esteem due to lack of employment. There are also personal losses resulting from the death of friends, siblings, or a spouse. Economic problems may be present, along with fears of being a burden to others. It is critical to remember that many individuals react to such losses *without* becoming clinically depressed; thus when a patient satisfies the criteria for depression, the diagnosis should be made. It is an error to refrain from making the diagnosis on the assumption that anyone in that situation should be depressed. Establishing the diagnosis forces the physician to establish a treatment plan, which may range from supportive psychotherapy to behavioral–cognitive therapy, tricyclic antidepressants, or hospital admission for electroconvulsive therapy.

Suicide risk must be assessed in depressed patients, who, by and large, will reveal their intentions to an empathic physician. Older men are particularly at risk according to figures from the National Center for Health Statistics, cited by Breed and Huffine (1979), which show that suicide rates for men almost double between ages 45 and 85 (27 and 51 per 100,000 respectively). By comparison, suicide rates for women over 65 are less than 10 per 100,000 and decline as age increases.

Table 5. Diagnostic Criteria for Major Depressive Episode

A. Dysphoric mood or loss of interest or pleasure in all or almost all usual activities and pastimes. The dysphoric mood is characterized by symptoms such as the following: depressed, sad, blue, hopeless, low, down in the dumps, irritable. The mood disturbance must be prominent and relatively persistent, but not necessarily the most dominant symptom, and it does not include momentary shifts from one dysphoric mood to another, e.g., anxiety to depression to anger, such as are seen in states of acute psychotic turmoil.

B. At least four of the following symptoms have each been present nearly every day for a period of at least 2 weeks.
   1. Poor appetite or significant weight loss (when not dieting) or increased appetite or significant weight gain.
   2. Insomnia or hypersomnia.
   3. Psychomotor agitation or retardardation (but not merely subjective feelings of restlessness or of being slowed down).
   4. Loss of interest or pleasure in usual activities or decrease in sexual drive not limited to a period when delusional or hallucinating.
   5. Loss of energy; fatigue.
   6. Feelings of worthlessness, self-reproach, or excessive or inappropriate guilt (either may be delusional).
   7. Complaints or evidence of diminished ability to think or concentrate, such as slowed thinking or indecisiveness not associated with marked loosening of associations or incoherence.
   8. Recurrent thoughts of death, suicide ideation, wishes to be dead, or suicide attempt.

C. Neither of the following dominate the clinical picture when an affective syndrome is absent (i.e., symptoms in all criteria above):
   1. Preoccupation with a mood-incongruent delusion or hallucination.
   2. Bizarre behavior.

D. Not superimposed on either schizophrenia, schizophreniform disorder, or a paranoid disorder.

E. Not due to any organic mental disorder or uncomplicated bereavement.

Depression is not always an easy diagnosis to make in the elderly, as the presenting problem may be difficult to distinguish from confusion or memory loss. It is also important to consider the possibility that dementia and depression coexist. In a series of cognitively impaired patients at our clinic, 23% (20 out of 88) met DSM III criteria for depression (Reifler et al., 1982). Of these 20 patients, only 3 were judged to have cognitive impairment due solely to depression; the rest had depression superimposed on an underlying dementia. Furthermore, the rate of coexisting depression decreased significantly with greater severity of cognitive impairment; 33% of the mildly impaired patients were depressed, compared to 23 and 12% of moderately and severely impaired patients. There was a nonsignificant trend for cognitively impaired women to have a greater likelihood of depression than similarly impaired men. We concluded that while it is important to distinguish dementia from depression, it is equally important to consider that the patient may have both.

Other Illness

We have emphasized dementia and depression because they are the two most common serious psychiatric problems in the elderly. There are other important diagnoses that we will mention only briefly.

Alcoholism occurs in 10–20% of geriatric patients seen in clinical practice, but the prevalence among the general population is not precisely known (Schuckit and Pastor, 1979). There is general agreement that it is frequently overlooked among the elderly.

Paranoid thinking can occur in virtually every psychiatric illness seen in the aged, as well as exist as a separate diagnosis. When the patient has persistent persecutory delusions in the absence of another psychiatric illness, the diagnosis of paranoid illness should be made.

There are geriatric patients with chronic schizophrenia, which usually began in early adulthood. It has also been noted that in some instances the illness begins in late life, and when this happens it is generally paranoid in type and may be called paraphrenia (Mensh, 1979).

Treatment of Mental Illness in the Elderly

Treatment for Depression

Depression is the most common reversible mental illness among the elderly, and the physician has several options for treatment once the diagnosis is made. In less severe cases, where the patient is not suicidal and is able to perform the activities of daily living, the physician may elect to treat the patient through behavioral programs designed to increase activities and encourage the patient to explore options for dealing with troublesome problems. Where the symptoms are interfering with daily function or where the above approach has not led to improvement after 1–2 months, an antidepressant might be prescribed. While selection of a specific antidepressant is a clinical decision, there are a few general guidelines to follow. The most important point is history of the patient's previous response to a given antidepressant. If this history is absent, the

Table 6. Features of Commonly Prescribed Antidepressants

More anticholinergic		Less anticholinergic	
More sedating	Less sedating	More sedating	Less sedating
Amitriptyline	Imipramine	Doxepin	Desipramine

major points to consider are potential problems with anticholinergic side effects (such as a history of cardiac arrhythmias or urinary retention) and desirability of sedation. Table 6 illustrates features of some of the most commonly prescribed antidepressants.

Dosage is a particular concern with geriatric patients. A common starting dosage with healthy young adults is 75 mg daily; in geriatric patients this should be reduced to 25–50 mg daily or even to 10 mg in very frail elderly. There are numerous reviews of the pharmacology and clinical use of antidepressants (Greenblatt and Shader, 1975; Hollister, 1978; Risch et al., 1979).

Hospitalization must be considered for severely depressed patients, such as those who are actively suicidal or unable to function at home. Despite its controversial nature, the research literature shows that electroconvulsive therapy remains an effective treatment for depressed patients who do not respond to an adequate trial of medication while in the hospital.

Treatment for Dementing Illness

Treatment for dementing illness is not as specific as that for depression, but there are many strategies that are helpful. As already noted, many patients will prove to have a reversible component to their illness; thus, establishing that accurate diagnosis is not only crucial but relieves the family of uncertainty and assures them that they have met their responsibility for identifying the problem. Furthermore, it allows the patient to assume the status of "patient" rather than "senile old person."

There are specific behavioral problems amenable to drug therapy. As noted earlier, demented patients often meet the criteria for depression, and antidepressant medication can improve their affect, and possibly improve cognitive function as well. Patients with prominent paranoid ideation or severe nighttime confusion and agitation often benefit from a low dose of antipsychotic medication such as haloperidol or thioridazine.

The class of drugs known as vasodilators seems to be of little value in most cases of dementia. Dilating blood vessels would not be particularly useful in Alzheimer's disease, where blood flow is already adequate, and may not be beneficial in patients who have suffered a stroke, since the normal physiological reflex mechanisms are presumably supplying the maximum possible perfusion to the affected area. The only drug in this class that seems to be superior to placebo is dihydroergotamine mesylate, which acts by improving the metabolism of individual brain cells (Yesavage et al., 1979). It seems to lead to subtle improvement in some patients with mild to moderate dementia.

Behavioral/Environmental Treatment Strategies

Psychological functioning involves a continuous interaction between an individual and his or her environment, with each influencing the other. Thus it is possible for the physician to provide incentives for increasing desirable behavior and diminishing undesirable behavior. Motivated behavior change through positive reinforcement, aversive control, or extinction (consistently ignoring maladaptive behaviors) is known as contingency management and is based upon applied or operant conditioning principles.

Ironically, persistent undesirable behavior on the hospital ward or in the nursing home is often maintained by the staff through intermittent positive reinforcement. Patients are usually more successful in gaining attention and caretaking from the staff by complaints related to an illness than by becoming more self-sufficient. The attention paid to such symptoms can function unwittingly to reinforce them and encourage dependency.

Contingency management has been employed with geriatric patients to increase many desirable behaviors. These include self-care (Sperbeck and Whitbourne, 1981; Baltes and Zerbe, 1976), ambulation (MacDonald and Butler, 1974; Sachs, 1975), exercise (Libb and Clements, 1979), verbal interaction (Wisocki et al., 1976; Hoyer et al., 1974; Mueller and Atlas, 1972), complex social interaction skills (Berger and Rose, 1977), memory improvement (Langer et al., 1979), attendance at a community-based nutritious meal program (Bunck and Iwata, 1978), and control of urinary incontinence (Hussian, 1981).

The use of operant conditioning techniques to increase desirable behaviors and reduce functional dependence of the staff was illustrated in a study by Baltes and Zerbe (1976), who instituted a behavioral program to increase self-feeding behavior in two nursing home residents. The first patient was a 67-year-old woman who had not fed herself for 5 months, despite the absence of physical impairments that would prohibit this. The second patient, a 79-year-old man who had had a cerebral vascular accident 9 months previously, was not feeding himself owing to both physical and environmental factors. For both patients, the treatment program consisted of a shaping procedure (successive approximations to the target behavior of self-feeding), reinforcement of appropriate responses, and selective inattention to inappropriate responses (e.g., dumping food). Both patients relearned appropriate eating behavior over a short period of time.

Another behavioral technique that has applications for the elderly is biofeedback, which involves conversion of physiological information into auditory or visual information "fedback" to the subject or patient. Employing this relatively immediate biofeedback, subjects have been able to learn to control a variety of biological responses, including those previously assumed to be involuntary (Shapiro and Schwartz, 1972). Engel (1978) utilized a biofeedback procedure to help subjects, including elderly ones, control fecal incontinence. The subjects were given feedback on muscular contractions and relaxations in the rectum and internal and external sphincters. Artificial distension was then produced in the rectum and sphincter areas, with ongoing biofeedback about muscular activity. Engel found that 40–50 distensions within a single session was sufficient to train 70% of the subjects to develop external sphincter control and maintain continence (at least a 90% decrease in incontinence). Patients who were followed over time (ranging from 4 months to 8 years) showed continued continence.

Motivation to increase desirable behaviors may be enhanced in ways other than through contingency management. Langer et al. (1979) manipulated motivation to practice "thinking" by varying the degree of reciprocal disclosure offered by interviewers in a series of dyadic interactions. The study was conducted to determine whether memory could be improved. The investigators hypothesized that cognitive abilities diminish in some older individuals (especially institutionalized elderly) because of disuse, and that practice in thinking over time may be successful in reversing the debilitations. However, they did not believe that a mere suggestion to increase cognitive activity would be enough to motivate patients to do so; therefore they attempted to motivate elderly nursing home residents to spend time thinking about various issues by providing them with the opportunity for reciprocal self-disclosure. Patients in the experimental group showed significant improvement on standardized tests of memory compared to controls.

A popular psychological treatment for confused, institutionalized elderly is reality orientation (RO) (Folsom, 1968). Reality orientation attempts to reduce confusion and promote autonomy and happiness through cues providing orientation and information about significant factors in the patients' environment. Cues are provided through a "reality orientation center" that includes items such as a clock, a calendar, and a chalkboard with the day's scheduled events, and through repeated verbal reminders to the patient by family or staff. A thorough review of the RO literature by Schwenk (1979) indicated few methodologically rigorous studies. Among those that exist, there is disagreement regarding the effectiveness of RO on reducing confusion. The data clearly do not support the hypothesis that RO increases autonomy or happiness in the elderly.

The importance of perceived personal control in the elderly on psychological, behavioral, and health factors has been demonstrated (Langer and Rodin, 1976; Rodin and Langer, 1977). Nursing home residents heard a communication emphasizing decision making and responsibility for themselves or one stressing the staff's responsibility for them. The experimental (self-directed) group was happier, more active, and more alert than the comparison group. Moreover, these beneficial effects were maintained 18 months later, and the mortality rate for the experimental group was significantly lower. By changing situational factors and restoring to the elderly the right to make decisions and a feeling of competence, it may be possible to retard or avert some of the physical, emotional, and intellectual decline so often observed.

Manipulating the environment can have positive effects on social interaction and activity level in institutionalized elderly (McClannahan and Risley 1973, 1975a,b; Sommer and Ross, 1958; Wisocki, 1977; Jenkins et al., 1977; Peterson et al., 1977). Simple environmental changes such as rearranging furniture in small groups rather than lined up along the walls and providing a lounge area with activity materials and refreshments can increase patient interactions, prosocial behavior, and the activity level. Some institutions have even established "pubs" for their residents, with beneficial results on prosocial interaction (MacDonald, 1972). Supportive environments that help promote socialization and the activity level in community-dwelling residents include senior citizens' centers and geriatric day centers.

Designing a supportive environment for the elderly also includes making the physical environment more congruent with the physical and cognitive capabilities of the older adult. Sensory–perceptual changes accompany advancing age, and the elderly cannot see, hear, touch, taste, or smell as well as they could when they were younger. Thus functional independence can be promoted through a "prosthetic" environment, with attention to such details as multiple cues (visual, auditory, tactile) that allow for easier orientation and navigation of the environment, and safety features (e.g., handrails and wheelchair ramps).

Community Services

A wide range of services for the elderly exists in most cities, including chore services, home-delivered meals, visiting nurse programs, telephone contact services, family support groups, and adult day centers. Frequently, family members are unaware of these community resources; information about available programs can be obtained by calling the local senior information and assistance program. This information can be of value even if none of these programs are used, as the family is reassured just by knowing they are there.

Case Examples

CASE 1

Mrs. A. was in her late 60s when she began to unjustly accuse her husband of trying to poison her. Although distressed by her comment, he thought back to problems he had noticed over the past few years.

While on vacation 2 years earlier, she had left their hotel to go out for a walk but became confused and could remember neither the name of her hotel nor how to get back to it. She considered calling her daughter in their hometown but decided that the daughter would be too alarmed, and finally approached a policeman, who found a hotel matchbook in her purse and directed her back. Her husband was worried when she explained what had happened, but did not know what, if any, action to take. She stayed near him for the rest of the trip and seemed fine when they returned home.

A year later, Mr. A. began to see other changes. Mrs. A forgot an invitation to her daughter's house, made uncharacteristic errors in the checkbook, began relying on lists, and even began to misplay cards at bridge, a game at which they excelled.

Mr. A. knew something was wrong, and decided to act when the accusations began. He took her to the family doctor, who commented that he could find nothing wrong except that she might be showing signs of "premature aging." A neurologist they consulted did an extensive workup, and then told Mr. A. that his wife had Alzheimer's disease and nothing could be done, offering little additional explanation but implying that a nursing home placement would soon be inevitable.

Mr. A. was confused and distraught. He had little idea as to the nature of the disease, how it would progress, or what he could do to help. After several months of trying to cope with his wife's accusations, including times when he felt his only option was to leave, he learned of a physician in his town who was interested in dementing illness. Dr. Z. reevaluated Mrs. A, and while he concurred with the basic diagnosis, he also felt that her paranoia was a treatable component.

There were three parts to Dr. Z's treatment plan: medication for her paranoia, counseling for Mr. A., and additional activities for Mrs. A. He began her on 1 mg of haloperidol at bedtime and within 2 or 3 days the paranoia subsided, changing from constant verbal attacks to only occasional references.

Over the next month or two Dr. Z. made it a point to spend some time alone with Mr. A. when he brought his wife in. They discussed current theories about the cause of Alzheimer's disease, common complications, clinical course, and the problems it causes for the caretaker. Dr. Z. reassured him that his feelings of frustration, guilt, and anger were normal reactions and urged him to discuss them.

When Mrs. A. improved, Dr. Z. suggested that she and her husband look into an adult day center program, where impaired elderly can spend several hours involved in constructive and therapeutic activities. She was hesitant but after a visit agreed to try it and quickly adjusted to going 3 days a week, thus allowing her husband some respite as well.

A year later, Mrs. A. had additional evidence of cognitive decline. Her paranoia had not returned as a major problem and she continued to go to the day center. New problems had come up, such as her inability to dress completely by herself and her lack of recognition of some of her old friends, but her husband felt able to manage and did not see the need to put her in a nursing home.

CASE 2

Mr. G. was in his early 60s when he began to have difficulty understanding visual information, but repeated visits to the ophthalmologist revealed no visual abnormalities. As his problems continued and he could learn no reason for them, he became quite depressed. The patient's wife was concerned not only about his mood, but also about his visual problems, which were evident to her. For example, when looking up a telephone number, he often "missed" some of the digits. He was also having trouble figuring out how to use tools with which he had been quite familiar.

Mrs. G. took her husband to a geriatric clinic for an evaluation. The medical evaluation revealed no significant health problems; however, psychological testing was strongly suggestive of right hemisphere impairment and in particular right parietal lobe dysfunction. A computerized tomographic (CT) scan of the brain was obtained and it confirmed the presence of a right brain cerebrovascular accident.

The diagnosis was explained to both Mr. and Mrs. G. Despite his problems, Mr. G. felt a great sense of relief at being "understood." Mr. G. was started on aspirin to reduce the likelihood of future strokes, along with an antidepressant medication because of his dysphoric mood and vegetative symptoms of depression (sleep disturbance and decreased appetite, interest, and energy level).

Mr. G. also participated in a cognitive remediation program consisting of repeated practice with scanning and tracking rows of visual information (e.g., windows on the face of building) to see whether his problem with left visual inattention could be ameliorated. He was also taught, when reading, to back across the page until he saw his left hand. The combined effect of these interventions was beneficial: His visual problem was better, his mood was greatly improved, and he and Mrs. G. were optimistic about the future.

References

American Psychiatric Association. 1980. Diagnostic and Statistical Manual of Mental Disorders, 3rd ed. Washington, DC: American Psychiatric Association.

Baltes, M. M., and M. B. Zerbe. 1976. Independence training in nursing home residents. Gerontologist 16:428–431.

Berger, R. M., and S. D. Rose. 1977. Interpersonal skill training with institutionalized elderly patients. Journal of Gerontology 32:346–353.

Blazer, D., and C. Williams. 1980. Epidemiology of dysphoria and depression in an elderly population. American Journal of Psychiatry 137:439–444.

Breed, W., and Huffine, C. L. 1979. Sex differences in suicide among older white Americans. In O .J. Kaplan, ed.: Psychopathology of Aging. New York: Academic Press; pp. 289–309.

Brody, E. M. 1977. Long-Term Care of Older People: A Practical Guide. New York: Human Sciences Press.

Bunck, T. J., and B. A. Iwata. 1978. Increasing senior citizen participation in a community-based nutritious meal program. Journal of Applied Behavior Analysis 11:75–86.

Eisdorfer, C. 1969. Intellectual and cognitive changes in the aged. In E. W. Busse and E. Pfeiffer, eds.: Behavior and Adaptation in Late Life. Boston, Massachusetts: Little, Brown; pp. 237–250.

Engel, B. T. 1978. Using Biofeedback with the Elderly (National Institute on Aging, Science Writer Seminar Series, National Institutes of Health). Washington, DC: Goverment Printing Office.

Estes, E. H. 1969. Health experience in the elderly. In E. W. Busse and E. Pfeiffer, eds.: Behavior and Adaptation in Late Life. Boston, Massachusetts: Little, Brown; pp. 115–128.

Filner, B., and T. F. Williams. 1981. Health promotion for the elderly: Reducing functional dependency. In A. R. Somers and D. R. Fabian, eds.: The Geriatric Imperative: An Introduction to Gerontology and Clinical Geriatrics. New York: Appleton-Century-Crofts; pp. 187–204.

Folsom, J. C. 1968. Reality orientation for the elderly mental patient. Journal of Geriatric Psychiatry 1:291–307.

Folstein, M. F., S. E. Folstein, and P. R. McHugh. 1975. "Mini-mental state." A practical method for grading the cognitive state of patients for the clinician. Journal of Psychiatric Research 12:189–198.

Ford, C. V., and R. J. Sbordone. 1980. Attitudes of psychiatrists toward elderly patients. American Journal of Psychiatry 137:571–575.

Goodstein, R. K. 1980. The diagnoses and treatment of elderly patients: Some practical guidelines. Hospital and Community Psychiatry 31:19–24.

Greenblatt, D. S., and R. I. Shader. 1975. Rational use of psychotropic drugs. IV. Antidepressants. American Journal of Hospital Pharmacy 32:59–64.

Growdon, J. H., and S. Corkin. 1980. Neurochemical approaches to the treatment of senile dementia. In J. O. Cole and J. E. Barrett, eds.: Psychopathology in the Aged. New York: Raven Press; pp. 281–294.

Gurland, B., L. Dean, P. Cross and R. Golden. 1980. The epidemiology of depression and dementia in the elderly: The use of multiple indicators of these conditions. In J. O. Cole and J. E. Barrett, eds.: Psychopathology in the Aged. New York: Raven Press; pp. 37–60.

Haug, M. 1979. Doctor patient relationships and the older patient. Journal of Gerontology 34:852–860.

Hollister, L. E. 1978. Tricyclic antidepressants. New England Journal of Medicine 299:1106–1109.

Hoyer, W. J., R. A. Kafer, S. C. Simpson, and F. W. Hoyer. 1974. Reinstatement of verbal behavior in elderly mental patients using operant procedures. Gerontologist 14:149–152.

Hussian, R. A. 1981. Geriatric Psychology: A Behavioral Perspective. New York: Van Nostrand Reinhold.

Issacs, B. 1971. Geriatric patients: Do their families care? British Medical Journal 4:282–286.

Jenkins, J., D. Felce, B. Lund, and L. Powell. 1977. Increasing engagement in activity of residents in old people's homes by providing recreational materials. Behavior Research and Therapy 15:429–434.

Langer, E. J., and J. Rodin. 1976. The effects of choice and enhanced personal responsibility for the aged: A field experiment in an institutional setting. Journal of Personality and Social Psychology 34:191–198.

Langer, E. J., J. Rodin, P. Beck, C. Weinman, and L. Spitzer. 1979. Environmental determinants of memory improvement in late adulthood. Journal of Personality and Social Psychology 37:2003–2013.

Lassen, N. A., and D. H. Ingvar. 1980. Blood flow studies in the aging normal brain and senile dementia. In L. Amaducci, A. N. Davison and P. Antuono, eds.: Aging of the Brain and Dementia. New York: Raven Press; pp. 91–98.

Libb J. W., Clements, C. B., 1969. Token reinforcement in an exercise program for hospitalized geriatric patients. Perceptual and Motor Skills 28:957–958.

Lowther, C. P., and J. Williamson. 1966. Old people and their relatives. Lancet 2:1459–1460.

MacDonald, M. J. 1972. Pub sociotherapy. Canadian Nurse, May:30–32.

MacDonald, M. L., and A. K. Butler. 1974. Reversal of helplessness: Producing walking behavior in nursing home wheelchair residents using behavior modification procedures. Journal of Gerontology 29:97–101.

McClannahan, L. E., and T. R. Risley. 1973. A store for nursing home residents. Nursing Homes 22:10–11.

McClannahan, L. E., and T. R. Risley. 1975a. Activities and materials for severely disabled geriatric patients. Nursing Homes 23:1–4.

McClannahan, L. E., and T. R. Risley. 1975b. Design of living environments for nursing home residents; Increasing participation in recreation activities. Journal of Applied Behavior Analysis 8:261–268.

Mensh, I. N. 1979. The older schizophrenic. In O. J. Kaplan, ed.: Psychopathology of Aging. New York: Academic Press; pp. 149–165.

Mueller, D. J., and L. Atlas. 1972. Resocialization of regressed elderly residents: A behavioral management approach. Journal of Gerontology 27:390–392.

Peterson, R. F., T. J. Knapp, J. C. Rosen, and B. F. Pither. 1977. The effects of furniture arrangement on the behavior of geriatric patients. Behavior Therapy 8:464–467.

Pfeiffer, E. 1975. A short portable mental status questionnaire for the assessment of organic brain deficit in elderly patients. Journal of the American Geriatrics Society 23:433–441.

Reifler, B. V., E. Larson, and R. Hanley. 1982. Coexistence of cognitive impairment and depression in geriatric outpatients. American Journal of Psychiatry 139:623–626.

Risch, S. C., L. Y. Huey, and D. S. Janowsky. 1979. Plasma levels of tricyclic antidepressants and clinical efficacy: Review of the literature. Journal of Clinical Psychiatry 40:4–16, 58–69.

Rodin, J., and E. J. Langer. 1977. Long-term effects of a control-relevant intervention with the institutionalized aged. Journal of Personality and Social Psychology 35:897–902.

Sachs, D. A. 1975. Behavioral techniques in a residential nursing home facility. Journal of Behavior Therapy and Experimental Psychiatry 6:123–127.

Schain, W. S. 1980. Patients' rights in decision making: The case for personalism versus paternalism in health care. Cancer 46:1035–1041.

Schuckit, M. A., and P. A. Pastor. 1979. Alcohol-related psychopathology in the aged. In O. J. Kaplan, ed.: Psychopathology of Aging. New York: Academic Press; pp. 211–227.

Schwenk, M. 1979. Reality orientation for the institutionalized aged: Does it help? Gerontologist 19:373–377.

Shanas, E. 1969. Living arrangements and housing of old people. In E. W. Busse and E. Pfeiffer, eds.: Behavior and Adapatation in Late Life. Boston, Massachusetts: Little, Brown; pp. 129–149.

Shapiro, D., and G. E. Schwartz. 1972. Biofeedback and visceral learning: Clinical applications. Seminars in Psychiatry 4:171–184.

Sommer, R., and H. Ross. 1958. Social interaction on a geriatric ward. International Journal of Social Psychiatry 4:128–133.

Sperbeck, D. J., and D. K. Whitbourne. 1981. Dependency in the institutional setting: A behavioral training program for geriatric staff. Gerontologist 21:268–275.

Stuart, M. R., and F. C. Snope. 1981. Family structure, family dynamics, and the elderly In A. R. Somers and D. R. Fabian, eds.: The Geriatric Imperative: An Introduction to Gerontology and Clinical Geriatrics. New York: Appleton-Century-Crofts; pp. 137–152.

Wells, C. E. 1977. Dementia. Philadelphia, Pennsylvania: F. A. Davis.

Williamson, J., I. H. Stokoe, S. Gray, M. Fisher, A. Smith, A. McGhee, and E. Stephenson. 1964. Old people at home. Their unreported needs. Lancet, May:1117–1120.

Wisocki, P. A. 1977. Sampling procedures: Tools for stimulating the activity and interest of institutionalized elderly. Paper presented at the American Psychological Association, San Francisco.

Wisocki, P. A., P. M. Mosher, and M. Korfhage. 1976. The effect of individual attention and recreational activities on improving the social skills of institutionalized geriatric men. Paper presented at the Tenth Annual Meeting of the Association For the Advancement of Behavior Therapy, New York City.

Yesavage, J. A., J. R. Tinklenberg, L. E. Hollister, and P. A. Berger. 1979. Vasodilators in senile dementias. Archives of General Psychiatry 36:220–223.

Index

A

Acetaldehyde levels, and alcohol, 424
Activity, and blood pressure, 252
Activity levels, and pain, 339, 341–342, 344
Adaptive value
    of conceptual systems, 138
    of depression, 362
Adolescents, behavioral problems of,
        326–329
Adrenal glands, and stress, 229–230, 231–232
Adrenaline, and stress, 229, 231
Adrenocorticotropic hormone (ACTH)
    and depression, 354
    and stress, 229, 231
Affective disorders; *see also specific disorder*
    and culture, 122–125
    incidence and prevalence of, in primary
        care patients, 107
    and neurotransmitters, 81
    and somatization, 106, 107–108, 122–125
    undiagnosed, 107–108
Aggression, and medial temporal injuries, 80
Aging. *See* Elderly
Alcoholism, 18, 419–441
    biochemical/constitutional factors in,
        423–426
    complications of, 27, 45, 430–431
    definition of, 419
    definitive treatment of, 434–438
    denial in, 431, 432
    detoxification in, 432–434
    diagnosis of, 426–432
    drug reactions in, 437–438
    in elderly, 453
    and genetics, 421, 422–423, 424, 425
    medication in treatment of, 433–434
    and mortality, 23, 26, 27, 28
    among physicians, 148, 419–420
    prevention of, 419
    primary, 421
    psychogenic etiology of, 420
    sex differences in, 419, 421
    secondary, 421–422
    treatment of, 432–438
    violence related to, 23, 26, 27
Allopathic medicine, 7
Alzheimer's disease, 75, 446
Amphetamine abuse, and psychosis, 407
Angina pectoris, and psychosocial features,
        253–254
Anorexia nervosa, 194–195
Antabuse, 424
Anthropology, applied contributions from,
        85–103
Antidepressants; *see also specific name; type*
    use of, among elderly, 453–454
Antipsychotic medications
    for dementia, 454
    for depression, 357–358
Anxiety, 16, 17, 385–395, 398–400
    acute, 386
    acute endogenous, 389
    acute exogenous, situational versus
        phobic, 389–390
    adaptive, 385–386
    biofeedback for, 297–298
    chronic, 386
    chronic endogenous, 390–394
    chronic phobic, 391
    chronic situational, 391–393
    and depression, 388, 391, 393, 394
    diagnosis of, 386–387
    and hypertension, 255, 256
    and insomnia, 395

and life change events, 242
medications for, 389–390, 392–393, 398
and negotiation, 387
normal versus pathological, 385–387
and paralinguistic communication, 145
and placebo effect, 390
psychotherapy for, 392, 393
reactions occurring during, 112, 113t
relaxation training for, 390
secondary to medical problems, 387–388
secondary to other psychiatric problems,
    388
social skills training for, 393
and somatization, 106, 107, 125–126
state, 386
systematic desensitization for, 390, 393
trait, 386
Aphasia
    Broca's, 72, 73
    receptive, 72
Apraxia
    constructional, 77
    dressing, 77
Arbitrary codes, 140–141, 142
Arieti–Bemporad approach to depression,
    368
Assertiveness skills, in stress management,
    243
Assessment
    in comprehensive health care, 166, 174t
    of sociocultural factors, 166
Asthma
    biofeedback for, 299
    and operant conditioning, 192–193
Asylums, 59–61
Attention, specific, and brain damage, 75
Attitude, and blood pressure, 252
Attribution
    process of, 116–119
    somatic, changing, 119–127
    and somatization, 112, 114–116
Auditory hallucinations
    in depression, 349
    in temporal lobe seizures, 79
Autogenic training
    limitations of, 293–294
    in stress management, 244
Autonomic functions, and brain, 80
Aversive conditioning
    for alcoholism, 436
    for ruminative vomiting in infants, 195
Aversive consequences, 206–208
Avoidance behavior, and stress, 233–234
Avoidance learning, and pain, 336, 339–342

B
Back pain
    costs of, 32

treatment of, 32–33, 292–293
Baroreceptor functions, and hypertension,
    272, 274–277, 278f, 279f
BASIC ID, 372
Behavior(s)
    acquisition of, 188–189
    basic concepts of, 186–191
    chained, 195–196
    culturally based, 99
    DA/TO, 317–326
    definition of, 186
    discriminated attention to, 315, 317–326
    escape, 339–340
    interaction of, with biological processes,
        186
    measuring, 186
    and misattributions, 186–187
    observing and analyzing one's own,
        208–209
    operant, 187, 188–189, 190–191
    respondent, 187, 188
    tactics to decrease frequency of, 316–318
    tactics to increase frequency of, 315–316
Behavior change
    and avoidance of change agent, 189
    and brain damage. See Brain damage
    and commitment, 204–205
    and motivation, 204, 205, 217, 219
    and negative reinforcement, 189
    and physician, 5
    and public education, 4–5
    and punishment, 189
Behavioral environment, analysis of, 208–209
Behavioral medicine
    basic concepts of, 186–191
    clinical application of, 191–196
    definition of, 185
    emergence of, 22–23
    historical considerations of, 6–9
    necessity of, 21–22
Behavioral problems, in pediatric practice,
    16, 311–330
    in adolescents, 326–329
    and chronic illness, 312
    and compliance, 328–329
    and experimental analysis of behavior,
        313–314
    and parental styles, 312–313
    and tactics used to decrease frequency of
        behavior, 316–318
    and tactics used to increase frequency of
        behavior, 315–316
    and therapeutic parsimony, 313
Behavioral sciences, 22
    and medical practices, 33–34
Behavioral system, 5–6
Benzodiazepines
    for anxiety, 390, 398
    for insomnia, 398, 399

Bicyclic antidepressants, 358
Biofeedback, 16, 197, 283–309
    for anxiety, 297–298
    for asthma, 299
    for cardiac symptoms, 295
    for chronic pain, 291–293
    cybernetic view of, 284
    definition of, 283
    for gastrointestinal disorders, 299,
        301–302, 456
    for headaches, 287–290
    for hypertension, 258, 296–297
    informational model of, 284
    for insomnia, 298–299
    modalities of, 197, 285–286
    for musculoskeletal pain, 290–291
    for pain, 286–293
    for peripheral vascular symptoms, 299–301
    for seizure disorders, 302–303
    skills acquisition model of, 284–285
    for skin rash, 299
    for speech disorders, 302
    in stress management, 244
    for stress reactions, 293–302
    for tinnitus, 299
    for ulcerative colitis, 299, 301
Biomedical model, 5
Biopsychosocial model
    and health care, 163–183
    interaction of components of, 177–179
Body image deficit, and brain damage, 77
Body–mind dualism, 6–7
    and chronic pain, 331–332, 336
    and conversion reactions, 106
Body–mind unity, 6, 7–8
    in antiquity, 48–50, 51
    in primitive medicine, 45, 47
Brain
    and alcoholism, 425
    blood flow in, 69
    and critical periods, 68, 82–83
    early study of, 69
    and hypertension, 251
    lateralization, 9, 69–70, 71–72, 74, 77
Brain–behavior relations, 9–11
    and delivery of health care, 67–84
    and learning versus innate mechanisms,
        67–68
Brain damage
    and behavioral changes, 68–69
    and emotions, 79–81
    and language, 71–74, 77
    and motor systems, 70–71
    and parallels with psychoses, 80–81
    and recovery of function, 69, 70
    and sensory systems, 76–79
    and treatment, lack of motivation for, 78
Bribery, in behavioral problems in children,
    315, 316

Broca's aphasia, 72, 73

C

Car accidents, as cause of death, 23, 26
Cancer; see also specific type
    and mortality, 26, 27t, 28t, 29t
    and pain, 335
    and stress, 240–241
Cardiac symptoms, biofeedback for, 295
Cardiovascular disease
    as cause of death, 26, 30–31
    factors associated with, 30–31
    and hypertension, 30–31
    and stress, 31, 239–240
    and type A personality. See Type A
        personality
Catecholamines, and hypertension, 251–252
Cell-mediated immunity, 11
Central nervous system, and immune
        system, 10–11
Central pain states, 332–333
Children. See Behavioral problems, in
        pediatric practice
Christianity, and interpretation and
        treatment of pathological behavior,
        51–54
Chronic illness
    costs of, 32
    supernatural explanations of, 45
Chronic pain, 16, 331–345
    versus acute pain, 16, 331, 335
    behavioral approaches to evaluation and
        management of, 342–344
    biofeedback for, 291–293
    of cancer versus benign, 335
    comprehensive treatment program for,
        291, 292
    and mind–body distinction, 331–332
    model of, 332–335
    and operant behavior, 187
    and respondent behavior, 187
    and role of learning/conditioning factors
        on, 16, 337–345
Cognitive compatibility, 135, 157–158
Cognitive disturbances, in depression, 349
Cognitive functioning, in elderly, 443–444,
        446–448, 452–453
Cognitive restructuring techniques, in
        stress management, 243
Cognitive testing, of elderly, 448–451
Cognitive therapy, for depression, 372–375
Communication; see also Language
    barriers to effective, 146–148
    and concept formation, 138
    and culture, 12–13
    and noncompliance, 134–135, 152–153
    nonverbal, 134, 139–143
    paralinguistic, 134, 144–146

and physician–patient relationship, 13,
36–38, 94, 100, 133–161
and social roles, 134, 148–152
verbal, 134, 135–137, 140
Community services, for elderly, 457–458
Compliance; see also Noncompliance
in children, 328–329
self-management in, 214–216
Computerized tomographic (CT) scan, 69
Concept formation, 138
Conceptual structure
and ecology, 138–139
and language, 137
Constructional apraxia, 77
Contingencies, in behavioral problems
in children, 315, 316, 322
Contingency management
in depression, 376
in elderly, 455
Contracts, 213, 217, 329, 369–370
Conversion reactions, 106
Coping strategies
and culture, 98–99
in protection against stress, 14, 15
sex differences in, and hypertension, 12
Cortisol, and depression, 354–355
Critical periods, and brain, 68, 82–83
Culture
and behavior, 99
and biomedical treatment, 99–101
and communication, 12–13
and coping, 98–99
definition of, 86
and depression, 122–125
and feeling, 99
influence of, 86–88
and language, 123
and pain, 34, 86
and physician–patient relationships, 99–
101
and plans, 169
and social support, 99
and stress, 98–101
Culture-bound disorders, 125

D

Data base, 164–166, 167f, 168f
Death; see also Mortality
leading causes of, 4, 23–31
Defense mechanisms; see also specific name
of family crisis, 174, 175t
Dementia, in elderly, 75, 446–448, 450t,
452, 454–455
Demonic possession, 45, 47, 52–53
Denial
in alcoholism, 431, 432
of emotions, 124
Depression, 16–17, 347–383; see also

Affective disorders
and alcoholism, 421
and anxiety, 388, 391, 393, 394
Arieti–Bemporad approach to, 368
behavior in, 349–350
biological correlates of, 354–355, 362
and cognition, 349
cognitive–behavioral perspectives on,
368–373
cognitive therapy for, 372–375
with dementia, 452
and dependency, 364
diagnosis of, 347–349, 350–351, 352, 452
and drug misuse and abuse, 353–354
drug treatment of, 354, 355–357, 366,
372, 374, 453–454
eclectic therapy for, 375–377
in elderly, 451–454
electroconvulsive therapy for, 357
family therapy for, 377
versus grief, 351–352
and insomnia, 395
and learned helplessness, 374–375
lifetime risk of developing, 347
and loss, 361, 367, 451
masked, 352
and medical conditions, 352–353
in medical setting, 352–353
multimodal therapy for, 372
and negative labeling, 364–365
and paralinguistic communication, 145
and parallels with symptoms of altered
brain function, 81
and parents, 365
physiological disturbances in, 350
psychoanalysis for, 363
psychosocial perspectives on, 17,
361–383
reactions occurring during, 112, 113t
running for, 355
self-control model of, 222, 370–371
severity of, assessing, 351
and Short-Term Interpersonal
Psychotherapy of Depression for,
365–368
sleep deprivation for, 355
and socialization, 365
and somatization, 106, 107–108, 122–125,
354
and stress, 241–242
and suicide, 377–379, 451
survival value of, 362
systematic desensitization for, 379
undiagnosed, 107–108, 120
vulnerability to, 362
Depressive Adjective Check List, 369
Dihydroergotamine mesylate, 455
Discrimination, in learning, 191
Disease(s); see also specific disease

and host characteristics, 3–4
versus illness, 88–90
interaction of, with illness, 89
and value sentiments, 89
Disease causation, theories of
in ancient Greece, 47–50
in ancient Rome, 50–51
in eighteenth century, 57–59
in medieval period, 51–54
in Mesopotamia and Egypt, 47
in primitive societies, 44–46
in sixteenth and seventeenth centuries,
55–57
Dissociation, 124
Doctor–patient relationship. See Physician–
patient relationship
Dopamine, and schizophrenia, 81
Dressing apraxia, 77
Drug(s); see also specific name; type
depression induced by, 352–353
and noncompliance. See Noncompliance
potency, and information seeking, 37
withdrawal of, and depression, 353–354
Drug misuse and abuse, 403–417
and choice of drug, 413–414
and classification of abusers, 413
definitions of, 403–405
diagnosis of, 414
iatrogenic, 414–415
initiation of, 412
and major clusters of drugs, 414
and panic reactions, 4–6, 407
patients at risk for, 415–416
pattern of, 405
and physical dependence, 407–408
physical sequelae of, 409
by physicians, 148
and psychological dependence, 408
and psychosis, 406, 407, 408–409
and self-medication–social/recreational
dichotomy, 413, 414
and streetwise–straight dichotomy, 413,
414
and tolerance, 407
toxic effects of, 406, 407
Dyslexia, developmental, 73–74, 77–78

E

Eclectic therapy, in depression, 375–377
Ecology, and conceptual structures,
138–139
Economics
of chronic illness, 32
of chronic low back pain, 32
Education
of health care providers, 74; see also
Medical education
public, 4–5

and self-management, 203, 205, 208
Egypt, ancient, interpretation and treatment
of pathological behavior in, 43, 47
Elderly, 18, 443–462
alcoholism in, 453
assessment of, 445
behavioral/environmental treatment
strategies for, 455–457
chronic schizophrenia in, 453
cognitive functioning in, 443–444, 446–
448, 452–453, 454–455
cognitive testing of, 448–451
community services for, 457–458
depression in, 451–454
family care of, 444
myths and stereotypes of, 443–444
multiple disabilities in, 445
and noncompliance, 445
paranoid thinking in, 453
physicial support of, 121–122
unmet need for medical care of, 110, 443,
445
Electrical stimulation mapping of brain, 69,
70–71, 72–73, 76, 81
Electroconvulsive therapy, for depression,
357
Electrolyte membrane potential
disturbance, and depression, 355
Emotions; see also specific emotion
and blood pressure, 252
and brain damage, 79–81
and pain, 34, 334–335
and paralinguistic communication, 144–
146
Empathic ability, as skill, 146
Employment status, and blood pressure,
254
Endocrine system; see also Hormones and
immune system, 11
Endorphins, 10
Enuresis, behavioral treatment of, 33
Environment
behavioral, analysis of, 208–209
and brain responses, 67–68; see also
Brain–behavior relations
changes in, and stress management,
242
and critical periods, 82–83
manipulating, for elderly, 457
and mortality, 4
Environmental restructuring, 210–214
Escape behavior, 339–340
Exercise
for depression, 355
for stress management, 243
for weight control, 221
Explanatory model (EM), 91–94, 100, 110,
126
of family, 91, 101, 174

Explanatory model [cont.]
  of patient, 91–94, 96, 100, 101, 174
  of physician, 91, 94, 96
  questions used to elicit, 94
Explanatory model of distress, 244
Extinction, 77, 326–327

F
Facial expressions, meaning of, 141–142
Family
  care of elderly by, 444
  and crisis, 173–174, 175
  definitions of, 171
  explanatory model of, 91, 101, 174
  in health, standard for, 171
  interaction, 165–166, 167f, 168f
  pathological defenses of, 174, 175t
  pathological equilibrium in, 175
  resources of, 172–173
  and stressful life events, 172, 180
  as support system, 99, 154, 166, 169–173
  terminal disequilibrium in, 175
Family APGAR, 166, 167f, 168f
Family function, cycle of, 170–176
Family medicine, 7
Family therapy, for depression, 377
Fears, childhood, 327–328
Fetal alcohol syndrome, 430–431
Fight–flight response, 10, 109, 228–233
Flashbacks, 406–407
Flexner report, 7
Folk healing practices, 101
Frustration, and blood pressure, 253

G
Gastric ulcers, and brain anatomy, 80
Gastrointestinal disorders
  behavioral treatment of, 195
  biofeedback for, 299, 301–302, 456
Gaze–gesture combinations, 142, 143t
Gender roles, 12
General adaptation syndrome, 15, 230–233
Generalization, in learning, 191
Genetics
  and alcoholism, 421, 422–423, 424, 425
  and hypertension, 264
  and psychosis, 81
Greece, ancient, interpretation and treat-
      ment of pathological behavior in 7,
      47–50
Grief
  versus depression, 351–352
  IPT for, 366–367
Guilt
  and depression, 365
  and hypertension, 254

H
Habit patterns; see also Life-style
  impact of, on mortality, 26–28, 30, 31
Hallucinations
  in depression, 349, 357–358
  in temporal lobe seizures, 78–79, 80–81
Hallucinogens
  and panic reactions, 406
  and psychosis, 408–409
  risks of, 410t
Handedness, and lateralization of language,
      71
Harmonia, 48
Headache, biofeedback for, 287–290
Healers
  folk, 101
  in primitive and ancient societies, 46, 47
  sensitivity of, to patient's behavior, 6
Healing systems
  efficacy of, factors in, 6
  non-Western. See Non-Western healing
      systems
Health, definition of, 31–32
Health belief model, 154
Health belief systems, 154, 155
Health care
  biopsychosocial approach to, 163–183
  comprehensive, 7, 163–164, 165f
  inadequacies in, and mortality, 4
  patient initiation of, 34–36
  quality of, 40
  and sex differences, 11
  unmet need for, in elderly, 110, 443, 445
Help-seeking, sex differences in, 11
Heroin
  addiction to, of American troops in
      Vietnam, 412
  withdrawal, 404, 407–408
Hippocratic theory, 48–50, 51
Homeopathic approach, 7
Homunculus, 71
Hormones; see also specific hormone
  and arousal, 112t
  and stress, 229–230, 231–232
Hostility, and hypertension, 254, 255, 256,
      259
Host characteristics; see also specific char-
      acteristic
  and disease phenomena, 3–4
Hyperactivity, treatment of, 33–34
Hypertension, 15, 249–282
  and brain anatomy, 80
  causes of, 250, 265–266
  complications of, 30–31, 253, 257–258,
      263
  definition of, 263
  essential, 250
  and genetics, 264

medications for, side effects of, 256, 266
and migration, 255
and mortality, 254, 255, 257–258, 263
mosaic theory of, 250, 265, 267
and noncompliance, 39, 139, 202, 204, 266
pathophysiology of essential, 15, 250–255, 266–282
and personality, 255–256
prevalence of, 250, 263
psychosocial–behavioral measures in management of, 256–260, 296–297
and race, 254–255, 264
renal, 265
sex differences in susceptibility to, 11–12
significance of, 250
and socioeconomic status, 254, 255
Hypnosis, 63–64, 65
Hypochondriasis, and panic attacks, 391
Hypothalamopituitary axis, and depression, 354–355
Hysteria, 63, 64–65

I

Iconic codes, 140
Illness
    versus disease, 88–90
    interaction of, with disease, 89
    meanings of, 91–94
    reinforcement of, 120–122
    and secondary gain, 121, 125
    social functions of, 91–94
    and stress, 4, 5, 112, 173, 239–242
Illness behavior, outcome of, biopsycho-social formula for, 177–179
Illness behavior problems, 176t
Illness experience problems, 94–95
Immune system
    and central nervous system, 10–11
    and stress, 240
Individual variability
    in brain mechanisms, 71, 77, 81–82
    in conceptual structure, 139
    in lateralization, 9, 71, 77
    in localization of brain functions, 9
    in pain, 34
    in spatial function lateralization, 77
    in stress, 234, 235–236
Infertility, and emotions, 80
Information seeking, and medication potency, 37
Insomnia, 395–399
    behavioral approaches to, 397–398
    benzodiazepines for, 398–399
    biofeedback for, 298–299
    causes of, 395, 396

cognitive–behavioral problems in, 396–397
    risk factors in, 395
Interferon, 11
Interpersonal Psychotherapy for Depression, Short-Term (IPT), 365–368
Intrinsic codes, 140

K

Korsakoff's disease, and recent memory loss, 75

L

Labeling; see also Attribution
    and pain tolerance, 114–115
    of symptoms, 34
Language; see also Communication
    biological capacity for, 136, 137
    of body, and metaphor, 12–13
    and brain damage, 71–74, 77; see also specific deficit
    and conceptual structure, 137
    and culture, 123
    development of, 136–137
    and electrical stimulation mapping, 81
    and handedness, 71
    and lateralization, 71–72, 77
    of pain, 334
    and physician–patient relationship, 100
    and social roles, 149
    and spatial abilities, 78
    versus speaking, 135
    structure of, 135
    and translators, 100
Learned helplessness model of depression, 374–375
Learning, and brain, 10, 67–68
Life changes
    and mental illness, 241, 242
    and stress, 112, 173, 237–239, 241, 242
Life expectancy, changes in, from 1900–1970, 22, 23
Life-style; see also Habit patterns
    behavioral approaches to change in, 196
    and cardiovascular disease, 31
    and mortality, 4
    somatization as, 110–111
Liver cirrhosis, 27
Locus of control, 236
Logical inference model of attribution, 117–119, 120
Lung cancer
    as cause of death, 26, 27t, 28t, 29t
    and smoking, 27–28
LSD psychosis, 408

M

Marijuana use, 405–406, 408
Meaning, versus message, 139–140
Medical education
    and alcoholism education, 420
    behavioral principles in, 7
    changes in, 133
    and cognitive compatibility, 158
    and socialization into subculture, 94
Medical practice, and behavioral science,
    33–34
Medical science, public's ignorance of, 35,
    36, 38
Medications. *See* Drug(s); *specific name; type*
Medicine, measure of quality care in, 40
Meditation
    for hypertension, 258, 296, 297
    in stress management, 244
Memory
    and brain damage, 74–75
    and language, 137
    and noncompliance, 39, 155, 214–216
    prosthetic, 215–216
Mental health, effect of, on physical health,
    13–14
Mesmerism, 62–63
Mesopotamia, interpretation and treatment
    of pathological behavior in, 43, 47
Message, versus meaning, 139–140
Methaqualone, 413–414
Methylphenidate, 414
Migraine headaches, biofeedback for, 287–
    288, 289
Migration, and hypertension, 255
Mini-Mental State (MMS), 450, 451
Minimal learning disability, 75
Minimization, 124
Miscommunication
    and noncompliance, 38
    and physician–patient relationship, 36–38
Misdiagnosis, of psychosocial problems,
    87–88
Modeling, 191, 196–197
Monoamine oxidase inhibitors, 354, 357
    for anxiety, 357, 389
    for depression, 357
    for panic attacks, 357
    for phobias, 357
Moral treatment, Pinel's, 57–58
Morality, and disease, in primitive society,
    46
Morbidity
    determinants of, 31–33; *see also specific*
        determinant
    sex differences in, 11–12
Mortality; *see also* Death
    from hypertension, and socioeconomic
        status, 254, 255

    infant, reduction in, 23
    sex differences in, 11–12
    slowdown in reduction in, 22, 23t
    and social ties, 14
Motor systems, and brain damage, 70–71
Movements, meaning of, 141
Musculoskeletal pain, biofeedback for, 290–
    291

N

Narcotics
    chronic pain caused by, 335
    and depression, 335
    toxic effects of, 407
    withdrawal, 407, 408
Naturalistic causation of disease
    in ancient Greece, 48–50, 51
    in primitive societies, 44
Negotiation, 203–204
    in anxiety, 357
    in physician–patient relationship, 95–97,
        98, 119, 126
Neurology, development of, 61
Neuropsychiatry, development of, 61
Neuroses
    hypnosis and suggestion for, 63–64
    repression in, 65
Neurotransmitters; *see also specific name*
    and affective disorders, 81, 354, 355
    and schizophrenia, 81
Nociception, 332, 333, 335, 336, 337
Non-Western cultures, and conversion re-
    actions, 106
Non-Western healing systems, 7, 43–46
Noncompliance, 38–39, 40, 152, 154; *see*
    also Compliance
    and communication, 134–135, 152–157
    definitions of, 152
    of elderly, 445
    and forgetting, 39, 115, 214–216
    of hypertensive patients, 39, 139, 202,
        204, 266
    management of, 154–156, 196, 214–216
    and physician–patient relationship, 153–
        157
    of psychiatric patients, 153
    self-management of, 214–216
Nonverbal communication, 134, 139–143
Norepinephrine, and affective disorders,
    81, 354

O

Object intrusion, 41–45
Olfactory hallucinations
    in depression, 349
    in temporal lobe seizures, 79

Operant behavior, 187, 188–189, 190–191
Oral cancer, causes of, 27–28

P

Pain
    and activity level, 339, 341–342, 344
    acute versus chronic, 16, 331, 335
    affective factors in, 34, 334–335
    biofeedback for, 286–293
    chronic. *See* Chronic pain
    and compliance, 38–39
    and culture, 34, 86
    definition of, 332
    individual differences in, 34
    language of, 334
    and stress, 34, 290–291
    tolerance to, and labeling, 114–115
Pain behavior, 335
    and attention factor, 336, 338–339
    and avoidance, 336, 339–342
    definition of, 334
    reinforcement of, 191–192, 336, 338–339, 340
Panic attacks, 389, 390–391
Panic reactions, in drug abuse, 406–407
Paralinguistic communication, 134, 144–146
    definition of, 144
    and emotional states, 144–146
Paranoid thinking, in elderly, 453
Pathological behavior, interpretation and treatment of; *see also specific type*
    in ancient Greece, 7, 47–50
    in ancient Rome, 50–51
    in eighteenth century, 57–59
    in medieval period, 51–54
    in Mesopotamia and Egypt, 47
    in nineteenth century, 59–61
    in primitive societies, 43–46
    in sixteenth and seventeenth centuries, 55–57
Patient(s)
    compliance of. *See* Compliance
    conflicts in orientation of, with physician, 90
    explanatory model of, 91–94, 96, 100, 101, 174
    informed, and adjustment, 156–157
    as initiator of medical care, 34–36
    knowledge of, and compliance, 154, 155
    labeling of symptoms by, 34–35
    noncompliance of. *See* Noncompliance
    –physician relationship. *See* Physician–patient relationship
    preparation of, for procedures, 196–197
    problems of, evaluating, 36–38
Perception, and language, 137

Perceptual disturbances, in depression, 349, 357–358
Peripheral vascular symptoms, biofeedback for, 299–301
Perseveration, 72
Personal knowledge model of attribution, 116–117
Personality
    and alcoholism, 420
    and hypertension, 254, 255–256
    split, 64–65
    type A. *See* Type A personality
Phencyclidine (PCP) psychosis, 407, 408–409
Phobias
    and chronic endogenous anxiety, 391
    biofeedback for, 298
    systematic desensitization for, 394
Physician(s)
    alcoholism among, 148, 419–420
    as authority figure, 37
    and behavior change, 5
    conflicts of orientation of, with patient, 90
    drug abuse among, 148
    explanatory model of, 91, 94, 96
    as poor patient, 148
    reinforcement of somatization by, 120–121
    suicide rate of, 148
    support of, 14, 121–122
    visits to, needs represented by, 348–349
Physician–patient relationship, 14–15, 39–40
    and communication, 12, 36–38, 94, 100, 133–161
    and culture, 12, 99–101
    and elderly, 444
    and language problems, 100
    and negotiation, 93–97, 98, 119, 126, 203–204, 387
    and noncompliance, 153–157
    and plans, 169
    and social roles, 134, 148–152
Placebo effect, 390
Plan, for patient care, 169
Planum temporale, asymmetries in size of, 71
Pleasant Events Schedule, 369
Pleasure, and hypothalamic lesions, 79–80
Positron emission tomography (PET), 69
Possession, and disease causation, 45, 47, 52–53
Practice thinking, 456
Presenile dementia, and recent memory loss, 75
Prevention, behavioral approaches to, 196

Primitive societies, interpretation and treatment of pathological behavior in, 43–46
Problem-oriented medical record (POMR), 164–169
Progressive relaxation; see also Relaxation therapy
  for hypertension, 258
  in stress management, 243–244
Psychiatric disorders; see also specific disorder
  alcoholism secondary to, 421–422
  anxiety secondary to, 388
  and stress, 241–242
  somatization in, 106–108, 122–126
Psychiatric patients, and noncompliance, 153
Psychiatry, dynamic, 61–66
Psychoanalysis, 65
  and depression, 363
Psychosis
  drug-induced, 406, 407, 408–409
  inheritability of, 81
  and parallels with symptoms of altered brain function, 80–81
Psychosocial problems; see also specific problem
  misdiagnosis and mistreatment of, 87–88
Psychosomatic disorders; see also specific disorder
  and brain anatomy, 80
Psychotherapy, for anxiety, 392, 393
Punishment, 189, 190
  physical, 316

R

Race
  and hypertension, 254–255, 264
  and response to alcohol, 424
Radioactive xenon tracers, 69
Rage, and hypothalamic lesions, 79–80
Raynaud's disease, biofeedback for, 299–300
Reality orientation, for elderly, 456–457
Recent life change questionnaire, 237
Receptive aphasia, 72
Reinforcement, 188–189
  in asthma, 192–193
  in behavioral problems in children, 315, 316
  continuous, 190
  and environmental change, 212
  fixed-interval, 190
  intermittent, 190
  negative, 189
  and pain behavior, 191–192, 336, 338–339, 340

  positive, 191–192, 326–327
  primary, 190
  and satiation, 190
  secondary, 190
  and shaping, 190
  in skin disorders, 193
  variable-interval, 190
Renin, and hypertension, 251, 277, 279–281
Relaxation therapy; see also Progressive relaxation
  for anxiety, 390
  with biofeedback, for hypertension, 296, 297
  limitations of, 293–294
Research Diagnostic Criteria, 369
Respondent behavior, 187, 188
Role changes, 151
Role expectations
  definition of, 149
  and physician–patient relationship, 149–152
Roles, and communication in physician–patient relationship, 134, 148–152
Rome, ancient, interpretation and treatment of pathological behavior in, 50–51
Ruminative vomiting, in infants, behavioral treatment of, 195

S

Salt, and hypertension, 281
Schedule of recent events, 237, 239
Schedule of recent experience, 237
Schizophrenias
  chronic, in elderly, 453
  and dopamine, 81
  and life change events, 242
  and parallels with symptoms of altered brain function, 80–81
Scratching behavior, behavioral treatment of, 193–194
SCREEEM, 172–173
Seditive-hypnotic drugs
  chronic pain caused by, 335
  and depression, 335
  recreational use of, 413–414
  risks of, 409t
  toxic effects of, 407
  withdrawal, 407, 408
Seizure disorders
  and hallucinations, 78–79
  treatment of, 195–196, 302–303
Self-control, 203–205; see also Self-management
  and depression, 370–381, 376
Self-management, 201–223
  and analysis of behavioral environment, 208–209

and commitment, 204–205, 217
and compliance, 214–216
definition of, 203
in depression, 222, 370–371
and environmental restructuring, 210–214
problems, 205–208
professional monitoring of, 222
and self-monitoring, 209–210, 212–213, 217, 219–220, 221
and skills, 203, 205, 208
and stopping smoking, 216–218
in weight control, 218–221
Self-monitoring, 209–210, 212–213, 217, 219–220, 221
Self-reports, and evaluation of patient's problem, 36–37
Self-treatment, 101
Sensationalist theory, 57
Sensory systems, and brain damage, 76–79
Serotonin, and affective disorders, 81, 354
Sexual dysfunctions, biofeedback for, 300–301
Shaping, 190, 194, 455–456
Short, portable mental status questionnaire, 448–450, 451
Short-Term Interpersonal Psychotherapy of Depression (ITP), 365–368
Skin disorders
    behavioral treatment of, 193–194
    biofeedback for, 299
Sleep deprivation, for depression, 355
Smoking
    addiction to, 409, 410
    and alcohol use, 28
    and antecedent stimulus control, 206
    and delayed negative consequences, 206
    and lung cancer, 26–27
    and oral cancer, 27
    stopping, self-management in, 216–218
Social group, in primitive medicine, 46
Social readjustment rating scale, 173, 237, 238t
Social skills training, for chronic anxiety, 393
Social structure
    definition of, 86
    influence of, 86–88
Social ties
    and morbidity, 14
    and risk of death, 14
Socioeconomic status
    and coronary heart disease risk factors, 12
    and hypertension, 254, 264
Sociopathic alcoholics, 421–422
Somatization, 13, 105–131
    and attribution, 112, 114–127

classic conversion as, 106
definition of, 105
and depression, 354
diagnosis of, 125–126, 127
and family conflicts, 165
as life-style, 110–112
and negotiation, 126
processes underlying, 111–116
in psychiatric disorders, 106–108, 122–125
and reinforcements, 120–121
and social support, 111
of stress, without major psychiatric disorder, 109–110
treatment of, 125–126, 127
Soul loss, as cause of disease, 45
Spatial abilities, and brain lateralization, 77–78
Speaking, versus language, 135
Speech disorders; see also specific disorder
    biofeedback for, 302
Spirit intrusion, as cause of disease, 45, 47
Stereotyping, 100
    of elderly, 443–444
Stimulants
    for hyperactivity, 33
    and panic reactions, 406
    risks of, 410t
    toxic effects of, 407
    withdrawal, 408
Stomach cancer, mortality from, decline in, 26, 27t, 28t
Stress
    appraisal of, 228, 233
    and behavior and illness, 10–11
    and cancer, 240–241
    and cardiovascular disease, 31, 239–240; see also Type A personality
    and culture, 98
    definitions of, 31, 227–228, 230–231
    and endorphins, 10
    and hypertension, 266–282
    and latent viruses, 11
    management of, 242–244
    measurement of, 237–239
    and mental illness, 241–242
    and pain, 34, 290–291
    physiological concomitants of, 111–112, 113t
    and smoking, 411
    somatization of, without psychiatric disorder, 109–111
    versus stressors, 237
    transactional model of, 233, 235–237
    vulnerability to, 244–245
Stress reactions, 10, 109, 228–234
    biofeedback for, 293–302
    cognitive–behavioral, 233–234
    physiological, 10, 109, 228–233

Stressful life events
  and family, 172, 180
  and family crisis, 174
  and illness, 173
  variation in response to, 173
Stressors
  categorization of, 237
  versus stress, 237
  types of, 228
Sturge–Weber syndrome, 72
Suffering, and pain, 333–334
Suggestion, 63–64
Suicide
  among physicians, 148
  prevention of, 377–379
  risk of, in elderly, 451
Supernatural
  and disease causation, 44–45, 47, 51–53
  and treatment, 45–46, 47
Support
  in acute exogenous anxiety, 389
  and culture, 99
  and extended family, 99
  of family, 99, 154, 166, 169–173
  lack of, and somatization, 111
  of physician, 14, 121–122
  and prevention, 121
  in stopping smoking, 218
  and stress, 236
  in weight control, 219, 221
Supportive therapy, for depression, 375–
    376
Susto, 125
Sympathetic nervous system, and high
    blood pressure, 251–252
Symptoms
  and culture, 99
  labeling of, by patients, 34–35
  meanings of, for patients, 91–94
  social functions of, for patients, 91–94
Systematic desensitization
  for anxiety, 390, 393
  for depression, 379
  limitations of, 293–294
  for phobias, 394–395

                                  T
Tension headaches, biofeedback for, 287,
    288–290
Testosterone, and development of spatial
    skills, 77
Tetracyclic antidepressants, 358
Thalamic alerting circuits, 75
Thalamic syndrome, 76

Thought(s) and thinking
  and blood pressure, 253
  and language, 137
  paranoid, among elderly, 453
  practice, 456
Thyroxine, and stress, 229
Timeout, in behavioral problems in chil-
    dren, 317–326
Tinnitus, biofeedback for, 299
Transactional model of stress, 233, 235–237
Treatment
  and culture, 99–101
  efficacy of, primary variables in, 133, 134
Translators, 100
Trepanation, 45
Tricyclic antidepressants, 354, 355–356,
    357, 358, 366
  for anxiety, 389
Tuberculosis, 3–4, 8–9
Type A personality, 15, 31, 239–240, 253,
    388

                                  U
Ulcerative colitis, biofeedback for, 299, 301
Unpleasant Events Schedule, 369

                                  V
Value sentiments, and disease 89
Verbal communication, 134, 135–137, 140;
    see also Language
Violence
  alcohol-related, 27
  and mortality, 26
Viruses, latent, and stress, 11
Visual hallucinations
  in depression, 349
  in temporal lobe seizures, 78–79
Visual systems, and critical periods, 82

                                  W
Weight control
  behavioral approach to, 194
  self-management in, 218–221
Whorfian hypothesis, 137
Witchcraft, 53
World view
  definition of, 42
  elements of, 43–44
  in medieval period, 52
  in primitive and ancient societies, 43–44,
    46, 47
  in seventeenth century, 55